Concepts of Alzheimer Disease

Concepts of Alzheimer Disease

BIOLOGICAL, CLINICAL, AND CULTURAL PERSPECTIVES

Edited by

Peter J. Whitehouse, M.D., Ph.D.
Konrad Maurer, M.D., Ph.D.
and Jesse F. Ballenger, M.A.

THE JOHNS HOPKINS UNIVERSITY PRESS
Baltimore & London

© 2000 The Johns Hopkins University Press
All rights reserved. Published 2000
Printed in the United States of America on acid-free paper
9 8 7 6 5 4 3 2 1

The Johns Hopkins University Press
2715 North Charles Street
Baltimore, Maryland 21218-4363
www.press.jhu.edu

Library of Congress Cataloging-in-Publication Data will be found
at the end of this book.
A catalog record for this book is available from the British Library.

ISBN 0-8018-6233-7

For Luigi Amaducci, 1932–1998

Luigi Amaducci was a key figure for the world neurological and psychiatric community. Like the great intellectuals of the Italian Renaissance before him, he not only looked back at history for inspiration but also produced ideas that will influence generations to come. Luigi was a clinician with sensitivity, a scholar of breadth, and a friend of considerable influence to many workers in this field. In our efforts to engage the ideas of the world and the world of ideas, few individuals have been as influential as Luigi. He was a politician and a diplomat in the finest senses of the words.

Luigi was led to studies of dementia by more than his formal education at the Medical School of the University of Padua and his postdoctoral studies in the United States. He was the son and the grandson of physicians who specialized in diseases of the brain. His maternal grandfather, Aleardo Salerni, was the neuropsychiatrist in charge of the Mental Hospital in San Servolo in Venice. In 1908 he published an article, "Di alcune analogie sintomatiche tra la demenza precoce e la demenza senile," referencing Kraepelin's studies and other reports. Luigi's father, Giovanni Amaducci, was a neuropsychiatrist in Verona, where Luigi was born. At Luigi's last working session with his close friend and frequent collaborator Katherine Bick, he showed her the black leatherette-covered notebook in which his father had written the directions for the Bielschowsky and Alzheimer methods for staining that he had received from Heidenhain on the latter's visit to Verona. Is it any wonder, then, that Luigi Amaducci had a deep, intuitive grasp of the flow of history in the discoveries that enlighten our lives?

Luigi will be honored and remembered in many different ways. We hope that the dedication of this book to him will gratify his family, his friends and colleagues, and his spirit. Although Luigi's illness made it impossible for him to attend the conference on which this book is based, his work was nonetheless a focal point and an inspiration for the participants. With gratitude for his contributions to both this book and our field, we honor his memory with this dedication.

— Peter J. Whitehouse & Katherine L. Bick

Contents

Preface

It is ironic that the professional and popular discourses surrounding Alzheimer disease (AD), whose most dreaded feature is the obliteration of memory, proceed with little awareness of its past. As with individuals, large-scale social enterprises such as the research, policy, and caregiving efforts that surround AD require a sense of history in order to situate themselves in the present and orient themselves toward the future. We hope that the essays in this volume, taken as a whole, will begin to address this irony — creating a fuller sense of the origins and development of the concept of Alzheimer disease, not simply to preserve the past for its own sake, but to better understand where we are and where we may be going.

The time is ripe for such an endeavor. At the end the twentieth century, knowledge about this "disease of the century" is in a state of flux. Biomedical and social scientists, policy makers, and caregivers are searching for new ways to think about AD as they grapple with information concerning its genetic basis, its relationship to aging, the problems and potential of developing effective drug treatments, and the ethical dilemmas surrounding the complex issues of the personhood of people with dementia. These issues are not entirely new, of course. As the historical chapters in this volume show, people concerned with this disorder have grappled with these issues for decades, though perhaps in different forms and with a different set of assumptions and resources. Likewise, though the development of science and society may change the particular form these issues take, people will continue to face versions of them for the foreseeable future.

We do not claim that this book will resolve these issues. There are, of course, as many perspectives on the past as there are on the present.

Thinking historically, which we suggest is a crucial aspect of thinking intelligently about any complex issue, does not involve reducing the past to an artificially stable narrative of inevitable progress that legitimates one particular point of view. Such abuse of the past is all too common in scientific discourse. Rather, thinking historically means creating a narrative that finds a meaningful pattern in the past without obliterating its contingencies and complexities. Our understanding of the past should be as complex and contestable as our understanding of the present. Historical thinking ultimately means re-creating a past that is real enough to argue about. Thus, if the reader finds much to argue with in the following chapters, this volume will have succeeded in its task of beginning to create a historical framework for thinking about the problem of AD.

History will not make the problems we face in AD today and tomorrow simpler or less daunting. But in its complexity, history can enrich our understanding and make our struggles more meaningful.

On a smaller scale, the power of history to affect the present and shape the future may be seen in the genesis of this book. A major impetus has been the interest of Konrad Maurer, his wife Ulrike, and his colleagues in the Department of Psychiatry and Psychotherapy at Johann Wolfgang Goethe University in Frankfurt, Germany, in uncovering historical data concerning Alois Alzheimer and his work. Their interest in history and their hard work led to the creation of a museum and conference site at Alzheimer's birthplace, the discovery of the clinical records for the first case of the disease that bears Alzheimer's name, and ultimately the symposium in November 1997 in which much of the material in this book originated. We expect that these important historical records will lead to further projects in the future.

The 1997 symposium was a celebration of the life and legacy of Alois Alzheimer and the neuroscientists of his generation. Alzheimer was born in Marktbreit, an idyllic German village in lower Frankonia situated on the river Main between Wurzburg to the north and Rothenburg to the south. Eduard Alzheimer, the father of Alois Alzheimer, was a notary public of the local royal court of justice. Eduard's first wife died of complications from childbirth a few days after their son Karl was born. Eduard married her sister and moved in the winter of 1863/64 to a substantially smaller, but attractive, house. This is the house in which Alois Alzheimer was born on June 14, 1864. More than a century later, it was the site of the symposium that drew distinguished scholars and scientists from many disciplines and many countries to discuss the past, present, and future of AD.

The Alzheimer family lived in the Marktbreit house for fourteen years. There Alois Alzheimer was baptized a Roman Catholic on the July 3, 1864. From 1870 to 1874 he attended the local Catholic primary school. Alzheimer's father had ambitions for the further education for his children and did not see such possibilities in Marktbreit itself. So when Alois was ten, he was sent to attend the gymnasium in Aschaffenburg, a city situated between Marktbreit and Frankfurt. The Alzheimer family moved to Aschaffenburg four years later, and after that very little is known about the history of the house.

Konrad and Ulrike Maurer rediscovered Alzheimer's childhood home in 1989. In July of that year, the house became the site of an international symposium marking the 125th anniversary of the scientist's birth. Alzheimer's oldest granddaughter unveiled a plaque commemorating the birthplace of her grandfather.

Also during the 1989 conference, American scientist R. J. Wurtmann honored Alzheimer's work and its importance for modern medicine in a lecture given in the historical city hall of Marktbreit. In his presentation, entitled "Some Philosophical Aspects of Alzheimer's Discovery: An American Perspective," Wurtmann said, "Dr. Alzheimer's contribution was considerably more than just medical; it also bore on a central concern of Western philosophers since the time of Plato and Aristotle, namely the 'mind-body problem.' The enunciation of Alzheimer's disease provided one of the best proofs then available that the distinctly human attributes of consciousness and cognition have their origins in specific components of the brain."

The first comprehensive textbook on AD (Maurer, Riederer, and Beckmann 1990) resulted from this conference, with contributions by the best-known Alzheimer researchers at that time.

In 1994 Eli Lilly and Company agreed to purchase the house. Ulrike Maurer was responsible for turning the house into a museum and conference site in Alzheimer's honor. On December 19, 1995, the eightieth anniversary of Alzheimer's death, the Lilly ZNS-Forum im Alzheimer Haus was established at a ceremony that included Alzheimer's five grandchildren as well as many influential researchers in the field. The Alzheimer Haus has the following mission:

— to commemorate the psychiatrist Alois Alzheimer and his important work.
— to promote academic interchange between researchers of psychiatric neurological and degenerative diseases.

— to promote collaboration among researchers, physicians, industry, and patients and their caregivers who are concerned with psychiatric and neurological diseases.

— to assist in the advancement of public understanding of neuropsychiatric diseases.

Two days after the dedication of the restored house in Marktbreit, Maurer and his colleagues made an even greater find: the clinical records of Auguste D., the first case described by Alzheimer, which ultimately was the basis for one of the most widely known medical terms of the twentieth century. The scientists had been conducting an exhaustive search for the file in the basement of the Johann Wolfgang Goethe University Hospital, where Maurer is director of the department of psychiatry. It was at this Frankfurt institution that Auguste D. spent her final days. The *Chicago Tribune* reported: "Maurer and two colleagues [Stephan Volk and Hector Gerbaldo] were again searching the basement when one of the other administrators randomly pulled out a handful of files, noticed that one was old, glanced at it and shouted 'That's Auguste D.!' " (Leroux 1997).

At the 1995 dedication of the Alzheimer Haus, plans were made for the 1997 symposium that led to this book. The generosity of Eli Lilly and Company made it possible to invite eighteen renowned experts on the historical development of the concept of Alzheimer disease; state-of-the-art contemporary research, ethics, and policy issues around the disease; and the social and cultural contexts in which the concept developed. Participants came from Germany, the Netherlands, and the United States and included biologists, clinicians, philosophers, social scientists, and historians. Communication across these national and disciplinary boundaries was not always easy. At conference end, the group certainly had not solved the problems of interdisciplinary and cross-cultural communication, but the intimate and richly historical atmosphere of the Alzheimer Haus fostered a sense of camaraderie and common purpose. This, in turn, allowed the participants to experience the stimulating possibilities inherent in working with individuals whose basic intellectual assumptions are radically different. All of the participants in the conference but one (a molecular biologist) supplied chapters for this volume. Luigi Amaducci, whose energy and interest in history were such an inspiration to many of the conference participants, was too ill to attend the conference. He contributed an essay, nonetheless, which was presented at the conference by Katherine Bick, but which could not be included in this volume (see dedication and introduction to Part I).

The book includes two historical sections that cover the major developments in the conceptual evolution of the concept of AD. Thematic sections follow on the way in which social and cultural factors have shaped the concept of the disease, on the perspectives of caregivers and patients, and on prospects and problems for the future. Detailed introductions of the chapters precede each of these sections.

We intend the volume to help a wide range of professionals who are committed to increasing knowledge of AD in both biomedical and social terms, to improving care for patients and their families, and to formulating policies to deal with the difficult issues the disease raises. Specifically, we intend the volume to be of use to: (1) biomedical researchers and clinicians who desire a historical perspective, a review of contemporary knowledge, and an assessment of future implications of the complex issues involved in the conception of AD; (2) scholars in the humanities and social sciences who require such a discussion of the past, present, and future in order to write broader accounts of social, cultural, and policy issues surrounding the disease itself and aging in general; and (3) caregivers, policy advocates, and others concerned with the disease and its victims. We hope that they will find these perspectives on scientific knowledge useful in coming to terms with the disease and its consequences. By amassing and organizing historical material and a review of contemporary research, the volume will serve as a basic reference tool for this broad audience. At the same time, by providing critical discussion, the book will serve as a challenging stimulus to further knowledge and exploration.

References

Leroux, Charles. 1997. The Case of Auguste D. *Chicago Tribune*, 22 July 1997, p. E1.

Maurer, K., P. Riederer, and H. Beckmann. 1990. *Alzheimer's Disease: Epidemiology, Neuropathology, and Clinics.* New York: Springer-Verlag.

Acknowledgments

In the two years that have passed since we first conceived this book, we have accumulated innumerable debts to many individuals without whose support this book could not have been produced.

First, we would like to thank Eli Lilly and Company for generous support at every stage of this project, and especially for providing the contributors of this book with the rich environment of Alois Alzheimer's birthplace to begin the process. In particular, we owe thanks to Robert Postlethwait, Jochen Becker, and John Lucas for their understanding and commitment to this project. Jennifer Stegemann made travel to and from the conference in Marktbreit remarkably easy and comfortable, and handled many other logistical details of the conference. We were also fortunate to have two researchers from Lilly, Larry Altstiel and Steve Paul, co-author a chapter for the book.

At the Johns Hopkins University Press, we would like to thank our editor, Wendy Harris, for her advice and understanding as this project slowly evolved into a book. The anonymous referee at Hopkins gave us many helpful suggestions that allowed us to improve this book. Elizabeth Yoder's copyediting of the final version smoothed out many rough edges.

In Cleveland, we would like to thank Barbara Juknialis for copyediting the entire manuscript at an early stage. Barbara Ballenger copyedited later versions of several chapters. Danielle DiBona helped with much of the laborious work of typing these revisions. Julia Rajcan of the Alzheimer's Center handled so many of the logistical details of producing this book that it surely would not have appeared without her help.

We would also like to thank a number of people at Case Western Reserve University. In the history department Alan Rocke, Jonathan

Sadowsky, and David Van Tassel provided helpful advice at various stages of this project. Jesse Ballenger would also like to thank his colleague and friend Patrick Ryan for understanding, enthusiastic support, and cogent advice on how to integrate this project into the larger journey we have shared in graduate school. Peter Whitehouse would like to thank the Department of Neurology in the School of Medicine, and in particular the chair of the department, Dennis Landis, for supporting the sort of broad intellectual pursuits that this book represents.

In Germany, Konrad and Ulrike Maurer and the staff of the Alzheimer-Haus worked especially hard to provide a gracious and inspiring atmosphere for the participants of the conference on which this book is based. The two days spent in the charming town of Marktbreit had a profound if intangible impact on this book.

We would also like to thank the many patients and their families who have long been a source of inspiration for us.

Finally, we would like to thank our families, without whose support this project would not have been possible.

Contributors

Larry Altstiel, M.D., Ph.D., *Lilly Research Laboratories, Eli Lilly and Company, Indianapolis, Indiana*

Jesse F. Ballenger, M.A., Ph.D. candidate, *Department of History, Case Western Reserve University, Cleveland, Ohio*

Katherine L. Bick, Ph.D., *Science Advisor, Charles A. Dana Foundation, Wilmington, North Carolina*

Eva Braak, Ph.D., *Professor, Department of Anatomy, Johann Wolfgang Goethe University, Frankfurt, Germany*

Heiko Braak, M.D., *Professor, Department of Anatomy, Johann Wolfgang Goethe University, Frankfurt, Germany*

Robert Mullan Cook-Deegan, M.D., *Director, National Cancer Policy Board, Institute of Medicine, National Academy of Sciences, Washington, D.C.*

Rob J. M. Dillmann, M.D., Ph.D., *Secretary of Medical Affairs, Royal Dutch Medical Association, Utrecht, Netherlands*

Hans Förstl, M.D., Ph.D., *Professor and Director, Department and Clinic of Psychiatry and Psychotherapy, Technical University, Munich, Germany*

Patrick J. Fox, Ph.D., *Co-director, Institute for Health and Aging; and Associate Professor, Department of Social and Behavioral Sciences, School of Nursing, University of California, San Francisco, California*

Hector Gerbaldo, M.D., *Department of Psychiatry and Psychotherapy I, Johann Wolfgang Goethe University, Frankfurt, Germany*

Manuel B. Graeber, M.D., *Max-Planck Institute of Neurobiology, Department of Neuromorphology, Martinsried, Germany*

Jaber F. Gubrium, Ph.D., *Professor, Department of Sociology, University of Florida, Gainesville, Florida*

Martha B. Holstein, Ph.D., *Research Scholar and Director, Program on Aging, Park Ridge Center for the Study of Health, Faith and Ethics, Chicago, Illinois*

Robert Katzman, M.D., *Research Professor of Neurosciences, Alzheimer Disease Research Center, Department of Neurosciences, School of Medicine, University of California, San Diego, La Jolla, California*

Konrad Maurer, M.D., *Professor, Head, Department of Psychiatry and Psychotherapy I, and Director, Clinic for Psychiatry, Johann Wolfgang Goethe University, Frankfurt, Germany*

Hans-Jurgen Möller, M.D., Ph.D., *Professor and Director, Psychiatric Hospital, Ludwig Maximillian University, Munich, Germany*

Steven Paul, M.D., *Lilly Research Laboratories, Eli Lilly and Company, Indianapolis, Indiana*

Daniel A. Pollen, M.D., *Department of Neurology, University of Massachusetts Medical Center, Worcester, Massachusetts*

Stephen G. Post, Ph.D., *Professor and Associate Director of Educational Ethics, Center for Biomedical Ethics, Case Western Reserve University, Cleveland, Ohio*

Stephan Volk, M.D., *Department of Psychiatry and Psychotherapy II, Johann Wolfgang Goethe University, Frankfurt, Germany*

Peter J. Whitehouse, M.D., Ph.D., *Professor of Neurology, Psychiatry, Neuroscience, Psychology, Nursing, Organizational Behavior, and Biomedical Ethics, Case Western Reserve University, Cleveland, Ohio*

PART I

The Cases of Auguste D. and Johann F.

Origins of the Modern Concept of Alzheimer Disease

As we enter a new millennium, neuroscience seems the most modern, forward-looking of endeavors in biomedicine, generating stunning insights into the molecular basis of brain function, which are then applied to problems of human behavior that have vexed humanity throughout history—problems such as age-associated progressive dementia. Over the past decade, research on Alzheimer disease (AD) has been on the cutting edge of the revolution in our understanding of the basic biologic mechanisms of the brain.

Yet, however promising its prospects appear, neuroscience and the particular field of AD research cannot afford to neglect the study of its origins. As master historian of medicine and psychiatry Erwin Ackerknecht argued, the question of origins is not merely of academic interest. If any science is to chart new and reliable paths, it must continually reexamine its essential premises, which can best be understood by studying its origins (Ackerknecht and Vallois 1956).

The two chapters in this section make an important contribution to our understanding of the origins of the concept of AD by providing newly uncovered historical evidence concerning the first two cases of the disease that Alzheimer described. Konrad Maurer's chapter presents evidence from the clinical records and recently recovered brain tissue of Auguste D., the 51-year-old woman whose case Alzheimer first described in 1907 (and which Gaetano Perusini described in greater detail in 1910). The clinical records were recovered by Maurer and his colleagues in Frankfurt in 1995, and the original histologic slides of Auguste D.'s brain that Alzheimer prepared were found by Hans-Jurgen Möller and his colleagues in Munich in 1998. In Chapter 2, Möller presents similar evidence concerning Johann F., the second case of the disease studied by Alzheimer and a crucial part of his important 1911 publication. Presenting this material in the context of the broader clinical and pathological work of Alzheimer, Perusini, Kraepelin, and others of this generation of pioneers, Maurer and Möller provide the reader with a thorough understanding of the clinical and pathological work that produced the modern concept of AD.

These two cases remain interesting and informative puzzles even from the perspective of contemporary neuroscience. Although, as later chapters in this volume will document, tremendous progress has been made in the understanding of AD, the basic pathological features of the disease, which were identified almost a century ago, remain mysterious enough to be open to differing interpretations. Although the specific proteins of which both the tangle (tau) and the plaque (beta amyloid) are composed have been identified, it remains a point of contention among researchers as to which of these is more important in the pathogenesis of dementia — a debate that has been caricatured as a fight between two groups of religious zealots, the "Baptists" (proponents of the beta amyloid protein of neuritic plaques) and "Taoists" (proponents of the tau protein of neurofibrillary tangles). Although researchers are perhaps not ready to burn each other at the stake — as the amicable coexistence of both points of view in this volume demonstrates — the issue remains beyond the ability of current neuroscientific knowledge to resolve.

The case of Johann F. is particularly interesting in connection with this issue because no neurofibrillary tangles were found in his brain, making it a case of "plaque-only AD." Plaques had been described in the brains of demented individuals even before Alzheimer by Fischer and Redlich. Alzheimer is credited with the discovery of neurofibrillary tangles and with providing, in the case of Auguste D., an account that associated the clinical signs of dementia with both plaques and tangles. In this light, it might even seem appropriate to refer to plaque-only dementia as Fischer's or Redlich's disease, rather than as AD. And in more recent times, there has been considerable controversy about whether we should call plaque-only progressive degenerative dementia AD or restrict the term *Alzheimer disease* to those cases in which both pathologic signatures are found. Most neuropathologists believe it is possible to label plaque-only and plaque-and-tangle dementia as the same entity, because other than this difference their pathological features are similar (i.e., neuronal loss and neurochemical changes). However, it is possible that in the future a distinction could be drawn between the two with important implications for different therapies.

Although neurofibrillary tangles are best known as a hallmark of AD, like plaques they are also found in a number of other neurological conditions. This has made it possible to question even the diagnosis of Auguste D., whose case serves as the classic description of AD. Luigi Amaducci, who has contributed so much to both contemporary research and historical understanding of AD (see dedication to this volume), argued forcefully that the clinical and neuropathologic picture of the case could reasonably be interpreted today as a metachromatic leukodystrophy (MLD), a very rare disorder that had not yet been defined and described in Alzheimer's time. MLD is among the other disorders in which tangles are found, and Amaducci thought that certain aspects of the clinical symptoms reported in the case of Auguste D. (early motor difficulties, schizophrenia-like symptoms, disturbances of visual short-term memory, and visuospatial perception) are, by today's standards, more typical of MLD than of AD. Similarly, he argued, the histopathology as described by Perusini showed some features that were characteristic of MLD (demyleination of central white matter and metachromatic deposits in the spinal cord) (Amaducci et al. 1991; Amaducci 1996).

Though Amaducci did not persuade many of his colleagues on this point, his argument was plausible enough that it had to be reckoned with. Though illness prevented him from attending in person, his MLD hypothesis was nonetheless one of the focal points of the conference at Alzheimer's birthplace in Marktbreit, Germany, from which this book evolved. Sadly, Amaducci did not live to see the discovery of the original slides of Auguste D.'s brain tissue prepared by Alzheimer. Tissue analysis of this material conducted by Möller's group in Munich conclusively settles the issue (Enserink 1998). The neuropathology first described by Alzheimer and Perusini in the case of Auguste D. is clearly that of what we today call AD. In light of this evidence, his closest colleagues feel certain that Amaducci would have dropped the MLD hypothesis, and we have thus chosen not to include the paper Amaducci prepared for the Marktbreit conference as a chapter in this book.

Reexamining these foundational cases from the perspective of contemporary neuroscience is, in the end, humbling. We are reminded of the difficult issues that were involved in defining the conceptual boundaries of this disease — issues that remain daunting despite the tremendous progress that has been made in the last few decades. From the perspective of contemporary neuroscience, the achievements of Alzheimer and his colleagues are all the more remarkable. As Amaducci put it in his paper for the Marktbreit conference, "We can be viewed as small children standing on the shoulders of a giant."

References

Ackerknecht, E., and H. Vallois. 1956. *Franz Joseph Gall, Inventor of Phrenology and His Collection.* Madison: Wisconsin Medical School.

Amaducci, L. A., S. Sorbi, S. Piacentini, and K. L. Bick. 1991. The first Alzheimer disease case: A metachromatic leukodystrophy? *Developmental Neuroscience* 13:186–87.

Amaducci, L. A. 1996. Alzheimer's original patient. *Science* 274: Letters, 18 October.

Enserink, M. 1998. First Alzheimer's diagnosis confirmed. *Science* 279:2037.

1

Auguste D.

The History of Alois Alzheimer's First Case

Konrad Maurer, Stephan Volk, and Hector Gerbaldo

The year 1997 marked the ninetieth anniversary of Alois Alzheimer's remarkable publication, "A Characteristic Disease of the Cerebral Cortex" (Alzheimer 1907). This two-page article, and the subsequent publications by Bonfiglio (1908), Perusini (1909), and again Alzheimer in 1911, led to the eponym *Alzheimer's disease* first used by Emil Kraepelin in his 1910 textbook of psychiatry. In his 1906 and 1907 papers, Alzheimer described Auguste D., a 51-year-old woman from Frankfurt who had exhibited progressive cognitive impairment, focal symptoms, hallucinations, delusions, and psychosocial incompetence. At postmortem she exhibited arteriosclerotic changes, senile plaques, and neurofibrillary tangles. Although the eponym *Alzheimer* was originally used to describe "presenile" dementia, it was later also applied to dementing processes of old age.

This chapter describes the discovery and the contents of the long-lost file of Auguste D. and provides some biographical data on Alois Alzheimer and information on the derivation of the eponym. The type of Auguste D.'s dementia will also be reviewed in this context. Parts of the file and its content have been published by Maurer, Volk, and Gerbaldo (1997).

ALOIS ALZHEIMER'S LIFE AND WORK

Alois Alzheimer was born on June 14, 1864, in Marktbreit, a small town in lower Franconia on the Main river in Bavaria, southern Germany. His father was a Royal Bavarian Notary. When he graduated from high school in the district capital of Aschaffenburg, Alzheimer's teachers certified that he was "excellent in the sciences." Science was also his hobby. Alzheimer studied medicine in Berlin, Würzburg, and Tübingen. He returned to Würzburg, where he graduated in 1888 after writing a doctoral dissertation, "On the Ceruminal Glands of the Ear." His doctoral adviser was the famous Swiss-born physiologist Albert Koelliker. Alzheimer completed his state medical exams in the same year.

After graduation Alzheimer worked for a short period in Koelliker's histologic laboratory in Würzburg. The young Alzheimer quite likely acquainted himself with the topical problems of the microscopic construction of the nervous system and was involved in the neurohistologic discussions of that time.

In 1888 Alzheimer went to Frankfurt to work in the Municipality Asylum for the Mentally Sick and Epileptics, directed by Dr. Emil Sioli, an open-minded, liberal psychiatrist. The young Alzheimer, at this time assistant house-officer, continued to be very fond of working with the microscope, a fascination that remained with him all his life. He was especially interested in researching the cortex of the human brain.

At the turn of the century, the number of mentally ill patients was increasing rapidly in Germany as elsewhere. Sexually transmitted diseases were widespread, and the number of patients with neuropsychiatric complications of progressive paralysis was increasing. In this atmosphere Alzheimer gained abundant clinical practice as a psychiatrist. He was in close contact with his patients and "wanted to help psychiatry with the microscope" (Kraepelin 1924).

Dr. Franz Nissl, Alzheimer's superior, who had arrived in Frankfurt in April 1889, discovered better tissue-staining techniques. Nissl and Alzheimer became friends and close colleagues. During the day they worked together in the hospital, and in the evening they sat side by side in the laboratory doing research and discussing their results. Alzheimer believed that clinical practice and laboratory research complemented each other. "Why should not the physician improve his competence by enlarging scientific knowledge of psychiatry besides doing his daily clinical practice?" he once wrote (Maurer and Maurer 1998).

In 1894 Alzheimer married Cecilie Geisenheimer, née Wallerstein,

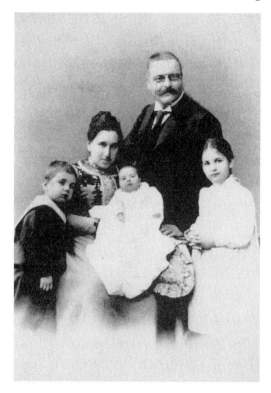

FIGURE 1.   Alois Alzheimer with his wife, Cecilie, and their children, Gertrude, Maria, and Hans.

a wealthy Jewish widow. They had three children: Gertrud (who married the psychiatrist Georg Stertz), Hans, and Maria (Figure 1). When his young wife died in 1901, Alzheimer's younger sister, Maria, came to take care of the three children. As a result of his marriage, Alzheimer had gained considerable financial independence.

While in Frankfurt, Alzheimer expressed the desire to have a position in which he could combine research and clinical practice. In 1895 Alzheimer's friend Nissl moved to Heidelberg, where Emil Kraepelin held the chair of psychiatry. Kraepelin heard of Alzheimer's application for the post of managing director of a mental asylum. Being exclusively a research scientist, Kraepelin did not think much of this idea. Instead, Kraepelin invited Alzheimer to come to Heidelberg to write his "Habilitationsschrift." Alzheimer accepted and completed his research project under Kraepelin's supervision. In 1903 Alzheimer followed Kraepelin to Munich, where Kraepelin had recently been appointed director of the Nervenklinik.

In Munich Alzheimer was appointed head of the neuroanatomic laboratory, which became an important center for brain research. He

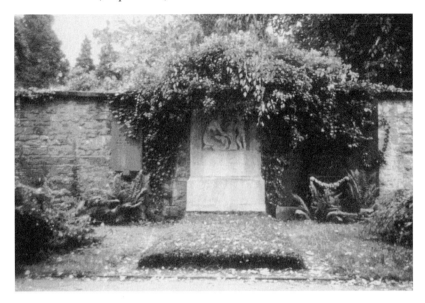

FIGURE 2.   The tomb of Cecilie and Alois Alzheimer in Frankfurt, Germany.

was joined by a number of renowned psychiatrists and neuropathologists, including Gaetano Perusini, Francesco Bonfiglio, Ugo Cerletti, Alfons Jakob, Hans Gerhard Creutzfeldt, Nicolas Achucarro, Karl Kleist, and Smith Ely Jeliffe. Alzheimer and his co-workers completed thousands of microscopic preparations.

Alzheimer's research interests were wide-ranging. During his years in Frankfurt and Munich, he published about seventy papers. He finished his inaugural dissertation, "Histological Studies on the Differential Diagnosis of Progressive Paralysis," in Munich in 1904. This work was based on 320 postmortem cases he had collected in Frankfurt. In addition to dementia of vascular and degenerative origins, Alzheimer was interested in areas such as forensic psychiatry, delirium, mental deficiency, indications for induced abortion in mentally ill women, and histopathology of psychoses.

The Friedrich-Wilhelm University of Breslau in Silesia appointed Alzheimer chair of the Department of Psychiatry and director of the University Psychiatric Clinic on July 16, 1912. He viewed the post as the fulfillment of his scientific and academic aims. On his way to Breslau, which was then in East Germany (though today it is Wroclaw, in Poland), Alzheimer caught a severe and persistent cold, which developed into subacute bacterial endocarditis. He never recovered completely. On December 19, 1915, during the second winter of World War I, Alois Alzheimer died in a uremic coma. He had not reached his fifty-second birthday. His body was transferred to Frankfurt and was laid to rest at the principal cemetery next to his wife, who had been buried there on February 28, 1901 (Figure 2).

AUGUSTE D. AND HER FILE

Until 1989 the whereabouts of Alzheimer's birthplace were largely unknown. That year, on the occasion of a symposium to celebrate Alzheimer's 125th birthday, the house, located in Marktbreit, was identified and fitted with a memorial plaque. On December 19, 1995, the 80th anniversary of Alzheimer's death, a symposium was held at the Marktbreit house. Purchased by the pharmaceutical firm Eli Lilly, the house was inaugurated as a museum and conference center. Ulrike Maurer has been responsible for its renovation (Figure 3).

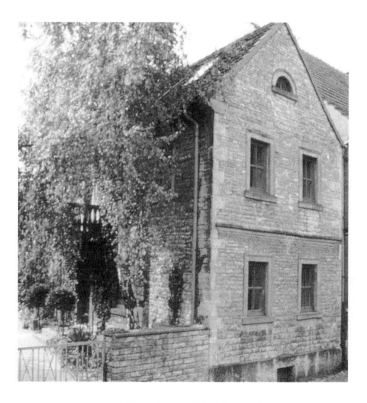

FIGURE 3.   Alois Alzheimer's birthplace, in Marktbreit, Germany.

Before this event, the authors had launched an intensive search for the file of Auguste D., which had been lost since Alzheimer's and Perusini's descriptions of the case in 1907 and 1909. The authors located the file in the archives of their department in Frankfurt on December 21, 1995 (Maurer et al. 1997).

After 90 years the blue cardboard file was still in pristine condition (Figure 4). It contained 32 pages, including the patient's admission report, several medical and administrative certificates, and three versions of the case history — one in Latin script and two in the now-outdated Germanic script "Sütterlin."

The case history begins with an interview of the patient's husband, followed by clinical findings and the details of the course of her disease. A report on her death includes an anatomopathologic diagnosis. A small sheet of paper with the handwriting of Auguste D., dated by Alois Alz-

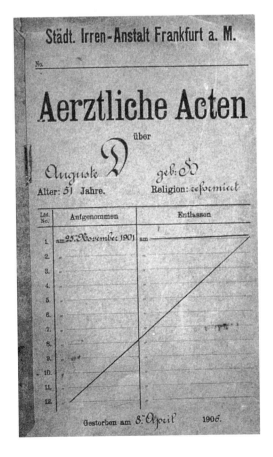

FIGURE 4.   Cover of the file of Auguste D.

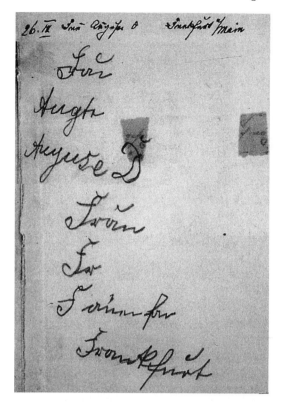

FIGURE 5.   Auguste D.'s
handwriting.

heimer, shows "anamnestic writing disorder" (Figure 5). Alzheimer's handwritten notes, also in Germanic script, document in detail his patient's symptoms from the first five days of her hospitalization on. In between Alzheimer's signatures are two hand-written notes by Auguste D., samples of Auguste's attempts to write her name. The file also contains four photographs of the patient, the most impressive of which is shown in Figure 6. The course of the disease is documented beginning in February 1902 until the day of her death, April 7, 1906. The file also includes a one-page case report from the Royal Psychiatric Department in Munich, in which Alzheimer summarizes the history and course of August D.'s disease.

AUGUSTE D.'S CASE HISTORY

Auguste D. was admitted to the clinic in Frankfurt on November 25, 1901. The case history in the file reads as follows:

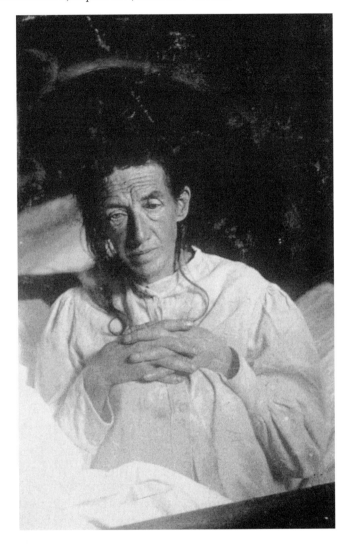

FIGURE 6.   Auguste D.

D., Auguste, wife of an office clerk, aged 51-and-a-half years. The patient's mother suffered convulsive attacks after menopause; it seems that she did not lose consciousness and did not drop objects that she was holding in her hands. Her mother died at the age of 64 of pneumonia; her father died at the age of 45 of anthrax of the neck. Three healthy brothers. No alcoholism or mental illness in the family history.

Previously, the patient had never been sick. She had been happily married since 1873, had borne a healthy daughter, and had had no abortions. Very diligent and tidy, slightly anxious and fearful, but polite. There seems to have been no syphilitic infection in either the patient or in her husband.

Until March 1901, nothing outstanding occurred. Around March 18, 1901, the patient suddenly asserted, without any reason, that her husband had gone for a walk with a neighbor. From then on she remained very cool toward him and the lady. Soon afterward, she started to have difficulty in remembering things. Two months later, she started making mistakes in preparing meals, paced nervously and without reason in the apartment, and was not careful with the household money. She progressively became worse. She asserted that a wagon driver who often came to her home might do something to her, and she assumed that all conversations of the people around her were about her. She had no language disturbances and no paralysis. Later she often had a fear of dying and nervous anxiety during which she started to tremble. She would ring all the bells of the neighbors and knock on their doors. She could not find certain objects that she had put away.

Alzheimer's Case Report

A full transcription of Alzheimer's questions and Auguste D.'s answers appears in previous publications as well as in a biography of Alzheimer (Maurer and Maurer 1998), and will not be printed here in their entirety. Alzheimer's notes in the file begin on November 26, 1901. He asked very simple questions and wrote down the dialogues systematically. His questioning continues on four handwritten pages, dated through November 30, 1901.

November 26, 1901
ALZHEIMER'S NOTE: She sat on her bed with helpless expression.
Alzheimer: What is your name?
Auguste D.: Auguste.
Alzheimer: Last name?
Auguste D.: Auguste.
Alzheimer: What is your husband's name?
Auguste D.: Auguste, I think.
Alzheimer: Your husband?
Auguste D.: Ah, my husband? [*She looks as if she doesn't understand the question.*]
Alzheimer: Are you married?
Auguste D.: To Auguste.

Alzheimer: Mrs. D.?

Auguste D.: Yes, Auguste D.

Alzheimer: How long have you been here? [*She seems to be trying to remember.*]

Auguste D.: Three weeks.

Alzheimer: What is this? [*I showed her a pencil.*]

Auguste D.: A pen.

ALZHEIMER'S NOTE: A purse, a key, a diary, a cigar are named correctly. At lunch she eats cauliflower and pork. Asked what she was eating, she answers "spinach." As she was chewing the meat and was asked what she was eating, she answered "potatoes" and then "horseradish." When objects were shown to her, after a short time she did not remember what objects had been shown. In between she always speaks about "twins." When she is asked to write, she holds the book in such a way that one has the impression that she has a reduction of the right visual field.

Asked to write "Mrs. Auguste D.," she tries to write "Mrs." and forgets the rest. It is necessary to repeat every word. Amnestic writing disorder ("Amnestische Schriftstörung"). In the evening her spontaneous speech is full of paraphrasic derailments and perseverations.

November 28

She continuously looks helpless, anxious, and says, "I do not want to be cut." She behaves as if blind, touching other patients on their faces while they fight her. When asked what she is doing, she replies: "I must put order." She had been brought into an "isolation room," where she behaved very quietly.

November 29

ALZHEIMER'S NOTE: Helpless, refuses everything.

Alzheimer: . . . What is your name?

Auguste D.: Mrs. D., Auguste.

Alzheimer: When were you born?

Auguste D.: Eighteen hundred and . . .

Alzheimer: Your birthday?

Auguste D.: This year, a past year.

Alzheimer: When born?

Auguste D.: Eighteen-hundred, I don't know.

Alzheimer: What did I ask you?

Auguste D.: Ah, D., Auguste.

Alzheimer: Do you have children?

Auguste D.: One daughter.

Alzheimer: What is her name?

Auguste D.: Thekla.

Alzheimer: How old is she?

Auguste D.: She is married in Berlin, Mrs. S.

Alzheimer: Where does she live?

Auguste D.: We live in Kassel.

Alzheimer: Where does your daughter live?

Auguste D.: Waldemarstreet, no different.

Alzheimer: What is the name of your husband?

Auguste D.: I do not know how I came to this. I cannot go on this way.

ALZHEIMER'S NOTE: She seems not to understand the question.

Alzheimer: What is the name of your husband?

Auguste D.: I don't know.

Alzheimer: What is your husband's name?

Auguste D.: My husband is not here at this time.

Alzheimer: What is the name of your husband?

ALZHEIMER'S NOTE: She suddenly and quickly answered, "August Wilhelm Carl. I don't know if I can say that."

Alzheimer: What is your husband?

Auguste D.: Office clerk. I am so wrong, so wrong. I cannot . . .

Alzheimer: How long have you been here?

Auguste D.: Rather long.

Alzheimer: Where are you now?

Auguste D.: But this is Wilhelmhöhe.

Alzheimer: Where is your flat?

Auguste D.: In Frankfurt am Main.

Alzheimer: Which street?

Auguste D.: Not the Waldemarstreet but another one. . . . Just wait, I am very, very . . .

Alzheimer: Are you ill?

Auguste D.: Well, more the spine.

Alzheimer: Do you know me?

Auguste D.: I think you have seen me two times. Please excuse me. . . . I cannot . . . in this way.

Alzheimer: What is the current year?

Auguste D.: 1800.

Alzheimer: Are you ill?

Auguste D.: Second month.

Alzheimer: What are the names of the patients? [*She answers quickly and correctly.*]

Alzheimer: Which month is it now?

Auguste D.: The eleventh.

Alzheimer: What is the name of the eleventh month?

Auguste D.: The last one, if not the last one.

Alzheimer: Which one?

Auguste D.: I don't know.

Alzheimer: What color is the snow?

Auguste D.: White.

Alzheimer: The soot?

Auguste D.: Black.

Alzheimer: The sky?

Auguste D.: Blue.

Alzheimer: The meadows?

Auguste D.: Green.

Alzheimer: How many fingers do you have?

Auguste D.: Five.

Alzheimer: Eyes?

Auguste D.: Two.

Alzheimer: Legs?

Auguste D.: Two.

Alzheimer: How many dimes are in a mark?

Auguste D.: 100.

Alzheimer: How many marks are in one thaler?

Auguste D.: One mark, yes, one mark.

Alzheimer: How much does an egg cost?

Auguste D.: Six or eight.

Alzheimer: Six or eight, what?

Auguste D.: Yes.

Alzheimer: Six or eight marks?

Auguste D.: Yes, mark.

Alzheimer: What does a pound of meat cost?

Auguste D.: Twenty.

Alzheimer: Twenty, what?

Auguste D.: I don't know.

Alzheimer: One roll?

Auguste D.: Three dimes.

Alzheimer: If you buy six eggs for seven dimes, how much does it cost?

Auguste D.: Differently.

Alzheimer: On what street do you live?

Auguste D.: I can tell you. I must wait a little bit.

Alzheimer: What did I ask you?

Auguste D.: Well, this is Frankfurt am Main.

Alzheimer: On which street do you live?

Auguste D.: Waldemarstreet . . . not . . . no . . .

Alzheimer: When did you get married?

Auguste D.: I don't know at present. The woman lives on the same floor.

Alzheimer: Which woman?

Auguste D.: The woman where we are living. [*The patient calls*] Mrs. G., Mrs. G., here a step deeper. She lives . . .

ALZHEIMER'S NOTE: I show her a key, a pencil, and a book and she names them correctly.

Alzheimer: What did I show you?

Auguste D.: I don't know, I don't know.

Alzheimer: It is difficult, isn't it?

Auguste D.: So anxious, so anxious.

Alzheimer: [*I show her three fingers.*] How many fingers?

Auguste D.: Three.

Alzheimer: Are you still anxious?

Auguste D.: Yes.

Alzheimer: How many fingers did I show you?

Auguste D.: Well, this is Frankfurt am Main.

ALZHEIMER'S NOTE: The patient was asked to recognize objects by touch, closing her eyes. A toothbrush, a sponge, bread, a roll, a spoon, a brush, a glass, a knife, a fork, a plate, a purse, a mark, a cigar, a key. She recognizes them quickly and correctly.

By touch, she calls a brass cup "a milk jug" and "a teaspoon," but when she opens her eyes she immediately says, "a cup." She writes as we have already described. When she has to write, "Mrs. Auguste D.," she writes "Mrs.," and we must repeat the other words because she forgets them. The patient is not able to progress in writing, and repeats, "I have lost myself."

Reading, she passes from one line to the other and repeats the same line three times. But she correctly reads the letters. She seems not to understand what she reads. She accents the words in an unusual way. Suddenly she says, "Twins." "I know Mr. Twin." She repeats the word *twin* during the whole interview.

The pupils accommodate to light without delay. The tongue has normal mobility and is dry, yellow-red-brown. No disturbance in speech articulation. She frequently interrupts herself about the pronunciation of words during the interview as if she would not know if she said something correctly. She carries a denture. No facial nerve differences. Muscular strength on the left side is considerably reduced in comparison with the right side.

Patellar reflex is normal. Radial reflex is a bit (but not relevantly) rigid. Cardiac ictus is not felt. Cardiac obtusity is not enlarged. The second pulmonary and aortic tones are not accentuated.

During the physical examination she cooperates and does not show anxiety. She suddenly says, "Just now a child called. Is he there?" She hears her calling . . .; she knows Mrs. Twin. When she was brought from the isolation room to the bed, she became agitated, screamed, and was noncooperative. She shows great fear and repeats, "I will not be cut." "I do not cut myself."

November 30
She frequently stays in the living room, touches the faces of other patients, and hits them. It is difficult to figure out what she wants. Therefore, she must be isolated. When we try to speak with her, she says, "I do not have either the will or the time. I don't want . . ."

Alzheimer: How are you?

Auguste D.: During the last days I was very good.

Alzheimer: Where are you?

Auguste D.: Here and everywhere. Here and now. You don't mind.

Alzheimer: Why are you here?

Auguste D.: We are going to live there.

Alzheimer: Where is your bed?

Auguste D.: Where should it be?

Alzheimer: How did you sleep?

Auguste D.: Very good.

Alzheimer: Where is your husband?

Auguste D.: In the clerk's office.

Alzheimer: How old are you?

Auguste D.: Fifty-seven years.

Alzheimer: Where are you living?

Auguste D.: Waldemarstreet.

Alzheimer: Did you already eat today?

Auguste D.: Soup and other things.

Alzheimer: What do you do now?

Auguste D.: To clean and something like that.

Alzheimer: Why didn't you put on your clothes?

Auguste D.: I had something to do.

Alzheimer: How long have you been here?

Auguste D.: You did write it, fifty-seven?

Alzheimer: Fifty-seven what?

Auguste D.: With the years.

ALZHEIMER'S NOTE: The behavior of the patient indicates that she is suspicious. She says to the doctor, "You do not have anything to do here." After that she greets him in a friendly way. "Please have a seat. I did not have time." She wants to live, screams terribly, like a small child. She shows signs of occupational delirium. She takes some bedspreads and folds them up or puts them under the bed. "I am making order." Sometimes she sweats profusely and calls, "Karl" or "Thekla" (the names of her husband and daughter). If she is asked to name her husband, she normally says, "Auguste." When asked where she is, she says, "at home" and after that, "at the hospital." When asked to knit, she pulls out the needles from the work and begins to pick up the single loops. When asked what a bedside table is, she answers, "This is a bedside chair, and needs a cover."

Alzheimer's hand-written report ends November 30, 1901. The other two copies, written in German old script and Latin, continue to document the course of the patient's disease from January 1902. The Latin copy contains a registration from 1902 to the beginning of 1906.

Shortly before Auguste D.'s death, the file states: "Tendency to decubitus since the beginning of 1906. Development of a sacral and left trochanteric ulcer. Very weak, high fever up to 40° C within the last days. Pneumonia of both inferior lobes."

The last documentation is dated April 8, 1906: "Within the morning, exitus letalis. Cause of death: Septicemia due to decubitus. Anatomical diagnosis: Moderate external and internal hydrocephalus. Cerebral atrophy. Arteriosclerosis of the small cerebral vessels(?). Pneumonia of both inferior lobes. Nephritis."

HOW DID THE EPONYM *ALZHEIMER'S DISEASE* COME INTO BEING?

In the autumn of 1903, Alois Alzheimer left Frankfurt. Following a short stay in Heidelberg, he moved to Munich to continue his scientific and medical activities at the Royal Psychiatric Clinic under director Emil Kraepelin. After Auguste D. died on April 8, 1906, Alzheimer asked that the record and the brain be sent to Munich. He immediately did a report on the admission formulas used in Munich at this time and wrote a full-page epicrisis. After this he made an entry to the autopsy book of the clinic under the number 181, dated 28 April 1906, Frankfurt, followed by the last name "D." and the source of the tissue as Frankfurt (Graeber et al. 1998). This proves that the brain had been analyzed in his famous neuropathologic laboratory. Within six months, on November 3, 1906, he presented his findings at the thirty-seventh meeting of the Southwest German Psychiatrists in Tübingen. In 1907 the lecture was published in *Allgemeine Zeitschrift für Psychiatrie und Psychisch-Gerichtliche Medizin* under the title, "A Characteristic Serious Disease of the Cerebral Cortex."

In this paper, Alzheimer described Auguste D.'s disease as follows:

The patient showed early clinical symptoms that deviated from the common ones and could not be classified under any well-known clinical patterns. The anatomical findings were also different from those of the usual disease processes. This disease started with a strong feeling of jealousy toward her husband. Very soon she showed rapidly increasing memory impairments. . . . She was disoriented as to time and place. Within half a year, Auguste developed symptoms typical for presenile dementia, later called Alzheimer's disease. Her neurological status was normal. There were no motoric disturbances in her gait or use of her hands. Her pupils reacted normally. . . . After four-and-a-half years of illness, the patient died. She was completely apathetic in the end and was confined to bed in a fetal position (with legs drawn up), was incontinent, and in spite of all the care and attention given to her, she suffered from decubitus. The autopsy showed an evenly affected atrophic brain without macroscopic foci. The larger cerebral vessels showed arteriosclerotic changes.

Concerning histopathology, Alzheimer wrote:

The Bielschowsky silver preparation showed very characteristic changes in the neurofibrils. However, inside an apparently normal-looking cell, one or more single fibers could be observed that became prominent through their striking thickness and specific impregnability. At a more advanced stage, many fibrils, arranged parallel, showed the same changes. Then they accumulated, forming dense bundles, and gradually advanced to the surface of the cell. Eventually the nucleus and cytoplasm disappeared, and only a tangled bundle of fibrils indicated the site where once the neuron had been located. As these fibrils can be stained with dyes different from the normal neurofibrils, a chemical transformation of the fibril substance must have taken place. This might be the reason why the fibrils survived the destruction of the cell. It seems that the transformation of the fibrils goes hand in hand with the storage of an as yet not closely examined pathological product of the metabolism in the neuron. About one-quarter to one-third of all the neurons of the cerebral cortex showed such alterations. Numerous neurons, especially in the upper cell layers, had totally disappeared.

Dispersed over the entire cortex, and in large numbers, especially in the upper layers, miliary foci could be found, which represented the sites of deposition of a peculiar substance in the cerebral cortex. It was even possible to recognize these without staining, but they were much more evident once stained.

The glia had abundant formed fibers; in addition, many glia cells showed large deposits. There was no infiltration of the vessels. Against this, focal lesions in the endothelium could be observed, and in some sites new vessel formation could also be seen.

Alzheimer concluded:

On the whole, it is evident that we are dealing with a peculiar, little-known disease process. In recent years these particular disease processes have been detected in great numbers. This fact should stimulate us to further study and analysis of this particular disease. We must not be satisfied to force it into the existing group of well-known disease patterns. It is clear that there exist many more mental diseases than our textbooks indicate. In many such cases, a further histological examination must be effected to determine the characteristics of each single case. We must reach the stage in which the vast, well-known disease groups must be subdivided into many smaller groups, each one with its own clinical and anatomical characteristics.

We learn more about Alzheimer's 51-year-old female patient in a 1909 article written by E. Perusini, "On Histological and Clinical Findings of Some Psychiatric Diseases of Older People." On the suggestion of Alzheimer, Perusini "examined four cases all characterized by clinical and especially anatomopathological signs." In this publication, Alzheimer's patient (case 1) was investigated again concerning her symptoms and histopathology. The initials of the surname, the complete Christian name, and the profession of her husband were mentioned for the first time ("D. Auguste, wife of an office clerk, aged 51½ years"). Perusini and Alzheimer thanked Dr. Sioli in Frankfurt for the use of the case history and the brain for microscopic research. These facts prove that Perusini's case 1 was identical to the case described by Alzheimer in 1907.

Concerning Auguste D's plaques, Perusini stated, "In preparations for myelin sheath, clear yellow-grey or yellow spots of different sizes are seen between the darkly colored fibers [Figure 7]. . . . It is difficult to count the number of those plaques. Many are seen in the preparations that show plaques." In another part of the paper, Bielschowsky's method is mentioned and described as "especially favorable for showing such formation; by this method the plaques are seen impregnated more or less intensely with silver nitrate" (Figure 8). Concerning neurofibrils, Perusini stated that "some cells are recognized only by their fibrillar skeletons: between the single fibrils that are clearly present there exists a particular myelin substance; this is colored metachromatically with toluidine blue" (Figure 9).

Perusini concluded that "the pathological process recalls the main

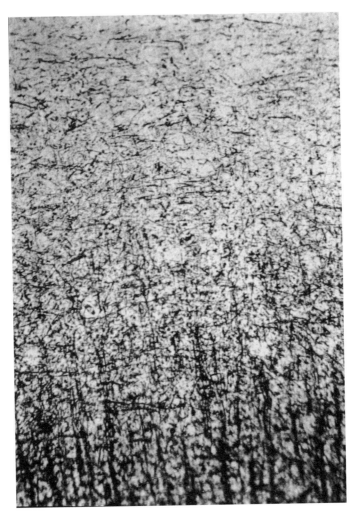

FIGURE 7.   Alzheimer's photo, showing plaques from the parietal lobes of Auguste D. The staining of the myelin sheaths is by Weigert's method. Miliary thinning can be seen in the plexus of the myelin sheaths.
Source: Perusini 1909

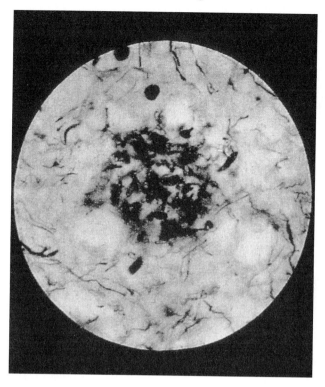

FIGURE 8.   A plaque using Bielschowsky's procedure.
Source: Perusini 1909

features of senile dementia. However, the alterations in the cases described are more far-reaching, although some of them represent presenile diseases. Regarding the clinical symptoms, those cases are peculiar as well. Apart from varying affective anomalies and varying psychotic symptoms, serious amnesia and rapid weakness of intelligence are present very early in the course of this disease."

Besides the two essential publications of Alzheimer (1907) and Perusini (1909), Kraepelin must have been familiar with the publications of Bonfiglio and Sarteschi. In 1908 Bonfiglio reported in Italian on the initiative of Alzheimer. Bonfiglio's 60-year-old patient exhibited similar symptoms and histopathologic findings. Sarteschi also published cases in Italian.

In the eighth edition of his *Handbook of Psychiatry* (1910), Kraepelin completely reorganized the chapter on senile dementia. Kraepelin mentioned Alzheimer disease for the first time in the following text:

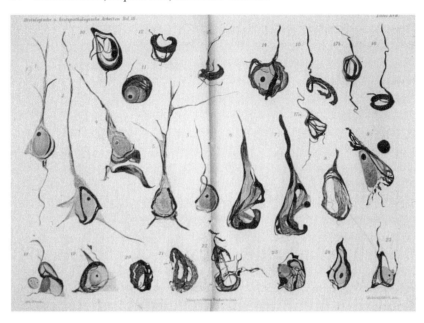

FIGURE 9.   Neurofibrils from all the four cases described by Perusini, 1909.
Source: Perusini 1909

The clinical interpretation of this Alzheimer's disease is still confusing. While the anatomical findings suggest that we are dealing with a particularly serious form of senile dementia, the fact is that this disease sometimes starts as early as the late 40s. In such cases we should at least assume a "senium praecox," if not rather a more or less age-independent peculiar disease process. The clinical picture involving an extraordinarily serious dementia, serious speech disorder, spastic signs, and seizures differs distinctively from "presbyophrenia," because pure senile cortical changes accompany this disease. Perhaps relations with one or more presenile diseases exist. (Kraepelin 1910)

In introducing the eponym *Alzheimer's disease*, Kraepelin likely knew only the few cases in Table 1. This was confirmed by Alzheimer himself in his 1911 paper, "Über eigenartige Krankheitsfälle des späteren Alters," pointing only to his own 1907 publication and those of Bonfiglio (1908) and Perusini (1909). One case from Sarteschi (1909), describing a 67-year-old female, does not fit into the scheme.

It is of some interest that Alzheimer's case of Auguste D. is, in fact,

Perusini's case 1. Some features have been changed (i.e., the postmortem results no longer showed arteriosclerosis). Besides that, the Perusini paper described Auguste D.'s histopathologic peculiarities in detail, with numerous plates showing pictures drawn with Abbe's camera lucida or photographs with Zeiss plana. Likewise, Perusini's fourth case (Leonhard Sch.) was the same as that described by Bonfiglio (1908).

Thus, Kraepelin had knowledge of only four cases (Auguste D., Leonhard Sch., R.M. male, and B.A. female) and knew their histopathologic findings.

The second case published by Alzheimer in 1911 involved Johann F., who had been admitted to the hospital on November 12, 1907, and died on October 3, 1910. (This case is described in Chapter 2 of this volume.) Certainly Kraepelin knew him from his ward rounds and was familiar with his history and clinical signs. However, it is unlikely that he knew the histopathologic findings of Johann F. when he was writing the eighth edition of his textbook and defining the term "Alzheimer's disease."

Why did Kraepelin, who introduced the eponym *Alzheimer disease*, use Alzheimer's name and not that of Perusini or Bonfiglio? Alzheimer was the editor of the journal in which Perusini published his 1909 paper, which starts as follows: "On the suggestion of Dr. Alzheimer, I examined the following four cases characterized by clinical and especially anatomo-pathological signs in common." Of interest is the fact that most of the papers in the series, *Histologische und histopathologische Arbeiten über die Großhirnrinde* (Histological and Histopathological Studies on the Cerebral Cortex), edited by Nissl and Alzheimer, had single authors. Thus, according to modern convention, Alzheimer was the senior author of the publication in which Perusini described the four cases. It was also common at this time for the editor of such an important journal to stay in the background.

TABLE 1 Published Cases of AD Available to Kraepelin in 1910

Case	Author/Year of Publication	Age (yr.)
Auguste D.	Alzheimer, 1907	51
Leonard Sch.	Bonfiglio, 1908	60
Auguste D.	Perusini, 1909	51
R.M.	Perusini, 1909	45
B.A.	Perusini, 1909	65
Leonard Sch.	Perusini, 1909	60

Of the four cases (Auguste D., Leonhard Sch., R.M., and B.A.) that had been verified histopathologically at the time the eponym was created, that of Auguste D. was the most prominent. Since that early start in 1907, the Auguste D. case has been cited numerous times and was used for introductions to publications and articles covering the field of AD. We are convinced that the eponym *Alzheimer disease* was based mainly on Alzheimer's 1907 report of Auguste D. and the few cases published by Perusini.

Several hypotheses have been suggested to account for the haste with which Kraepelin created the eponym. Beach (1987) says that Kraepelin did so for scientific reasons (i.e., because he believed that Alzheimer had discovered a new disease). Another reason might have been the existing rivalry between Kraepelin's department and that of Pick in Prague and Kraepelin's desire for prestige for his Munich laboratory. Also plausible is Kraepelin's wish to show the superiority of his school over psychoanalytical theories and to show (vis-à-vis Freud) that some mental disorders were organically based. The most likely explanation, however, is the close collaboration that existed between Kraepelin and Alzheimer, and Kraepelin's awareness of Alzheimer's clinical and scientific work on presenile cases.

AUGUSTE D.'S DEMENTIA

In addition to Alzheimer disease, other hypothetical diagnoses of Auguste D.'s disease have been put forward, especially arteriosclerosis and, astonishingly, metachromatic leukodystrophy. Many postmortem diagnoses listed arteriosclerosis at this time. In Auguste D.'s file, Alzheimer himself noted "Arteriosklerotische Gehirnatrophie(?)." The question mark is interesting and also appeared in the autopsy report: "Arteriosklerose der kleinen Hirngefäße(?)." However, the histopathologic details in the 1907 and 1909 publications always pointed to vessels without arteriosclerosis: Perusini found "that the large vessels, the arterial circle of Willis, and the Sylvian arteries showed no significant sign of arteriosclerosis"; only "some regressive alterations of the arterial walls" were described. In both papers the presence of the neuritic plaques and neurofibrillary tangles was confirmed.

There are a number of convincing arguments against the assumption of a metachromatic leukodystrophy in Auguste D.'s case, as suggested by Amaducci (Amaducci et al. 1991). The clinical picture of Auguste D. bears only a limited resemblance to the symptoms of metachromatic leukodystrophy. In particular, key symptoms caused by in-

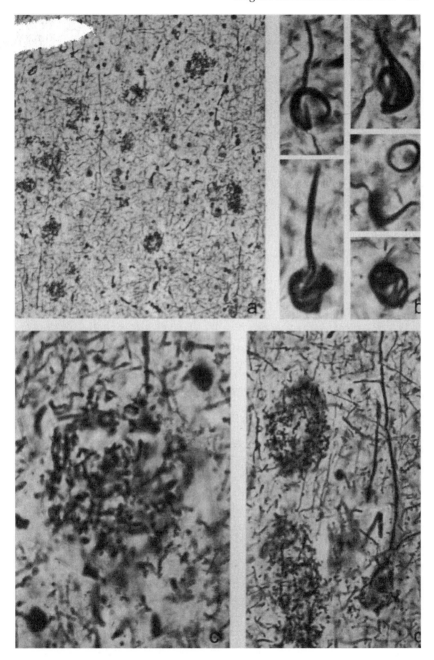

FIGURE 10.   Histological examination of Auguste D.'s brain, showing neurofibrillary tangles and amyloid plaques.
Source: Graeber et al. 1998

volvement of the peripheral nervous system are lacking. Alzheimer was an experienced neuropsychiatrist, and it is unlikely that he would have missed clear symptoms concerning the disease.

All discussions about Auguste D.'s illness should end now that the tissue sections from Auguste D., discovered by Graeber and co-workers in 1998, have been examined (Figure 10). "There were numerous neurofibrillary tangles and many amyloid plaques, especially in the upper cortical layer of this patient. Yet, there was no microscopic evidence for vascular — i.e., arteriosclerotic lesions (Graeber et al., 1998). Thus, considering the publications and the file of Auguste D., it becomes more and more evident that she is the initial case of Alzheimer's disease."

Acknowledgments

We dedicate this publication to Dr. Hector Gerbaldo, who was so helpful in finding the file and investigating the published results. Tragically, he died in April 1998.

Parts of this chapter are based on an article by the authors published in *The Lancet* 349 (1997): 1546–49.

All translations from the German are by Konrad Maurer.

References

Alzheimer, A. 1904. Histologische Studien zur Differentialdiagnose der progressiven Paralyse. Jena: Fischer.

——. 1906. Über einen eigenartigen schweren Erkrankungsprozeß der Hirnrinde. *Neurologisches Centralblatt,* Leipzig 23:1129–36.

——. 1907. Über eine eigenartige Erkrankung der Hirnrinde. In *Allgemeine Zeitschrift für Psychiatrie und Psychisch-Gerichtliche Medizin,* ed. E. Schultze and G. Suell, 64:146–48. Berlin: Georg Reimer.

——. 1910. Beiträge zur Kenntnis der pathologischen Neuroglia und ihre Beziehungen zu den Abbauvorgängen im Nervengewebe. In *Histologische und histopathologische Arbeiten zur Großhirnrinde,* ed. F. Nissl and A. Alzheimer, 3:401–562. Jena: Gustav Fischer.

——. 1911. Über eigenartige Krankheitsfälle des späteren Alters. *Z Ges Neurol Psychiatr* 4:356–85.

Amaducci, L., S. Sorbi, S. Piacentini, and K. L. Bick. 1991. The First Alzheimer Disease Case: A Metachromatic Leukodystrophy? *Dev Neurosci* 13:186–87.

Barret, A. M. 1911. Degenerations of Intracellular Neurofibrils with Miliary Gliosis in Psychoses of Senile Period. *Am J of Insanity* 67:503–16.

Beach, T. G. 1987. The History of Alzheimer's Disease. *J Hist Med Allied Sci* 42:327–249.

Berrios, G. E. 1987. Alzheimer's Disease: A Conceptual History. *J Geriat Psychiatr* 5:355–65.

Bleuler, E. 1916. *Lehrbuch der Psychiatrie.* Berlin: Springer.

Bonfiglio, F. 1908. Di Speciali Reperti in un Caso di Probabile Sifilide Cerebrale. In *Rivista Sperimentale di Freniartria e Medicia Legale delle Alienazioni Mentali,* ed. A. Tamburini, 34:196–206. Reggio Emilia.

Fischer, O. 1907. Miliare Nekrosen mit drusigen Wucherungen der Neurofibrillen, eine regelmäßige Veränderung der Hirnrinde bei seniler Demenz. *Monatsschr Psychiatr Neurol* 22:361–72.

Graeber, R. B., S. Kösel, E. Grasbon-Frodl, H. J. Möller, and P. Mehraein. 1998. Histopathology and APOE Genotype of the First Alzheimer Disease Patient, Auguste D. *Neurogenetics* 1:223–28.

Kahlbaum, K. L. 1863. *Die Gruppierung der psychischen Krankheiten und die Einteilung der Seelenstörungen.* Danzig: A. W. Kafemann.

Kraepelin, E. 1910. *Psychiatrie: Ein Lehrbuch für Studierende und Ärzte.* 2 Band. Leipzig: Barth.

———. 1924. Aloys Alzheimer, 1864–1915. In *Deutsche Irrenärzte,* ed. T. Kivelhoff, 2:299–307. Berlin: Springer.

Maurer, K., S. Volk, and H. Gerbaldo. 1997. Auguste D. and Alzheimer's Disease. *Lancet* 349:1546–49.

Maurer, K., and U. Maurer. 1998. *Alzheimer: Das Leben eines Arztes und die Karriere einer Krankheit.* München: Piper.

Perusini, G. 1909. Über klinisch und histologisch eigenartige psychische Erkrankungen des späteren Lebensalters. In *Histologische und Histopathologische Arbeiten,* ed. F. Nissl and A. Alzheimer, 297–351. Jena: Verlag G. Fischer.

Redlich, E. 1898. Über milliare Sklerosen der Hirnrinde bei seniler Atrophie. *Jahrb Psychiatr Neurol* 17:208–16.

Sarteschi, G. 1909. Contributo all' istologia patologica della presbiofrenia. In *Revista Sperimentale di Freniartria,* Vol. 35. Reggio Emilia.

2

Johann F.

THE HISTORICAL RELEVANCE OF THE CASE FOR THE CONCEPT OF ALZHEIMER DISEASE

Hans-Jurgen Möller and Manuel B. Graeber

After the short report on Auguste D. (Alzheimer 1907), Alois Alzheimer left the task of producing a more detailed publication on the disease later named after him to Perusini (Perusini 1910). In 1911 Alzheimer turned his attention back to the disease and published a long paper of his own on the clinical picture and the neuropathologic background of the disease (Alzheimer 1911). This chapter describes the 1911 paper in detail and analyzes its significance for the conceptualization of the disease. In this context the rediscovery of the neurohistopathologic stains of the patient Johann F., whose description is the center of the 1911 publication, is of special interest.

THE CASE RECORD OF JOHANN F.

In contrast to Alzheimer's brief report published in 1907, his 1911 paper describes fully his conceptualization of the disease and contains numerous illustrations, mainly drawings, which include several examples of the histopathology of the first case together with a second case report, that of Johann F. This case report seemed most important to Alzheimer. It is not known whether Kraepelin ever saw Auguste D., but Kraepelin was probably familiar with Johann F., because after Alzhei-

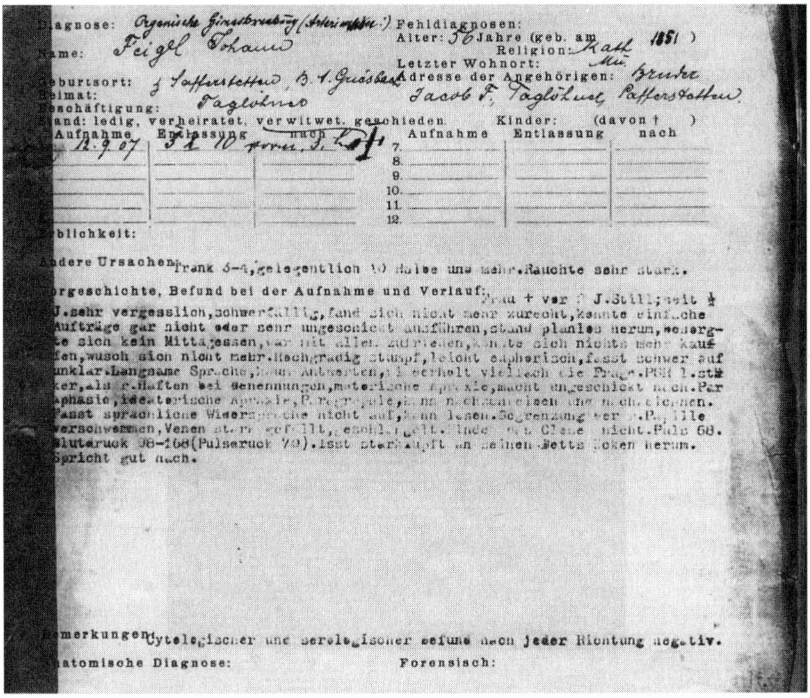

FIGURE 11.   Epicritical report of Johann F.
Source: Archives of the Psychiatric Hospital, Munich; Graeber et al., 1997

mer moved to Munich, Kraepelin and Alzheimer used to work together very closely, as Kraepelin gratefully acknowledged in the introduction to the second volume of his textbook (Kraepelin 1910).

Alzheimer provided ample clinical, biographical, and neuropathologic data on this patient, which allowed us not only to find the short case record of this patient in the archives of the Psychiatric Hospital of the University Munich but also to identify neurohistopathologic stains found among archives at the Institute of Neuropathology of the University of Munich (Graeber et al. 1997).

According to the epicritical report (Figure 11), the patient, a 56-year-old laborer, was admitted to the Psychiatric Hospital on September 12, 1907. The report further states:

> Wife died two years ago. Quiet; since half year very forgetful, clumsy, could not find his way, was unable to perform simple tasks or carried these out with difficulty, stood around helplessly, did not provide himself with lunch,

was content with everything, was not capable of buying anything by himself and did not wash himself. Very dull, slightly euphoric, slow in comprehension, unclear. Slowed speech, rare answers, frequent repetition of the question. PTR (patellar tendon reflex) l. more pronounced than r. Sticking when naming things, motor apraxia, imitates in a clumsy way. Paraphasia, ideational apraxia, paragraphia, able to copy writings and drawings. Does not realize contradictions in speech, can read. Blurred demarcation of the r. optic disk, veins very filled, wavy. Does not find the toilet. Heart rate 68. Blood pressure 98–168. Eats a lot. Is tugging at his sheets. Repeats sentences without problems.

The patient died on October 3, 1910, of pneumonia after three years of hospitalization in the Psychiatric Hospital of the University of Munich.

Interestingly, Johann F. was admitted under the diagnosis of possible vascular dementia. The initial clinical diagnosis, probably written by Alzheimer, reads "organische Hirnerkrankung (Arteriosklerose?)" (organic brain disease [arteriosclerosis?]). But the autopsy book states "Alzheimersche Krankheit" (Alzheimer disease). The notation of the patient's diagnosis in the autopsy book was apparently written by Alzheimer (Figures 12 and 13). In the publication from 1911, Alzheimer gave a detailed description of the clinical history of Johann F. (Alzheimer 1911, 358–61). Because of the special relevance of this case in the conceptualization of AD, the case report is presented here nearly in full — not only to show the individual history of the case but also to demonstrate Alzheimer's clinical diagnostic approach (trans. Förstl and Levy 1991).

> The 56-year-old laborer Johann F. was admitted to the psychiatric clinic on 12 November 1907. There was no history of excessive drinking. Two years

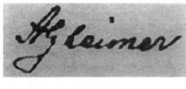
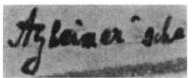

Figure 12.   Alzheimer's signature *(upper part of the figure)* taken from his curriculum vitae, which was written after he had joined the Psychiatric Hospital in Munich. For comparison, the diagnosis written in the autopsy book has been enlarged *(lower part of the figure)*.
Source: Graeber et al. 1997

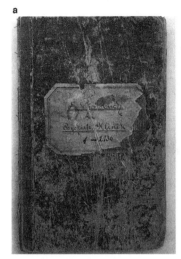

FIGURE 13. *(a)* Autopsy book of the psychiatric clinic in Munich. *(b)* Entry 784 lists a male bearing the name "Feigl" who died on October 3, 1910, in the psychiatric hospital ("Klinik München"). The diagnosis reads "Alzheimer'sche Krankheit" (Alzheimer disease).
Source: Graeber et al. 1997

before admission his wife died, since when he became quiet and dull. In the previous six months he had become forgetful, could not find his way, could not perform simple tasks or carried these out with difficulty. He stood around, did not appear to bother about food, but ate greedily whatever was put before him. He was not capable of buying anything for himself and did not wash. He was admitted by the service for the poor.

14 November 1907. Pupillary reaction normal. Patellar-reflex a little brisk. No signs of nervous palsy. Language strikingly slow, but without articulatory disturbance. Dull, slightly euphoric, impaired understanding. Echoes questions put to him frequently and repeatedly instead of giving a reply. Can only solve very simple calculations after a long delay.

When asked to point to different parts of his body, he hesitates. After having spoken about the knee-cap, he calls a key a knee-cap. Does the same with a matchbox, which he rubs against his knee-cap when asked what one would do with it. He then does the same with a piece of soap. He finally responds correctly to other commands to unlock a door or to wash his hands but only does so extraordinarily slowly and clumsily.

20 September 1907. To the question, what is the color of blood? "red"; snow? "white"; milk? "good"; soot? . . .

Counts correctly to ten, does the same with days of the week and months of the year. Gives half of the "Our Father" but cannot continue. $2 \times 2 = 4$, $2 \times 3 = 6$, $6 \times 6 = 6$. Reads the time correctly. Unbuttons his frock correctly. Takes a cigar in his mouth, strikes a match, lights the cigar and smokes: everything in the correct manner. Takes coins in his hands and checks each side. "That is, that is, we have got a, here, here. . . ." Similarly, he cannot name a matchbox.

He knows how to use a mouth organ, bell, purse, but cannot name them. When asked to do so, he selects a matchbox and a light from a number of objects but not a brush or a corkscrew. When asked to bend his knees, he makes a fist. Repetition is unimpaired.

How many legs has a calf? "four." A man? "two."

Where does a fish live? In the forest up in the trees? "In the forest up in the trees."

Lumbar puncture: No increased cell count. No alteration in complement in blood and cerebrospinal fluid.

Ophthalmoscopy: blurring of the right papilla, veins well filled, normal findings on the left.

23 September 1907. Gets up and urinates by the bed.

8 October 1907. When asked to write, he does not take the pencil but picks a matchbox and tried to write with it. Otherwise focal symptoms show striking changes in severity.

15 November 1907. Happy, laughs a lot, eats an extraordinary amount. Sits around looking dull but moves his hands constantly, picking his blanket or his shirt. At times he tears pieces of cloth, which he pushes into his mouth.

Repetition still good. He often uses objects in the wrong way (e.g., tries to brush his frock with his comb). When he is given a key and is asked to unlock the door, he approaches the door but does not know what to do. When writing his name, he sticks to letters. He cannot be persuaded to write anything but his name. When he is asked to name objects, he does not respond promptly or echoes the question without understanding it, at times repeatedly. He does not speak spontaneously. When teased (e.g., by trying to take away a cloth, which he is uncoiling), he sometimes curses. When asked to carry out a movement, he often repeats the question. When the movement is demonstrated to him, he usually looks without appearing to understand. He imitates some of the demonstrated movements with his right or left hand. When asked to touch his nose with his right hand, he holds the extended fingers to his chin. When asked to blow a kiss, he holds out his hand in a peculiar way. Then when a threatening gesture and a military salute are demonstrated to him, he puts his hand to his mouth as though blowing a kiss.

8 December 1907. Obviously further deterioration. Keeps leaving his bed, fusses around with his sheets. Wassermann's test in blood and serum negative. 1 cell per mm^3 cerebrospinal fluid.

2 March 1908. Asked to wash his hands, he starts correctly but then keeps on washing endlessly. Asked to close a tap, he holds his hands under it. Asked to seal a letter, he tries to light the candle with the seal, then he warms up the sealing-wax and applies it against the seal. Asked to light a cigar, he strikes it against the matchbox.

4 March 1908. Restless, appears as though delirious. Keeps rolling his sheets into a bundle and wants to walk out with them. He often keeps working away for days on end without a break, his face sweating. Gets more and more reluctant. Does not obey when summoned. When given a hair-brush, he licks it. Almost no spontaneous speech.

5 May 1908. Other patients have taught him how to sing. When asked, he sings: "We sit so happily together." He has to be prompted again and again with the words but does rather well with the tune.

12 May 1908. Physical examination does not yield any abnormal results in either of the pupils or the reflexes. Papillae look normal (right papilla shows a slightly abnormal configuration).

When asked for something, he usually answers with a "yes" and laughs idiotically, or he repeats the question without understanding. He is still quite capable of repetition, and at times he keeps repeating the word several times. He generally imitates individual movements, like extension of hands, swearing [*Schwurfinger,* holding up three fingers to indicate swearing an oath] correctly, but clumsily.

12 June 1908. He walks in the garden and will not let anyone stop him. Although completely soaked with sweat, he walks round and round continuously, constantly winding the long coat-tails of his frock round his hand which he clenches occasionally. In his bed he does the same thing with his blanket. When pricked with a needle or tickled on his soles, he does not react for a long time but finally hits the physician. Hardly utters a word.

It is striking that his gross motility appears unimpaired in spite of his profound imbecility. No ataxia or weakness of limb movements are to be seen.

14 December 1908. Incontinent of feces and urine wherever he is. Does not say anything anymore; is permanently occupied with his bed or shirt. Does still sing, "We are sitting so happily together," when others start him off.

3 February 1909. Epileptiform seizure lasting a few minutes. Twitching of his face.

6 February 1909. Right-sided facial palsy.

9 February 1909. No obvious facial weakness anymore. Repeat tests of blood and serum yield the same negative results as before. Very reluctant to cooperate. Always busy with his blanket or shirt. Does not speak anymore; does not obey any commands.

31 May 1910. His body-weight falls slowly and steadily. Still fidgeting with his sheets in the same manner.

28 July 1910. Epileptiform seizure of two minutes duration.

1 September 1910. Temperature increased to 38.5 C. Rhonchi over his lung.

3 October 1910. Death with features of pneumonia.

ALZHEIMER'S NEUROPATHOLOGIC FINDINGS AND THEORETICAL REFLECTIONS

In the introduction of the 1911 publication, Alzheimer refers to Auguste D., the first case of AD, discussing not only the clinical picture but also the typical neuropathologic characteristics. Then he provides some theoretical reflections. Alzheimer states that Kraepelin, in the eighth edition of his textbook on psychiatry (1910), gave a short summary of this disease and called it Alzheimer disease. Alzheimer refers to the scientific findings concerning this topic since 1906 (Bonfiglio, Fischer, Hübner, Myake, Perusini, Pick, Redlich, Sarteschi, Simchowicz) and discusses whether or not the cases he and Perusini (1910) reported should be separated clinically or histologically from senile dementia. In this context he makes special reference to the plaques and tangles, specifying AD as a presenile disease as opposed to a presenile dementia:

> The patches in the cortex had in the meantime been observed in presbyophrenia by Fischer who described them in detail in a number of papers and considered them as a characteristic feature of that disorder. Redlich had also demonstrated them by different methods. I had myself already observed and described them in Dementia senilis using Nissl and Weigert staining. I had not, however, realized that they corresponded to the images seen in Bielschowsky-stained preparations. Perusini has pointed out that the fibrillary changes in nerve cells which I had described are also seen in severe cases of Dementia senilis, and Fischer has expressed the same view. The question therefore arises as to whether the cases of disease which I considered peculiar are sufficiently different clinically or histologically to

be distinguished from senile dementia or whether they should be included under that rubric. (Alzheimer 1911, 356)

Then Alzheimer focuses his argument more on the clinical picture and course of these cases:

Perusini felt that these cases represented a separate disease, partly for clinical and partly for histological reasons. The clinical differences were the early onset and the presence and severity of focal symptoms which were not thought to be a feature of Dementia senilis, the anatomical differences being the greater severity of the histological changes, although they develop at an earlier age. Kraepelin still considers that the position of these cases is unclear. Even if the anatomical findings might suggest severe mental impairment, the early onset (one would have to assume a "senium praecox"), the profound language disturbance, spasticity and seizures are very different from those of presbyophrenia, which is usually associated with purely cortical senile changes. The disease may, therefore, be related to one or another of the pre-senile conditions which he described. Fischer has written an exhaustive discussion of Perusini's cases in his paper, "The presbyophrenic dementia, its anatomical basis and clinical differentiation." He considered the patches as characteristic of a specific disorder and saw no objections to including in the same category cases occurring at an early age, both because of the histological changes and because the paralysis of adults and young people, which represent the disease at a different age, share all the essential features of later cases.

It seems to me that a simple inclusion of these cases with presbyophrenia does not take sufficient account of several interesting features, and that Perusini's and Kraepelin's reservations against this integration have not been convincingly eliminated by Fischer's arguments. After all, we are dealing with the case of a 56-year-old woman and of Perusini's 46-year-old man, in whom nobody would have made a clinical diagnosis of senile dementia. (Alzheimer 1911, 356–58)

After the broad description of the case history of Johann F. (see above), Alzheimer gives a short summary of the clinical findings:

Thus we see a 54-year-old man who, slowly and imperceptibly and with no impairment of consciousness or seizures, develops a state of profound mental impairment with prominent agnostic, aphasic, and apractic disturbances. A more accurate analysis of these focal symptoms presents various problems because the impairment of recognition, language comprehension

and expression, as well as praxis, the general mental impairment and reluctant behavior, make the interpretation of individual verbal capacities and
acts difficult. It is, however, certain that the language disturbances of the
patients have to be considered as transcortical aphasias because of the long-
preserved ability for repetition. Since there was an early impoverishment of
word production which progressed to a complete loss of spontaneous language, we have to assume a mixed motor and sensory aphasia in spite of
gross signs of paralysis. Of the apractic disturbances, although these were
sometimes purely motor, ideational apraxia was more prominent. In contrast to the severe disturbances of language and of praxis, disturbance of
motility was slight, and the absence of real signs of paralysis of the ex-
tremities was striking. In the late stages of the condition and toward the
end of his life, repeated epileptic attacks and a transient right-sided facial
nerve paralysis occurred.

The clinical analysis of this case raises several difficulties. Senile dementia was never considered because of the onset at the age of 54 and the fact
that, even on first examination, a profound mental impairment with a hint
of aphasic agnostic and apractic disturbances was found. After physical
examination had apparently established a right-sided papilledoema, one
had to consider a tumor. Because of the lack of other signs of increased
intracranial pressure and the profound general mental impairment with
multiple localizing signs, one would have to postulate a diffuse tumor in-
vading nervous tissue without occupying much space. Since repeated examination yielded only a slight abnormality of the right papilla which did
not progress, this could not be considered as papilledoema, and the diagnosis of a tumor was no longer supported. (pp. 361–62)

Alzheimer offers some differential diagnostic reflections on this
case, excluding especially the diagnosis of a vascular brain disease. He
then describes in detail the neuropathologic features of the case found at
autopsy, especially the details of the amyloid plaques:

The gyri of the frontal, parietal, and temporal lobes were considerably
narrowed on both sides, and the sulci enlarged, while the central gyri did
not appear particularly atrophic. There were no softened areas in cortex or
white matter, nor were any other circumscribed alterations to be found
anywhere. The rest of the autopsy findings were without importance. Thus
although the macroscopic observation of the brain revealed a diffuse atrophic process which has been established as the cause of the disorder, it did
not clarify the nature of the underlying process. (p. 362)

Microscopic investigation showed the cortex to be filled in varying degrees of Fischer's plaques. Their number in general corresponded with the macroscopically recognizable amount of brain atrophy. They were numerous in the frontal lobe, scarce in the central gyri, present in enormous numbers in the parietal and partly also in the temporal lobes, and again less numerous in the occipital lobe. There were no obvious differences between left and right sides. In the striatum, lentiform nucleus, and thalamus, they were also present in abundance. Within the cerebellum they occurred abundantly in individual lobuli, while they were completely absent in other large parts of the brain. Single plaques were also visible in the gray matter of the pons and in different nuclei of the medulla oblongata. In the spinal cord I only saw a solitary one in the posterior horn of a slice at the thoracic level.

Among the plaques in the cerebral cortex, many were of an extraordinary size, such as I have never seen, even in the cornu ammonis of senile dementia. They often extended through several layers. Some evidently arose from the fusion of smaller ones, since they contained several central cores; but others had one exceptionally big central core and an uncommonly large halo. Very frequently it was noticeable that the number of plaques at the surface and center of the gyrus was smaller than at the sides. In places where they were particularly numerous, the plaques were very rarely located in the first cortical layer. They usually started in the region with a sudden increase of glial reticulum at the transition to the first microcellular layer. There were sometimes a few particularly small ones at the very edge of the first to the second layers. They tended to accumulate in the second and third layers, were rarer in deeper layers, but were still fairly numerous in the white matter. (p. 363)

Then Alzheimer discusses the observation that the degeneration of fibrils apparently is not found in this case:

Rather remarkably, numerous preparations produced from very many different areas of the brain did not show a single cell with the peculiar fibrillary degeneration I have previously described. This form of cell change, which occurred very frequently in the other case descriptions of this peculiar disease and which is not infrequently also to be found in severe cases of senile dementia, was missing here, although the plaques were of a size and frequency never seen before in the other cases. So, although one might be tempted to do so, one cannot relate plaques to fibrillary changes or vice versa. (p. 369)

Later he discusses the relationship of the amyloid plaques in senile and presenile dementia:

I believe that the results of the microscopic examination of this case allow us to address a general pathological question which has been of interest in anatomico-pathological research, as far as it is concerned with the psychoses since Fischers's papers. It cannot be doubted that the plaques in these specific cases do, in all relevant aspects, correspond to those which we find in Dementia senilis. This is evident from the description which other investigators have given about the plaques in Dementia senilis and from the comparisons which Perusini, Simchowicz, and I myself have undertaken in quite large amounts of material. (p. 371)

As I have pointed out in connection with other histological findings, Dementia senilis and arteriosclerosis of the brain are in principle different disease processes. This has been proved even more conclusively because of the presence of senile plaques (Fischer, Simchowicz).

If we now return to our case, we must of course still have reservations in asserting its attribution to the senile disease process solely on the basis of the presence of particularly numerous plaques. This is because, according to our previous thoughts, we can only consider the plaques as an accompanying feature of the senile cortical alterations, and one must first establish how the other alterations which we find in this case relate to those of senile dementia. The fibrillary degeneration of the ganglion cells is absent in this case, while in the cases of such presenile diseases described up to now it was particularly common. We now know that the same cellular degeneration had been observed frequently in cases of severe senile dementia, but sometimes it is absent altogether. On the other hand, up to now it has not been found in any disease of younger people. The particularly frequent occurrence in most of the presenile cases might support their relationship to senile dementia. Moreover, we see in this case an extraordinarily heavy accumulation of lipoid substances in the ganglion cells, glial cells, and the walls of the vessels, and especially in the numerous fibre-forming glial cells of the cerebral cortex and indeed in the whole central nervous system.

Therefore, we observe that all elements are altered in the same manner and direction as in senile dementia; but in this case, as in the others described by Perusini, the alterations exceed in their severity the average to be found in Dementia senilis. . . .

. . . A further peculiarity of the present case was the localization of the alterations. Even if we were dealing with a diffuse disease of the cortex alone, the parietal and temporal lobes bilaterally were unmistakably especially affected, and much more so than the frontal brain. In ordinary cases of senile dementia, the frontal brain is the most severely diseased, as has been found only recently by Simchowicz. . . .

. . . However, the differences of the localization of the disease process cannot be used as an argument against relating these forms of dementia to Dementia senilis. After all, we know that the disease process of progressive paralysis allows for the emergence of numerous cases with an atypical localization as well as the majority of cases with a typical one.

Further essential facts, which support the membership of such cases to the category of senile dementia, came out of the observations in two cases which I have investigated recently.

. . . Hence there appear to be a variety of intermediate forms between these presenile diseases and the typical cases of senile dementia. As similar cases of disease obviously occur in the late old age, it is therefore not exclusively a presenile disease, and there are cases of senile dementia which do not differ from these presenile cases with respect to the severity of disease process.

There is, then, no tenable reason to consider these cases as caused by a specific disease process. *They are senile psychoses, atypical forms of senile dementia.* Nevertheless, they do assume a certain separate position, so that one has to know of their existence, just as one has to know about Lissauer's paralysis, in order to avoid misdiagnosis. It will therefore have to be the task of future research to collect a larger number of such cases, which, as the observations in this department show, should not be too rare in order to establish the symptomatology of this group even more clearly, and to substantiate their position with respect to senile dementia on an even firmer basis by proving the existence of further transitional cases. (pp. 376–78)

MODERN HISTOPATHOLOGIC AND MOLECULAR GENETIC ANALYSIS OF THE CASE OF JOHANN F.

As mentioned above, the histologic sections were found among archives at the Institute of Neuropathology of the University of Munich (Graeber et al. 1997).

Light microscopic examination of the histologic sections from Johann F.'s brain yielded morphologic results that are in complete agreement with Alzheimer's paper (Alzheimer 1911). Although many amyloid plaques were visible in the cerebral cortex of this patient (Figure 14b–d), neurofibrillary tangles could not be detected. It is interesting to note that sections of the hippocampus and the entorhinal region were not available. Silver impregnations performed over two days in Alzhei-

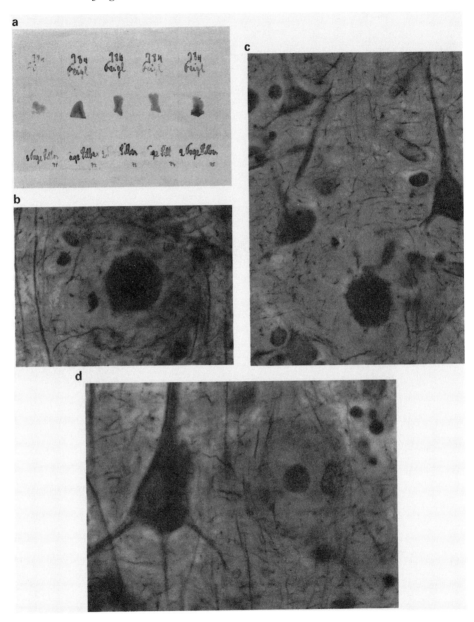

FIGURE 14.   (a) Bielschowsky-stained tissue section processed for two days ("2 Tage Silber"). (b–d) Staining of classical amyloid plaques (with core) in the cerebral cortex of Alzheimer's patient. Pyramidal neurons and neurites within the plaque do not show neurofibrillary change. Magnification ×700 (b), ×1000 (c), ×500 (d).
Source: Graeber et al., 1997

mer's laboratory using Bielschowsky's method (Figure 14a) were found together with a number of Nissl-stained specimens. In addition, numerous sections apparently prepared according to the methods of Mann, Herxheimer, and Weigert were discovered.

Using direct nonradioactive sequencing of polymerase chain reaction (PCR) products (Kösel and Graeber 1993; Kösel et al. 1997), mutations at codons 692, 693, 713, and 717 or at other nucleotides within exon 17 of the APP gene could be excluded. The apolipoprotein E genotype of Alzheimer's patient Johann F. was determined as e3/e3. In addition, screening for mutations in the presenilin genes is planned. But given the limited amount of tissue available, the latter study was postponed until our knowledge of the genetics of AD is more comprehensive.

HISTORICAL AND MODERN PERSPECTIVES

Much speculation exists (Hoff 1991) as to why Kraepelin so readily accepted Alzheimer's clinical and histopathologic description. One reason may have been the competition between Munich and the group in Prague headed by Arnold Pick, whose co-worker Fischer had published interesting findings on amyloid plaques (Fischer 1907). However, the case of Johann F. may provide a better explanation. Alzheimer submitted his report on this patient together with a detailed description of the cellular pathology of AD in January 1911, only a few months after the autopsy. This suggests that the studies on Johann F. became part of a long-planned manuscript that eventually comprised 30 printed pages. It also implies that Johann F., who was admitted with a diagnosis of possible vascular dementia (Figure 11), was observed very closely during his stay in the psychiatric clinic. Finally, publication of the new eponym *Alzheimersche Krankheit* by Kraepelin (Alzheimer 1911; Kraepelin 1910) practically forced Alzheimer to write his own name as the patient's diagnosis in the autopsy book (Figures 12 and 13), only three years after his first description of the disease.

The tissue sections discussed in this chapter, as well as those of Auguste D. (Graeber et al. 1998), are likely to represent the only histologic material that is left from Alzheimer's own research on the disease that was named after him. The material and the stains are well-preserved and of high quality, documenting once again Alzheimer's high technical standards (Meyer 1961). Examination of the histologic sections with the light microscope found many amyloid plaques but not neurofibrillary tangles. So far, the results are in complete concordance with Alzheimer's results in this case as well as the modern examination of the histologic sections of the first case (Auguste D.). In contrast to the case of Johann F., the neurohistopathology of Auguste D. is characterized by tangles as well as plaques.

As already stated by Alzheimer himself, the case of Johann F. is remarkable from a histopathologic point of view since numerous plaques but no neurofibrillary tangles are detectable in the cerebral cortex of this patient. A substantial fraction of Alzheimer cases apparently belong to this type, and it has been suggested by modern neuropathologists that "plaque dementia" may comprise a separate subgroup of the disorder (Terry et al. 1987). Concerning the question of whether AD should be considered as a variant of senile dementia or a separate disease entity, there is growing agreement that AD is only a variant of senile dementia.

At the end of this chapter, it seems appropriate to quote Förstl and Levy (1991) on Alzheimer's case report and its theoretical implications:

> The neuropathological description includes important points which have subsequently been "rediscovered" and are currently much debated (Förstl and Levy 1991). This applies to Alzheimer's detailed account of the changes in white matter to which Brun et al. (1986) have more recently drawn attention and to the lack of any close correlation between the number of plaques and the number of tangles. Alzheimer also devotes a great deal of space to the changes in glial cells and speculates about the possible role that these may have played in the formation of plaques. His careful distinction between the "core" and the rest of the plaque which he refers to as the "halo" also strikes a notable modern note, as does his emphasis on the different variety of plaques seen both in his case and in others (Hansen et al. 1983).
>
> Although many of the changes reported by him had previously been described both singly and collectively by others, notably Fischer, Redlich, and Simchowicz — to whom Alzheimer always pays generous tribute — it is the 1911 paper which clearly establishes Alzheimer's central role and which fully justifies the attachment of his name to this intriguing disease. (Förstl and Levy 1991, 72)

Acknowledgments

This historical research on Alzheimer's scientific work was supported by a grant of the pharmaceutical company Hoechst, Germany.

References

Alzheimer, A. 1907. Über eigenartige Erkrankung der Hirnrinde. *Allg Zschr Psychiat u Psychisch-gerichtl Med* 64:146–48.

———. 1911. Über eigenartige Krankheitsfälle des späteren Alters. *Zbl ges Neurol Psych* 4:356–85. Translated and with an introduction by H. Förstl and R. Levy. 1991. On Certain Peculiar Diseases of Old Age. *Hist Psychiatry* 2:71–101.

Brun, A., and Englund, E. 1986. A white matter disorder in dementia of the Alzheimer type: A pathoanatomical study. *Ann Neuro* 19:253–62.

Fischer, O. 1907. Miliare Nekrosen mit drusigen Wucherungen der Neurofibrillen, eine regelmässige Veränderung der Hirnrinde bei seniler Demenz. *Monatsschr Psychiatr Neurol* 22:361–72.

Förstl, H., and R. Levy. 1991. On certain peculiar diseases of old age. *Hist Psychiatry* 2:71–101.

Graeber, M. B., S. Kösel, R. Egensperger, R. B. Banati, U. Müller, K. Bise, HP. Hoff, H. J. Möller, K. Fujisawa, and P. Mehraein. 1997. Rediscovery of the case described by Alois Alzheimer in 1911: Historical, histological, and molecular genetic analysis. *Neurogenetics* 1:73–80.

Graeber, M. B., S. Kösel, E. Grasbon-Frodl, H. J. Möller, and P. Mehraein. 1998. Histopathology and *APOE* genotype of the first Alzheimer disease patient, Auguste D. *Neurogenetics* 1:223–28.

Hansen, L. A., E. Maslia, R. D. Terry, and S. S. Mirra. 1983. A neuropathological subset of Alzheimer's disease with concomitant Lewy body disease and spongiform change. *Acta Neuropathol* 9:134–201.

Hoff, P. 1991. Alzheimer and his time. In *Eponymists in Medicine: Alzheimer and the Dementias*, ed. G. E. Berrios and H. L. Freeman, 29–124. London: Royal Society of Medicines Services Limited.

Kösel, S., and M. B. Graeber. 1993. Non-radioactive direct sequencing of PCR products amplified from neuropathological specimens. *Brain Pathol* 3:421–24.

Kösel, S., C. B. Lücking, R. Egensperger, and M. B. Graeber. 1997. Nonradioactive PCR sequencing using digoxigenin. In *PCR Sequencing Protocols: Methods in Molecular Biology*, ed. R. Rapley, 81–89. Totowa, N.Y.: Humana Press.

Kraepelin, E. 1910. *Psychiatrie: Ein Lehrbuch für Studierende und Ärzte.* II. Band, Klinische Psychiatrie. Leipzig: Verlag Johann Ambrosius Barth.

Meyer, J. E. 1961. *Alois Alzheimer: 50 Jahre Neuropathologie in Deutschland.* Stuttgart: Thieme.

Perusini, G. 1910. Über klinische und histologische eigenartige psychische

Erkrankungen des späteren Lebensalters. In *Histopathologische Arbeiten über die Grosshirnrinde unter besonderer Berücksichtigung der pathologischen Anatomie der Geisteskrankheiten*, III. Band, ed. F. Nissl and A. Alzheimer, 297–352.

Terry, R. D., L. A. Hansen, R. DeTeresa, P. Davies, H. Tobias, and R. Katzman. 1987. Senile dementia of the Alzheimer type without neocortical neurofibrillary tangles. *J Neuropathol Exp Neurol* 46:262–68.

PART II

From Alzheimer to the Present

The concept of disease begins with people and their minds. First, the notion of disease, or "dis-ease," implies that we start with the suffering of an individual human being. Lay concepts of illness are critical to understanding the behavior of patients and their families, and it is these ideas that largely determine what sort of cases come into the view of the clinician. However, once the patient appears before the clinician, it is the professional's identification of a condition as a disease that dominates society's models of illness (or at least the public discourse about disease). Thus the scientific concept of Alzheimer disease (AD) begins with the clinical characterization of a pattern of progressive cognitive impairment. This pattern occurring in the elderly has been described in a literature extending back for centuries.

The second critical aspect of the development of the initial concept of AD was the application of labels to characterize the disease state. The term *dementia*, implying loss of mentation, predates AD. Perhaps fifty years before Alzheimer's time, other clinicians had characterized this loss of cognitive abilities and had begun to differentiate it from other clinical conditions. For example, dementia was differentiated from *amentia*, or mental retardation; that is, dementia requires normal intellect and a deterioration to an impaired level of thinking ability. Dementia was also differentiated from *delirium*, which was defined as changes in cognition occurring often acutely in response to medical illness.

Thus, the initial characterization of neuropsychiatric diseases depended on the skills of clinicians (or others) to observe individuals and to cluster their symptoms into certain categories. However, the development of methods to examine brain tissue allowed the concept of clinical pathological entities — of which AD is one — to emerge. When that conceptual level has been reached, it becomes possible to develop theories about etiology and corresponding strategies for therapeutic intervention.

The chapters in this section describe the twists and turns in the development of AD as a clinicopathologic entity from Alzheimer's time to the present. Certain issues have consistently been at play in this development: the related problems of differentiating the normal from the pathological, and aging from disease; and of sorting out the various roles that psychosocial, environmental, and genetic factors play in producing dementia. Before the late nineteenth century, the techniques to preserve the brain for examination and to process tissue in a way that microscopic evaluation could be conducted did not exist. Alzheimer, however, was practicing at a time when a revolution was occurring in our ability to examine pathological material from patients who suffered from dementia. Moreover, while Alzheimer was applying the techniques of the new field of neuropathology to understanding disease, the rudimentary concepts that would lead to future work on understanding the neurochemical basis of the neurotransmitter alterations in dementia also emerged.

The chapter by Heiko and Eva Braak describes the development of effective silver staining techniques in Alzheimer's time — crucial to Alzheimer's discovery of neurofibrillary tangles. The chapter goes on to describe recent developments in knowledge about the nature of the neurofibrillary tangles, including the selective vulnerability to degeneration of particular neurons at specific locations within the brain.

Hans Förstl's chapter describes how the concept of AD was handled in the German neuropsychiatric literature from Alzheimer's time through the early 1930s. One of the issues that faced clinicians, and continues to face them today, was the differentiation of disease from normality. As they age, many individuals develop changes in cognitive abilities, but for most the changes are fortunately not as severe as for those suffering from AD. Clinicians had a difficult time differentiating normal age-related problems from pathological states. AD was originally conceptualized as a presenile dementia, meaning it occurred in individuals younger than 65. When a person who is 50 — Auguste D.'s age was when she started with her symptoms — develops a progressive dementia, this state appears to be more obviously a disease than when it occurs in a person who is 85. But histopathologic study of brain tissue failed to establish solid ground for this distinction.

Jesse Ballenger's chapter describes how the difficulty of establishing a firm basis in brain pathology for the clinical expression of dementia led

American psychiatrists to emphasize the role of psychosocial factors in dementia. Following the work of the German Gellerstedt, David Rothschild observed that some individuals who had plaques and tangles did not develop dementia. Thus, the determinism of those who thought that all psychiatry should be based on an understanding of the brain was challenged when the brain changes did not match the clinical condition. Throughout the 1940s and 1950s, this psychodynamic theory of senile dementia was, in fact, dominant in the American literature. Although the psychosocial approach to dementia all but disappeared in the resurgence of biological models since the 1970s, a similar approach to AD was developed in the 1980s by the late Tom Kitwood in the United Kingdom (Kitwood 1997). Reexamining this period is thus of considerable interest to those who have been critical of the narrow bioligization of the concept of AD.

The "rediscovery" of AD in the 1970s, as described in the chapter by Katzman and Bick, occurred as a result of several converging factors. First, the aging of the population in western Europe and the United States focused attention on those conditions that occurred more frequently in this population, including dementia. Katzman's famous editorial claiming that the changes found in senile dementia were the same as those found in AD allowed a redefinition of this problem around the eponym *Alzheimer disease*. This eponym did not have any of the social and linguistic baggage associated with terms such as *senility* and *dementia*. Moreover, lumping all presenile and senile dementias of the Alzheimer type together created an aura of an epidemiological crisis.

This identification of AD as a social disaster might not have achieved the prominence it did except for the fact that new developments in biology were changing the conceptualization of the disease. Electron microscopy allowed researchers to see the plaques and tangles with a degree of detail not possible with a microscope. The evolution of neurochemistry, particularly as it related to the characterization of neurotransmitters, allowed new conceptualizations. The success in Parkinson disease was modeled by those working in AD. In Parkinson disease, cell loss in the substantia nigra was linked to the neurotransmitter dopamine, and most importantly, compounds that increased the level of dopamine were found to be effective in treating clinicopathologic symptoms. In AD, loss of chemical markers for the neurotransmitter acetylcholine were identified. In animal studies, this neurotransmitter was found to be important for learning and memory. Thus emerged a new concept of AD as a cholinergic deficiency dementia. It took a number of years, but eventually medications to increase acetylcholine levels were approved by regulatory bodies and led to some modest benefits for patients. Thus AD moved from being a clinical entity to being a pathological entity and now to being a neurochemical entity.

Today, however, AD has come to be regarded as a genetic disease — a development described in the chapter by Daniel Pollen. Shortly after Alzheimer's original description, families in which AD appeared to be inherited were described. The original techniques of genetics, such as observing familial cases, could not connect inheritance to basic biological mechanisms. Nor were techniques available to identify where the genetic problem existed on the human genetic map. A clue to the chromosomal location of genes that could cause AD emerged when it was found that plaques and tangles occurred in the brains of individuals suffering from Down syndrome if they lived beyond the age of 40 or so. It was further found that a certain number of individuals, although not all, developed a dementia superimposed on their mental retardation. The fact that Down syndrome was caused by an extra copy of the 21st chromosome led to the search for clues to the genetic basis of autosomal dominant AD on the 21st chromosome. Eventually a large protein, which is the precursor to the amyloid protein found in senile plaques, was identified on the 21st chromosome, and mutations in this chromosome were found to cause AD in certain rare families. The discoveries concerning genetic linkage and amyloid led to the identification of other mutations, including the presenilins.

The excitement associated with understanding AD at the genetic level is tied to the hope that such knowledge will allow more powerful therapies to be developed. Molecular biology offers the promise not only for symptomatic relief but also for slowing the formation of senile plaques and thus slowing the clinical deterioration as well. This genetic information even allows the possibility of considering interventions that might prevent or cure the disease.

From a diagnostic point of view, genetic tests, at least for the autosomal dominant forms, offer great ability to predict future clinical states. Individuals who suffer from a mutation in the amyloid gene or one of the related presenilin genes can find out when they are still asymptomatic whether they are carrying the gene and are therefore likely to come down with the disorder if they live long enough. Thus, these genetic tests have allowed considerable increase in the power for diagnosis in autosomal dominant disease. Genetics is also contributing to understanding other nonautosomal dominant forms. For example, the gene for apolipoprotein E (APOE), located on chromosome 19, has been associated with the disorder. Individuals who are homozygote for the

APOE-4 allele are more at risk for the disease (and those with APOE-2 less so).

In summary, the history of the concept of AD has developed as an interaction among biological, clinical, and social factors. Biology has been the dominant force in reconceptualizations of dementia. The characterizations of AD at an anatomic/pathologic level, followed by a neurochemical/neurotransmitter level of description, and now, finally, at the molecular/genetic level, have changed the way we think of the disease. However, social factors have been critical in modulating the power of this biology to completely dominate our conceptions of the disease. The power of biology lies in its creating expectations that research will improve diagnosis and treatment. However, current treatments have been limited in the impact they have had on individuals suffering from AD. It remains to be seen how biological and social factors will interact to modulate our conceptions of AD in the future.

Reference

Kitwood, Tom. 1997. *Dementia Reconsidered: The Person Comes First.* Buckingham: Open University Press.

3

Neurofibrillary Changes

The Hallmark of Alzheimer Disease

Heiko Braak and Eva Braak

Neurofibrillary Tangles and Neuropil Threads

A major criterion essential for postmortem diagnosis of Alzheimer disease (AD) is the presence of somatic neurofibrillary tangles (NFTs) and dendritic neuropil threads (NTs) in specific subsets of nerve cells. Individuals who have a history of cognitive decline but no NFTs or NTs are classified in the heterogeneous group of the non-Alzheimer dementias (Braak and Braak 1997). NFTs and NTs consist mainly of abnormal microtubule-associated tau protein. In healthy individuals, the main function of this protein is to stabilize microtubules, which, in addition to other functions, play an important role in transporting substances among a nerve cell's individual compartments, which may be located at great distances from each other. Increasing aggregation of the abnormal tau protein results in impairment of this transport function and could ultimately lead to the death of the afflicted neurons.

An initial turning point in the pathologic process is a marked hyperphosphorylation of the tau protein. Hydrophilic material emerges, which, at the onset, is still nonargyrophilic in nature. Cross-linkages occur in a second step. Because the resulting insoluble and argyrophilic fibrils cannot be degraded by the parent cell, they accumulate, fill large portions of the cytoplasm, extend occasionally into the proximal dendrites, and eventually crowd the nucleus into an eccentric position (Bancher et al. 1989; Iqbal et al. 1994; Goedert, Trajonowski, and Lee 1997).

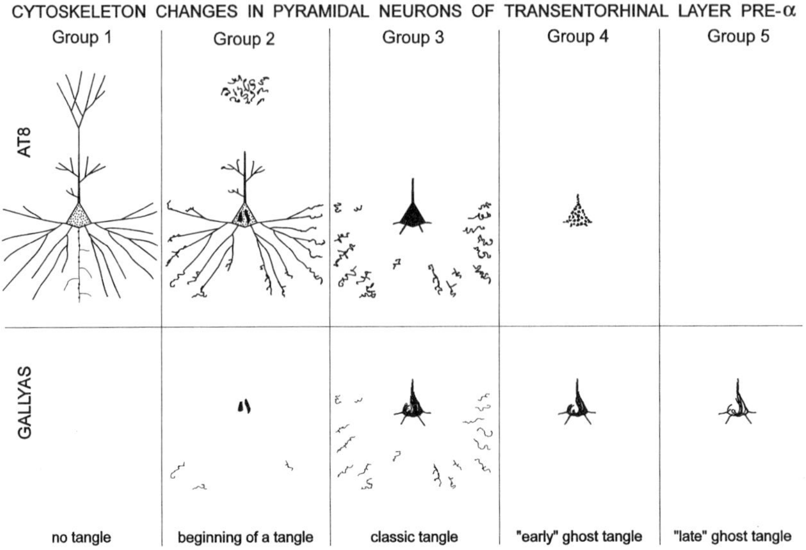

CYTOSKELETON CHANGES IN PYRAMIDAL NEURONS OF TRANSENTORHINAL LAYER PRE-α

FIGURE 15. Schematic drawing summarizing immunostaining with the phosphorylation-dependent anti-tau antibody AT8, compared with the corresponding Gallyas silver staining of developing neurofibrillary tangles and neuropil threads. The progression of pathological alterations of the neuronal cytoskeleton is shown from the group 1 neuron to the group 5 structure.
Source: Braak et al., 1994

Recently developed antibodies that react with the abnormally phosphorylated tau protein permit a demonstration of the evolution of the cytoskeletal changes. The still-soluble and nonargyrophilic tau protein fills the perikaryon and all of the neuronal processes, a picture closely resembling the result of a successful Golgi impregnation. If that crosslinking and aggregation of the abnormal protein to insoluble and argyrophilic NFTs or NTs have not yet occurred, the neurites of such cells maintain their normal shape. Nerve cells in such a "pretangle phase" first appear at the typical cortical induction site of AD-related lesions (i.e., the transentorhinal region). Studying this region in brains of comparatively young individuals provides evidence of the very first changes in the cytoskeleton in the absence of beta-amyloid deposits, vascular changes, or any other overt pathologic lesions (E. Braak, H. Braak, and Mandlekow 1994, 3–23). Cells in the pretangle phase represent the earliest detectable stage in the development of lesions, when the potential for reversibility is theoretically at its highest (Figure 15).

Sooner or later, however, cross-linked and argyrophilic precipitates begin to appear. As the distal segments of the dendrites become twisted and dilated, they develop short appendages and probably become detached from the proximal stem (E. Braak, H. Braak, and Mandlekow 1994). Within the changed dendritic segments, the formation of slender NTs begins, and shortly thereafter a stout NFT appears in the cell body (Figure 15). The first traces of the argyrophilic abnormal material are generally associated with the intraneuronal deposits of lipofuscin or neuromelanin granules (see Alzheimer 1911, 380). The central portions of larger NFTs form a dense feltwork around the pigment granules. It is possible that these granules provide initiation sites supporting oxidative cross-linking reactions. In any event, other neuronal inclusions, such as Lewy bodies, Hirano bodies, or granulovacuolar bodies, have no close association with the initial NFTs. After the final deterioration of the parent cell, the NFT material remains visible in the tissue for years as an extraneuronal "ghost" or "tombstone" tangle, marking the site at which the neuron was destroyed. In the course of this transformation, the NFT gradually becomes less densely twisted and loses much of its argyrophilia. Finally, even the extraneuronal NFT remnants completely disappear (Simchowicz 1911; Grünthal 1930; von Braunmühl 1957; Probst, Langui, and Ulrich 1991; Braak and Braak 1994).

DEPOSITS OF BETA-AMYLOID AND NEURITIC PLAQUES

Accompanying changes that generally develop later in the course of the disease include extracellular depositions of beta-amyloid protein and the formation of neuritic plaques (NPs). NFTs and NTs, on the one hand, and beta-amyloid precipitations and NPs, on the other, develop independently of each other; their distribution patterns barely overlap (Braak and Braak 1994).

Cortical deposits of the hydrophobic self-aggregating beta-amyloid protein appear as patches or cored plaques of variable size and generally globular form (Grünthal 1926, 1930; Divry 1927; von Braunmühl 1957; Beyreuther and Masters 1991; Selkoe 1994). They are encountered frequently, though not inevitably, in the brains of aged individuals. Despite a great deal of research, there is currently no clear evidence that deposits of insoluble ß-amyloid protein are capable of inducing the formation of NFTs and/or NTs (Hardy and Higgins 1992).

NPs consist of spherical aggregations of swollen neurites containing argyrophilic tau protein, dystrophic nonargyrophilic neurites, changed astrocytes, and activated microglial cells. Deposits of beta-amyloid are generally present in the form of peripheral infiltrations and, occasionally, as a compact core. NPs occur at much lower densities than mere beta-amyloid deposits (Friede 1965; Dickson 1997). We do not know how they are formed or why they disappear from the tissue. A few cortical areas and layers remain virtually devoid of NPs, while others exhibit high densities quite early in the disease. The cortex that covers the depths of the sulci generally exhibits a higher NP-density than that covering the crests of the gyri (see, among others, Alzheimer 1911, 363).

THE DISCOVERY OF NEURITIC PLAQUES AND THEIR SUBSEQUENT ASSOCIATION WITH DEMENTIA IN OLD AGE

Before the publication of his report on Auguste D., Alzheimer knew that spherical aggregations (now known as NPs) frequently appeared in the neocortex of older persons afflicted by cognitive decline. In 1892 Blocq and Marinesco reported glial nodules in the brain of an aging woman with epilepsy ("véritables nodules des scléroses neurogliques"). Redlich (1898) drew attention to the wealth of such nodules (miliary sclerosis) in the neocortex of individuals who had senile dementia. Blocq, Marinesco, and Redlich recognized that the proliferation of glial cells was a decisive factor in the formation of plaques. At approximately the same time, Alzheimer was preoccupied with finding the neuropathologic corollary to progressive dementia in older patients (Alzheimer 1899). Initially, he devoted himself to the relatively well-defined diseases of the central nervous system associated with syphilis. Until the turn of the century, and thereafter until well into the 1960s, the non-syphilitic decline of intellectual capacities in elderly persons was attributed primarily to sclerotic changes of cerebral blood vessels — an assumption often referred to under the misnomer "cerebral sclerosis." In his early studies Alzheimer based his findings on sections that required pretreatment in a Weigert mordant (for glial cells) and subsequent processing in Mann's methylblue-eosin solution. Portions of the NPs could be delineated fairly well with this technique, and Alzheimer was able to confirm the frequent occurrence of miliary plaques in the neocortex in cases of senile dementia detected by his predecessors (see also Fischer 1907; Oppenheim 1909; Alzheimer 1911; Lafora 1911; Schönfeld 1914). Alzheimer then began to question the thesis that the genesis of nonsyphilitic senile dementia generally resides in the aftereffects of sclerotic damage to brain vessels (Nissl 1916; Spielmeyer 1916; Kraepelin 1924; Meyer 1959, 1961; Torack 1978; Thomas and Isaac 1987; Kreutzberg and Gudden 1988; Hoff and Hippius 1989).

THE SEARCH FOR A SUITABLE SILVER TECHNIQUE

A convincing delineation of the grievous alteration in the neuronal cytoskeleton (the true hallmark of AD-related pathologic changes) cannot be achieved with general tissue stains. Distinct viewing of NFTs and NTs requires the application of a silver method. There are two different types of silver methods: precipitation methods, which use chromate solutions to transform soluble silver salts to virtually insoluble silver chromate deposits; and reducing methods, which are based on the reduction of soluble silver salts to metallic silver (Braak and Braak 1985). The silver precipitation technique was discovered by Camillo Golgi (1873). Further groundbreaking work in the silver reduction technique was done by Santiago Ramon y Cajal and Max Bielschowsky.

In addition to being an outstanding neuroscientist, Ramon y Cajal was an avid and superb photographer who had an important role in the technical evolution of color photography (Albarracin 1982). Using his detailed knowledge of photographic processes, Ramon y Cajal developed histologic silver techniques. The tissue was first impregnated in a solution of silver nitrate and then developed in strong reducing agents used in photographic developers (e.g., hydrochinone) (Ramon y Cajal 1903). Still, inconsistent results prevented the widespread adoption of these methods in the field of routine diagnostics. Numerous modifications of Ramon y Cajal's procedures failed to gain a foothold apart from their application in specialized settings.

Ramon y Cajal's methods were superseded by a more reliable working technique developed by Bielschowsky (1902) and his predecessor Fajerszatjn (1901). By introducing an ammoniacal silver solution, exceptionally fine silver precipitations could be acquired with weak reducing agents such as formaldehyde. Bielschowsky improved and modified his method repeatedly (1903, 1904, 1905, 1909). A short time later the colloid chemist Liesegang developed a fundamental theory of histologic silver staining that decisively influenced the further evolution of these methods (Liesegang 1911).

Alzheimer used modern staining techniques and research methods. To examine the famous case of Auguste D., he used both the methylblue-eosin modification and the novel silver method developed a few years previously by Bielschowsky. The new technique enabled Alzheimer to describe the NFT, the essential hallmark of the degenerative illness that Kraepelin named "Alzheimer's disease" (1910, 627).

In this context, Carl Weigert should be cited. In a publication honoring the fiftieth anniversary of the Frankfurt Physicians Association, he somewhat acridly remarked:

> There are people who regard the invention of a new method as though it were a scientific achievement of inferior quality, and who look down upon the inventors themselves. Upon closer scrutiny, however, it is precisely these people who resort with the utmost zeal to the methods of the inventors whom they so disdain in order to erect their own scientific constructs with technical competence. Similarly, many a journeyman mason may have a low opinion of the architect whose blueprints he is following because the architect does not personally lay the tiles one upon the other. There has to be room for such odd people in the world! (Weigert 1895, v; author's translation)

Although Alzheimer did not think like those whom Weigert pillories, Weigert's lament is not unfounded even in our own times. Accordingly, the achievement of Max Bielschowsky (1869–1940) should be duly emphasized. This pathbreaking pioneer of the neurosciences was descended from an old, established Jewish family of merchants in Breslau. Upon completing medical school, the musically gifted and versatile young man was admitted, at the invitation of Ludwig Edinger, to the Dr. Senckenberg Institute of Pathology and Anatomy in Frankfurt under the direction of Carl Weigert. Over the course of three years (1893–6) of close collaboration with Edinger and Weigert, Bielschowsky developed the impulses and ideas that decisively marked his later work. During this time he must also have encountered Alzheimer, who had been working since 1888 in the Frankfurt Hospital for the Mentally Ill under the directorship of Sioli. Max Bielschowsky, who was five years Alzheimer's junior, also became acquainted with Alzheimer's close friend Franz Nissl, who served as assistant medical director in the Frankfurt Asylum until 1895 (Weil 1953). Krücke probably characterized the situation correctly when he declared in his essay commemorating the 100th birthday of Ludwig Edinger: "Owing to the contributions of Edinger and Weigert, Nissl, and Alzheimer, there emerged in Frankfurt at the close of the last century the foundation of our present-day histopathology of the nervous system" (Krücke 1959; see also Krücke 1961).

After completing his study in Frankfurt, Bielschowsky moved to Berlin and initially worked with the neurologist Mendel. Beginning in 1904, he worked with Korbinian Brodmann and Oskar Vogt in the neurologic laboratory that subsequently became the Kaiser Wilhelm

Institut für Hirnforschung. The initial report of Bielschowsky's silver technique appeared in print in 1902. The method quickly attained international recognition and remains an indispensable methodologic tool of neuropathologists (Perusini 1910; von Braunmül 1929; Yamamoto and Hirano 1986; Lamy et al. 1989).

THE FIRST DETAILED DESCRIPTION OF NEUROFIBRILLARY TANGLES

Because of his longstanding preoccupation with dementing disorders, Alzheimer promptly recognized the peculiarities of a case characterized by particularly rapidly progressing memory impairment. The 51-year-old Auguste D. was admitted to the Frankfurt Hospital for the Mentally Ill in 1901 (Lewey 1970; Berrios 1987; Bick, Amaducci, and Pepeu 1987; Bick 1994; Maurer, Volk, and Gerbaldo 1997). Following an invitation by Kraepelin, Alzheimer left Frankfurt the following year and moved, after a brief sojourn in Heidelberg, to the Royal Psychiatric Clinic in Munich, which opened on November 4, 1904. After Auguste D.'s death and autopsy in 1906, Alzheimer arranged for the consignment of the patient's brain tissue and clinical records. Alzheimer succeeded in demonstrating that Auguste D. had not suffered from syphilitic or arteriosclerotic brain changes (Alzheimer 1906, 1907, 1911). O'Brien's interpretation (1996) that arteriosclerotic changes lay the root of Auguste D.'s illness cannot be substantiated in the patient's clinical record or in Alzheimer's publications (Alzheimer 1911, 356. For summaries of the first case and succeeding cases, see Bonfiglio 1908; Perusini 1909; Bielschowsky 1911; Fuller 1912).

At the turn of the century, researcher-physicians represented a broad spectrum of the modern specialties of neuroscience. Alois Alzheimer and Max Bielschowsky performed all the functions of psychiatrists, neurologists, neuroanatomists, and neuropathologists (Alzheimer 1913; Kraepelin 1983). As Alzheimer put it at one point, both wanted to help the field of psychiatry on its way with the assistance of the microscope. To the degree that both men were engaged in clinical work and basic research, it is tempting to ask why it was not Bielschowsky who discovered the thoroughgoing changes of the neuronal cytoskeleton in presenile and senile dementia. Like Alzheimer, Bielschowsky initially studied syphilitic diseases of the brain. He then turned his attention to the normal development of the cytoskeleton in diverse types of nerve cells. Moreover, he was fascinated by both the chronology of the maturing cytoskeleton and deviations from this sequence (Bielschowsky 1910). Bielschowsky outlined the significance of his silver technique for histopathology and illustrated several disease-related changes (Biels-chowsky 1904, 184ff.). It seems that Bielschowsky missed discovering the neuropathologic hallmarks of a most important dementing disorder by a hair's breadth.

STRENGTHS AND WEAKNESSES OF THE BIELSCHOWSKY METHOD AND THE INTRODUCTION OF THE GALLYAS TECHNIQUES

The Bielschowsky technique is superior to other silver methods and to general histologic stains. Despite its weaknesses, it is significant that the method is still in use worldwide some ninety-five years after its development. Only in the hands of a master such as Alzheimer, however, does Bielschowsky's silver technique results in richly detailed specimens (Alzheimer 1911, 372). Sections were discovered recently in connection with a case studied by Alzheimer in Munich: Johann F., a 56-year-old male with progressive dementia (Graeber et al. 1997). Bielschowsky specimens stemming from routine manufacture, on the other hand, often display the disadvantages associated with this technique. In par-ticular, the production of the ammoniacal silver solution calls for experi-ence and considerable meticulousness. In addition, solutions of this kind tend to explode suddenly, particularly after long periods of exposure to the light (Schlemmer 1908; Wallington 1965). A crucial disadvantage of using the Bielschowsky technique to detect related neurofibrillary changes is that many normal tissue elements are also depicted, making it difficult to differentiate altered components of the brain from unin-volved structures.

In contrast, the modern silver methods of Ferenc Gallyas (1971) detect the changes with notable clarity. The roots of the Gallyas tech-niques go back to basic colloid-chemical considerations that were pub-lished by Liesegang in 1911. It is important to mention that the Gallyas techniques do not require the somewhat cumbersome production of an ammoniacal silver solution. This step is replaced by an easily performed and reproducible procedure. The Gallyas techniques enjoy the further advantage of applying a light-insensitive physical developer to visualize the nucleation sites, thereby permitting tight control of the entire pro-cedure. The Gallyas techniques are simpler to use and more reliable than the Bielschowsky method or other conventional silver stains. When the Gallyas technique is used to detect AD-related pathologic changes, lesions are made visible without distracting background staining (Braak et al. 1988; Braak and Braak 1991b). Small abnormal elements such as neuropil threads, which are not easily recognized in Bielschowsky-stained sections, have been detected using the Gallyas method for neurofibrillary changes (Braak et al. 1986). Gallyas techniques can be applied to routinely fixed autopsy material even if it has been stored for decades in formalin solutions. They facilitate the processing of large numbers of sections and permit staining of large sections such as double hemispheres. Both 5 to 15 μm thin paraffin sections and 50 to 150 μm thick frozen or polyethylenglycol-embedded sections can be processed. For easy recognition of architectonic units, it is possible to counterstain the paraffin sections for lipofuscin deposits, Nissl material, or other structures (Braak et al. 1988). As compared to the results of using immunoreactions, a more homogeneous staining is achieved throughout the entire thickness of sections. The methods are remarkably inexpensive and can be applied anywhere in the world.

THE GRADUAL EVOLUTION OF NFT/NT-RELATED PATHOLOGIC CHANGES IN THE COURSE OF ALZHEIMER DISEASE

Following the comprehensive account of 1911, Alzheimer no longer devoted himself to further studies of the disease bearing his name. A pathoarchitectonic analysis (an inventory of all the subdivisions of the brain and spinal cord that undergo the typical degenerative changes in the course of the disease) is missing. For understandable reasons, Alzheimer did not conduct systematic studies entailing serial sections through the entire central nervous system comparable to those performed by his contemporaries, Brodmann and the Vogts, in Berlin. It is particularly difficult for the neuropathologist or neuroanatomist to explain why the pathologic process underlying AD produces a specific and peculiar pattern of lesions (Kemper 1978). Given the circumstances, why the Vogts refrained from studying the pathoarchitectonics of AD in detail remains inexplicable. At any rate, Bielschowsky was an important member of their staff and worked, more or less harmoniously, with the Vogts from 1904 until 1933. At that point the friendship with Oskar Vogt became strained, and Bielschowsky not only lost his position at the Kaiser Wilhelm Institute but also left Germany (Weil 1953; Peiffer 1997).

Based on more recent findings, it is known that the destructive process underlying AD begins in predisposed induction sites (transentorhinal region); it then invades other portions of the cerebral cortex and specific sets of subcortic nuclei in a predictable, nonrandom sequence,

transentorhinal stages
I -II

limbic stages
III - IV

neocortical stages
V - VI

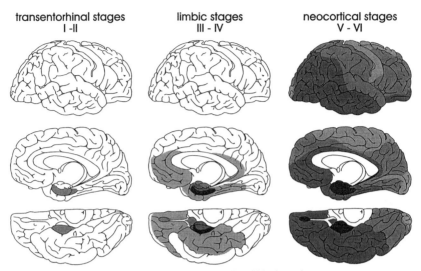

Neurofibrillary changes of the Alzheimer type

FIGURE 16.   Sequence of changes in the distribution pattern of neurofibrillary tangles and neuropil threads in the course of AD. Six stages can be distinguished. Stages 1 and 2 show alterations that are virtually confined to a single layer of the transentorhinal and entorhinal regions. Stages 3 and 4 show severe affection of the entorhinal territory and additional involvement of many related limbic structures. Stages 5 and 6 are marked by a devastating destruction of the neocortex. Increasing density of shading indicates an increasing density of neurofibrillary tangles and neuropil threads.
Source: Braak and Braak, 1991a

with very little variation (Figure 16). This sequence provides a basis for distinguishing stages in the evolution of the lesions (Braak and Braak 1991a, 1994; Hyman and Trojanowski 1997).

Transentorhinal Stages.   Specific projection cells in the transentorhinal region (temporal lobe) are the first neurons to show the development of NFTs and NTs in the cerebral cortex (stage I). From here, the lesions extend into the entorhinal region proper (stage II). The transentorhinal stages represent a preclinical phase of AD. The initial changes preferably develop in the absence of beta-amyloid deposits and may commence at a surprisingly young age. Thus, advanced age is not a prerequisite for the development of NFTs and NTs (Braak and Braak 1997).

Limbic Stages.   The key characteristic of limbic stage III is a severe destruction of the entorhinal cortex, accompanied by mild changes in the hippocampus and temporal proneocortex. The mature neocortex is virtually devoid of lesions. At stage IV, the pathologic changes make inroads into the temporal and insular neocortex. Stage III or IV cases frequently exhibit mild to modest impairment of cognition as well as subtle personality changes. They are considered to represent incipient AD.

Neocortical Stages. Fully developed AD is represented by stages V and VI, which are characterized by a widespread destruction of neocortical association areas (stage V) that eventually include even primary neocortical fields (stage VI). Stages V and VI generally are accompanied by a marked macroscopically detectable atrophy of the cortex and a corresponding loss in brain weight. During the entire course of AD, intraneuronal NFTs develop either in isolation or in combination with a variable number of extraneuronal "ghost" tangles. "Ghost" tangles alone cannot be observed.

The appearance of the first traces of abnormal intraneuronal material signals the beginning of a degenerative process that continues inexorably until death. An extended period of time elapses between the beginning of histologically verifiable lesions and the appearance of initial clinical symptoms (Ohm et al. 1995; Braak and Braak 1997). Once initiated, the destruction progresses relentlessly, and neither remission nor recovery is observed. A continuum of intraneuronal changes starts with the first tangle and extends to the high density of lesions seen in fully developed AD. No single feature permits definition of a specific form of intraneuronal changes exclusively related to age (Braak and Braak 1997).

SELECTIVE VULNERABILITY OF DISTINCT NEURONAL TYPES IN ALZHEIMER DISEASE

AD-related destruction focuses on specific types of nerve cells, while adjoining ones may remain unscathed or suffer only secondary damage. Only a very small number of the many neuronal types that make up the human central nervous system are susceptible to the development of NFTs and NTs. Accordingly, AD is a suitable model for studying the problem of selective vulnerability. NFT-bearing cells within the cerebral cortex all belong to the class of pyramidal cells. Projection neurons that furnish long ipsilateral corticocortical connections are particularly susceptible to the accumulation of the argyrophilic tau protein, while cortical local circuit neurons that generate a short axon are resistant (Morrison and Hof 1997). Most of the vulnerable cells in the subcortical nuclei also stand out, thanks to their lengthy axons.

The causes of this selective vulnerability and the consistence in the spread of the pathologic changes are still unknown.

A key to deciphering these peculiarities may reside in the surprising observation that the gradual spread of NFTs and NTs throughout the cortex turns out to be a mirror image of the early development of myelin: the progression is the same, but the order is reversed. Late-myelinating cortical areas and layers develop NFTs and NTs earlier in the course of AD and at higher densities than those that commence myelination early (McGeer et al. 1990; Braak and Braak 1996). Myelination is considered a final process in maturation of the brain. The functional maturity of most cortical and subcortical projection cells is achieved only after myelination of their axons. Myelination of the human cerebral cortex is a particularly late-onset and prolonged process, and follows a predetermined sequence. The first traces of myelin appear in the primary motor area of the neocortex, followed by the sensory core areas. Thereafter, the process continues via the border fields into the related association areas. The result is exceptionally dense myelination of the neocortical core fields in the human adult. Because a gradual decrease in the average density of myelin is observed with increasing distance from the core fields, the temporal proneocortex and the transentorhinal region are extremely sparsely myelinated (Figure 17).

This consideration has to be supplemented by the finding that the human adult brain is particularly richly endowed with intraneuronal deposits of lipofuscin or neuromelanin. In this respect it differs markedly from the brain of subhuman primates. The pigment deposits vary from one type of nerve cell to another. It is important to note in this context that the average density of cortical pigmentation bears an enigmatic likeness to the negative image of cortical myelination (Figure 17). Richly myelinated cortical areas, such as the primary sensory fields and the primary motor area, as well as cortical layers endowed with a thick plexus of myelinated fibers, are, in general, sparsely pigmented; the temporal proneocortex and the transentorhinal region, which are the last to myelinate, are among the most richly pigmented territories of the human cerebral cortex (Braak 1980).

The first areas to show NFT and NT changes are in the transentorhinal region and adjoining areas. Involvement of the neocortical belt and core areas is observed only late in the course of the disease. The primary motor area is the last to show the changes (Figure 17). Subcortical nuclei that are prone to developing NFTs and NTs include components of the magnocellular nuclei of the basal forebrain, the tuberomammillary nucleus of the hypothalamus, the locus coeruleus, and the

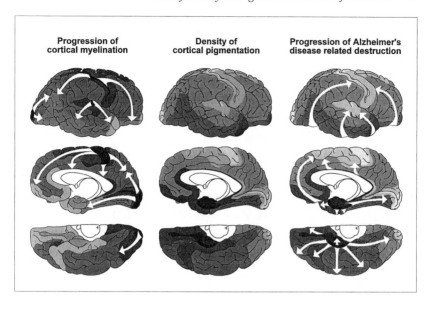

FIGURE 17. *Left,* the outward progression of myelination from the neocortical core fields via belt areas into the associated higher-order processing areas. The central column points to the fact that the average density of cortical pigmentation bears an enigmatic likeness to the negative image of cortical myelination. *Right,* the gradual progression of neurofibrillary tangle/neuropil thread-related lesions from the transentorhinal/entorhinal regions into the core fields via neocortical higher-order processing areas and belt areas. Note that the spread of AD-related pathology mirrors the process of cortical myelination: the progression is the same, but the order is reversed.

nuclei of the anterior raphe complex. All give rise to diffuse projections to the cerebral cortex (German, White, and Sparkman 1987; Saper 1987). An important feature shared by these subnuclei is that they generate remarkably thin axons that remain unmyelinated or only sparsely myelinated even in adulthood (Nieuwenhuys 1996). A further characteristic common to the projection cells of these nuclei is that they contain conspicuous amounts of lipofuscin or neuromelanin granules.

In this context, it is important to point out that all of the cortical or subcortical projection neurons that develop a long and thick axon enclosed in a thick myelin sheath are protected against the development of NFTs and NTs, regardless of which features their pigment deposits display. Should it turn out that pigment-laden neurons endowed with long, sparsely myelinated or unmyelinated axons are characteristic of all cells that gradually become involved in the course of AD, there are still many unanswered questions. It can only be hoped that answers to these questions will bring us closer to an understanding of the conditions that trigger the process underlying AD. Such answers will possibly point the way toward developing new and effective therapeutic strategies.

Acknowledgments

This work was supported by the Deutsche Forschungsgemeinschaft and the Bundesministerium für Bildung, Wissenschaft, Forschung und Technologie; the Alzheimer Research Center Frankfurt (AFZF); and Degussa, Hanau. The skillful assistance of Ms. Szasz (drawings) is gratefully acknowledged. The authors would further like to thank Ms. Grell and the Cecile and Oskar Vogt Institute for Brain Research (Düsseldorf) for help in details of biographical data.

References

Albarracin, A. 1982. Santiago Ramón y Cajal o la pasión de españa. Barcelona: Editorial Labor.

Alzheimer, A. 1899. Beitrag zur pathologischen Anatomie der Seelenstörungen des Greisenalters. *Neurologisches Centralblatt* 18:95–96.

——. 1906. Über einen eigenartigen schweren Erkrankungsprozeß der Hirnrinde. *Neurologisches Centralblatt* 23:1129–36.

——. 1907. Über eine eigenartige Erkrankung der Hirnrinde. *Allgemeine Zeitschrift für Psychiatrie und Psychisch-Gerichtliche Medizin* 64:146–48. (For English translations, see Fuller 1912 and Bick et al. 1987.)

——. 1911. Über eigenartige Krankheitsfälle des späteren Alters. *Zeitschrift für die gesamte Neurologie und Psychiatrie* 4:356–85.

——. 1913. 25 Jahre Psychiatrie: Ein Rückblick anlässlich des 25jährigen Jubiläums von Prof. Dr. Emil Sioli als Direktor der Frankfurter Irrenanstalt. *Archiv für Psychiatrie und Nervenkrankheiten* 52:853–66.

Bancher, C., C. Brunner, H. Lassmann, H. Budka, K. Jellinger, G. Wiche, F. Seitelberger, I. Grundke-Iqbal, and H. M. Wisniewski. 1989. Accumulation of abnormally phosphorylated precedes the formation of neurofibrillary tangles in Alzheimer's disease. *Brain Research* 477:90–99.

Berrios, G. E. 1987. Alzheimer's disease: A conceptual history. *International Journal for Geriatrics and Psychiatry* 5:355–65.

Beyreuther, K., and C. L. Masters. 1991. Amyloid precursor protein (APP) and ßA4 amyloid in the etiology of Alzheimer's disease: Precursor product relationships in the derangement of neuronal function. *Brain Pathology* 1:241–52.

Bick, K. L. 1994. The early story of Alzheimer's disease. In *Alzheimer's Disease*, ed. R. D. Terry, R. Katzman, and K. L. Bick, 1–8. New York: Raven Press.

Bick, K. L., L. Amaducci, and G. Pepeu. 1987. *The Early Story of Alzheimer's Disease*. New York: Raven Press.

Bielschowsky, M. 1902. Die Silberimprägnation der Axenzylinder. *Neurologisches Centralblatt* 13:579–84.

———. 1903. Die Silberimprägnation der Neurofibrillen. *Neurologisches Centralblatt* 21:997–1006.

———. 1904. Die Silberimprägnation der Neurofibrillen: Einige Bemerkungen zu der von mir angegebenen Methode und den von ihr gelieferten Bildern. *Journal für Psychologie und Neurologie* 3:169–89.

———. 1905. Die Darstellung der Axenzylinder peripherischer Nervenfasern und der Axenzylinder zentraler markhaltiger Nervenfasern: Ein Nachtrag zu der von mir angegebenen Imprägnationsmethode der Neurofibrillen. *Journal für Psychologie und Neurologie* 4:228–31.

———. 1909. Eine Modifikation meines Silberimprägnationsverfahrens zur Darstellung der Neurofibrillen. *Journal für Psychologie und Neurologie* 12:135–37.

———. 1910. Allgemeine Histologie und Histopathologie des Nervensystems. In *Handbuch der Neurologie*, ed. M. Lewandowsky. 1:3–90. Berlin: Springer.

———. 1911. Zur Kenntnis der Alzheimerschen Krankheit (präsenilen Demenz mit Herdsymptomen). *Journal für Psychologie und Neurologie* 18:273–92.

Blocq, P., and G. Marinesco. 1892. Sur les lésions et la pathogenie de lépilepsie dite essentielle. *Sémaine Médicale* 12:445–46.

Bonfiglio, F. 1908. Di speciali reperti in un caso di probabile sifilide cerebrale. *Rivista Sperimentale di Freniatria e Medicina Legale Delle Alienazioni Mentali* 34:196–206.

Braak, E., H. Braak, and E. M. Mandelkow. 1994. A sequence of cytoskeleton changes related to the formation of neurofibrillary tangles and neuropil threads. *Acta Neuropathologica* 87:554–67.

Braak, H. 1980. *Architectonics of the Human Telencephalic Cortex*. Berlin: Springer.

Braak, H., and E. Braak. 1985. Golgi preparations as a tool in neuropathology with particular reference to investigations of the human telencephalic cortex. *Progress in Neurobiology* 25:93–139.

———. 1991a. Neuropathological staging of Alzheimer-related changes. *Acta Neuropathologica* 82:239–59.

———. 1991b. Demonstration of amyloid deposits and neurofibrillary changes in whole brain sections. *Brain Pathology* 1:213–16.

———. 1994. Pathology of Alzheimer's disease. In *Neurodegenerative Diseases*, ed. D. B. Calne, 585–613. Philadelphia: Saunders.

——. 1996. Development of Alzheimer-related neurofibrillary changes in the neocortex inversely recapitulates cortical myelogenesis. *Acta Neuropathologica* 92:197–201.

——. 1997. Frequency of stages of Alzheimer-related lesions in different age categories. *Neurobiology of Aging* 18:351–57.

Braak, H., E. Braak, I. Grundke-Iqbal, and K. Iqbal. 1986. Occurrence of neuropil threads in the senile human brain and in Alzheimer's disease: A third location of paired helical filaments outside of neurofibrillary tangles and neuritic plaques. *Neuroscience Letters* 65:351–55.

Braak, H., E. Braak, T. G. Ohm, and J. Bohl. 1988. Silver impregnation of Alzheimer's neurofibrillary changes counterstained for basophilic material and lipofuscin pigment. *Staining Technology* 63:197–200.

Dickson, D. W. 1997. The pathogenesis of senile plaques. *Journal of Neuropathology and Experimental Neurology* 56:321–39.

Divry, P. 1927. Etude histo-chimique des plaques séniles. *Journal of the Belge Neurology and Psychiatry* 27:641–57.

Esiri, M. M., B. T. Hyman, K. Beyreuther, and C. Masters. 1997. Aging and dementia. In *Greenfield's Neuropathology*, ed. D. L. Graham and P. I. Lantos, 153–234. London: Arnold.

Fajerztajn, J. 1901. Ein neues Silberimprägnationsverfahren als Mittel zur Färbung der Axencylinder. *Neurologisches Centralblatt* 20:98–106.

Fischer, O. 1907. Miliare Nekrosen mit drusigen Wucherungen der Neurofibrillen, eine regelmässige Veränderung der Hirnrinde bei seniler Demenz. *Monatsschrift für Psychiatrie und Neurologie* 22:361–72.

Friede, R. L. 1965. Enzyme histochemical studies of senile plaques. *Journal of Neuropathology and Experimental Neurology* 24:477–91.

Fuller, S. C. 1912. Alzheimer's disease (senium praecox): The report of a case and review of published cases. *Journal of Nervous and Mental Disorders* 39: 440–55, 536–57.

Gallyas, F. 1971. Silver staining of Alzheimer's neurofibrillary changes by means of physical development. *Acta Morphologica Academiae Scientiarum Hungaricae* 19:1–8.

German, D. C., C. L. White, and D. R. Sparkman. 1987. Alzheimer's disease: Neurofibrillary tangles in nuclei that project to the cerebral cortex. *Neuroscience* 21:305–12.

Goedert, M., J. Q. Trojanowski, and V. M. Y. Lee. 1997. The neurofibrillary pathology of Alzheimer's disease. In *The Molecular and Genetic Basis of Neurological Diseases*, 2d ed., ed. R. N. Rosenberg, 613–27. Boston: Butterworth-Heinemann.

Golgi, C. 1873. Sulla struttura della sostanza grigia dell cervello. *Gazzetta Med-*

ica Italiana Lombarda 33:244–46. (Reprinted 1903 in *Opera Omnia* 1:91–98. Milano: Hoepli).

Graeber, M. B., S. Kösel, R. Egensperger, R. B. Banati, U. Müller, K. Bise, P. Hoff, H. J. Möller, K. Fujisawa, and P. Mehraein. 1997. Rediscovery of the case described by Alois Alzheimer in 1911: Historical, histological, and molecular genetic analysis. *Neurogenetics* 1:73–80.

Grünthal, E. 1926. Über die Alzheimersche Krankheit: Eine histopathologische Studie. *Zeitschrift für die gesamte Neurologie und Psychiatrie* 101:128–57.

———. 1930. Die pathologische Anatomie der senilen Demenz und der Alzheimerschen Krankheit: Mit besonderer Berücksichtigung der Beziehungen zur Klinik. In *Handbuch der Geisteskrankheiten*, ed. O. Bumke, 11:638–72. Berlin: Springer.

Hardy, J. A., and G. A. Higgins. 1992. Alzheimer's disease: The amyloid cascade hypothesis. *Science* 256:184–85.

Hoff, P., and H. Hippius. 1989. Alois Alzheimer, 1864–1915: Ein Überblick über Leben und Werk anläßlich seines 125. Geburtstages. *Nervenarzt* 60: 332–37.

Hyman, B. T., and J. Q. Trojanowski. 1997. Editorial on consensus recommendations for the postmortem diagnosis of Alzheimer disease from the National Institute on Aging and the Reagan Institute Working Group on diagnostic criteria for the neuropathological assessment of Alzheimer disease. *Journal of Neuropathology and Experimental Neurology* 56:1095–97.

Iqbal, K., A. C. Alonso, C. X. Gong, S. Khatoon, T. J. Singh, and I. Grundke-Iqbal. 1994. Mechanism of neurofibrillary degeneration in Alzheimer's disease. *Molecular Neurobiology* 9:119–23.

Kemper, T. L. 1978. Senile dementia: A focal disease in the temporal lobe. In *Senile Dementia: A Biomedical Approach*, ed. E. Nandy, 105–13. Amsterdam: Elsevier.

Kraepelin, E. 1910. *Psychiatrie, ein Lehrbuch für Studierende und Ärzte*. Leipzig: Barth. (Alzheimer disease: see 2:619ff.).

———. 1924. Alzheimer, Aloys (1864–1915). In *Deutsche Irrenärzte: Einzelbilder ihres Lebens und Wirkens*, ed. T. Kirchhoff, 299–307. Berlin: Springer.

———. 1983. Lebenserinnerungen. In *Emil Kraepelin: Lebenserinnerungen*, ed. H. Hippius, G. Peters, and D. Ploog, 1–220. Berlin: Springer.

Kreutzberg, G. W., and W. Gudden. 1988. Alois Alzheimer. *Trends in Neuroscience* 11:256–57.

Krücke, W. 1959. *Ludwig Edinger 1855–1918*, 1–97. Wiesbaden: Steiner.

———. 1961. Carl Weigert (1845–1904). In *50 Jahre Neuropathologie in Deutschland 1885–1935*, ed. W. Scholz, 5–19. Stuttgart: Thieme.

Lafora, G. R. 1911. Beitrag zur Kenntnis der Alzheimerschen Krankheit oder präsenilen Demenz mit Herdsymptomen. *Zeitschrift für die gesamte Neurologie und Psychiatrie* 6:15–20.

Lamy, C., C. Duyckaerts, P. Delaère, C. Payan, J. Fermanian, V. Poulain, and J. J. Hauw. 1989. Comparison of seven staining methods for senile plaques and neurofibrillary tangles in a prospective series of fifteen elderly patients. *Neuropathology and Applied Neurobiology* 15:563–78.

Lewey, F. J. 1970. Alois Alzheimer. In *The Founders of Neurology*, ed. W. Haymaker, 165–68. Springfield, Ill.: C. C. Thomas.

Liesegang, R. E. 1911. Die Kolloidchemie der histologischen Silberfärbungen. *Kolloidchemische Beihefte* 3:1–46.

Maurer, K., and Maurer, U. 1998. *Alzheimer.* München: Piper.

Maurer, K., S. Volk, and H. Gerbaldo. 1997. Auguste D. and Alzheimer's disease. *Lancet* 349:1546–49.

McGeer, P. L., E. G. McGeer, H. Akiyama, S. Itagaki, R. Harrop, and R. Peppard. 1990. Neuronal degeneration and memory loss in Alzheimer's disease and aging. *Experimental Brain Research* Suppl. 21:411–26.

Meyer, J. E. 1959. Alois Alzheimer (1864–1915). In *Große Nervenärzte*, 2d ed., ed. K. Kolle, 2:32–28. Stuttgart: Thieme.

———. 1961. Alois Alzheimer. In *50 Jahre Neuropathologie in Deutschland, 1885–1935*, ed. W. Scholz, 67–78. Stuttgart: Thieme.

Morrison, J. H., and P. R. Hof. 1997. Life and death of neurons in the aging brain. *Science* 278:412–19.

Nieuwenhuys, R. 1996. The greater limbic system, the emotional motor system, and the brain. *Progress in Brain Research* 107:551–80.

Nissl, F. 1916. Alois Alzheimer. *Deutsche medizinische Wochenschrift* 14:1116–20.

O'Brien, C. 1996. Auguste D. and Alzheimer's disease. *Science* 273:28.

Ohm, T. G., H. Müller, H. Braak, and J. Bohl. 1995. Close-meshed prevalence rates of different stages as a tool to uncover the rate of Alzheimer's disease-related neurofibrillary changes. *Neuroscience* 64:209–17.

Oppenheim, G. 1909. Über "drusige Nekrosen" in der Großhirnrinde. *Neurologisches Centralblatt* 8:410–13.

Peiffer, J. 1997. Hirnforschung im Zwielicht: Beispiele verführbarer Wissenschaft aus der Zeit des Nationalsozialismus. *Abhandlungen zur Geschichte der Medizin und der Naturwissenschaften* 79:1–112. Matthiesen Verlag.

Perusini, G. 1909. Über klinisch und histologisch eigenartige psychische Erkrankungen des höheren Lebensalters. *Histologische und histopathologische Arbeiten* 3:297–351.

———. 1910. 3. Über Gliabilder mittels der Bielschowsky'schen Neurofibrillenmethode. *Neurologisches Zentralblatt* 22:1256–59.

Probst, A., D. Langui, and J. Ulrich. 1991. Alzheimer's disease: A description of the structural lesions. *Brain Pathology* 1:229–39.

Ramon y Cajal, S. 1903. Über einige Methoden der Silberimprägnierung zur Untersuchung der Neurofibrillen, der Achsencylinder und der Endverzweigungen. *Zeitschrift für wissenschaftliche Mikroskopie* 20:401–8.

Redlich, E. 1898. Über miliare Sklerose der Hirnrinde bei seniler Atrophie. *Journal für Psychologie und Neurologie* 17:208–11.

Saper, C. B. 1987. Diffuse cortical projection systems: Anatomical organization and role in cortical function. In *Handbook of Physiology*. Vol. 5, *The Nervous System*, ed. F. Plum, 169–210. Bethesda, Md.: American Physiological Society.

Schlemmer, A. 1908. Über die Herstellung der ammoniakalischen Silbersalzlösung bei der Imprägnationsmethode von Bielschowsky. *Zeitschrift für wissenschaftliche Mikroskopie* 27:22–23.

Schönfeld, A. 1914. Über Vorkommen und Bedeutung der drusigen Bildungen (Sphaerotrichie) in der Hirnrinde. *Monatsschrift für Psychiatrie* 36:342–78.

Selkoe, D. J. 1994. Alzheimer's disease: A central role for amyloid. *Journal of Neuropathology and Experimental Neurology* 53:438–47.

Simchowicz, T. 1911. Histologische Studien über die senile Demenz. *Histologische und histopathologische Arbeiten* 4:267–444.

Spielmeyer, W. 1916. Alzheimers Lebenswerk. *Zeitschrift für die gesamte Neurologie und Psychiatrie* 33:1–41.

Thomas, M., and M. Isaac. 1987. Alois Alzheimer: A memoir. *Trends in Neuroscience* 10:306–7.

Torack, R. M. 1978. 1. Historical overview of dementia. In *The Pathologic Physiology of Dementia*, ed. R. M. Torack, 1–16. Berlin: Springer.

Von Braunmühl, A. 1929. Eine einfache Schnellmethode zur Darstellung der senilen Drusen. *Zeitschrift für die gesamte Neurologie und Psychiatrie* 122:317–22.

———. 1957. Alterserkrankungen des Zentralnervensystems. Senile Involution. Senile Demenz. Alzheimersche Krankheit. In *Handbuch der speziellen pathologischen Anatomie und Histologie*, ed. O. Lubarsch, F. Henke, and R. Rössle. 13/1A:337–539. Berlin: Springer.

Wallington, E. A. 1965. The explosive properties of ammoniacal-silver solutions. *Journal of Medical Laboratory Technology* 22:220–23.

Weigert, C. 1895. Beiträge zur Kenntnis der normalen menschlichen Neuroglia. Festschrift zum fünfzigjährigen Jubiläum des ärztlichen Vereins zu Frankfurt a.M., 3. November 1895. In *Abhandlungen der Senckenbergischen naturforschenden Gesellschaft* 19:1–149.

Weil, A. 1953. Max Bielschowsky (1869–1940). In *The Founders of Neurology*, ed. W. Haymaker and K. A. Baer, 169–71. Springfield, Ill.: C. C. Thomas.

Yamamoto, T., and A. Hirano. 1986. A comparative study of modified Bielschowsky, Bodian, and thioflavine S stains on Alzheimer's neurofibrillary tangles. *Neuropathology and Applied Neurobiology* 12:3–9.

4

Contributions of German Neuroscience to the Concept of Alzheimer Disease

Hans Förstl

During the first half of the twentieth century, the concept of Alzheimer disease was written about entirely in German. A new staining method described by Bielschowsky (1903) allowed Alois Alzheimer to demonstrate a new kind of argentophilic intraneuronal fibrillary tangle (1906, 1907) in his first patient with the severe form of presenile dementia that came to be known as Alzheimer disease (AD). This short story of a serendipitous observation has a prehistory that may clarify why a single brief case study on a degenerative form of dementia made history, while whole monographs written at the same time about closely related topics are almost forgotten (Leri 1906; Pick 1898).

Research on progressive paralysis had led to a number of important discoveries during the previous decade. A. Pick (1892, 1898, 1901, 1906) observed a number of presenile and senile patients with focally accentuated neocortical atrophy and associated neuropsychological deficits. O. Binswanger (1894) and A. Alzheimer (1895, 1898, 1902, 1904) had described a variety of vascular brain changes associated with severe cognitive impairment that could be distinguished clinically and neuropathologically from progressive paralysis. The clinicopathologic paradigm led to the delineation of several new diseases. The exploration of progressive paralysis itself led beyond the realms of clinical and pathological description, etiology, and therapy. The combination of more specific diagnostic methods and therapeutic success led to a steep decrease in the number of patients with progressive paralysis. During the same period old diseases were on their way up, and new diseases were born.

Senile dementia (*Altersblödsinn*) was considered the most common mental disorder and gained increased attention (Alzheimer 1898). E. Redlich (1898) found extraneuronal plaques (miliary sclerosis) in patients with dementia. Blocq and Marinesco (1892) had observed similar plaques in patients with temporal lobe epilepsy. Beljahov (1889) had even seen plaques in senile dementia. Cortical atrophy and ventricular enlargement in senile dementia had been known for some time (Kraepelin 1899; Marce 1863).

In the sixth edition of his textbook of Psychiatry, E. Kraepelin (1899) listed macroscopic brain atrophy, neuronal atrophy, and pigmentation as the typical postmortem findings in senile dementia, referring to Campbell's study published in the *Journal of Mental Science* (1894, 638). Kraepelin mentioned that senile dementia usually begins between the ages of 65 and 75, "sometimes earlier (senium praecox)" (1899, 356). This senium praecox is nosologically unrelated to Dementia praecox and Dementia paralytica, which were considered in separate chapters.

In the famous eighth edition of his textbook (1910), Kraepelin singles out a peculiar (*eigentümlich*) group of cases with severe neuronal changes. Clinically, these are characterized by "immensely severe mental disease with fuzzy (*verwaschene*) signs of an organic brain disease" (624). Kraepelin gives a vivid account of characteristic psychopathological and neurological findings and goes on to elaborate clinicopathologic correlations and differential diagnostic issues. Alzheimer disease (*Alzheimersche Krankheit*; p. 627) was characterized by severe dementia, profound aphasia, spasticity, and seizures; whereas presbyophrenia represented a simple deterioration of mental capacity (*geistiger Besitzstand*) without further physical and psychopathological disturbances. Of 183 patients who were between the ages of 65 and 80 and who had senile dementia, 23 percent were diagnosed as having presbyophrenia, 63 percent as having simple senile dementia (*einfacher Altersblödsinn*), 8 percent as having severe arteriosclerotic forms, and the rest as having senile paranoia (*seniler Verfolgungswahn*; p. 629). Kraepelin hypothesized that a neuronal degeneration with a deposition of pathological material was the anatomical correlate of presbyophrenia. On the other extreme, focal vascular change would lead to a mosaic of individual disturbances in the arteriosclerotic group of senile dementia. Kraepelin discussed the difficulties of drawing clear lines between (1) arteriosclerotic and primary degenerative forms of senile dementia, clinically and neuropathologically; (2) senile dementia — particularly presbyophrenia — and normal aging; and (3) presenile AD and senile dementia.

Kraepelin concluded: "At present the clinical importance of Alzheimer's disease is still unclear. While the anatomical findings would suggest that it represents a particularly severe form of senile dementia, the fact that it may start in the 40s argues against that view. One would have to assume at least a senium praecox, if it was not perhaps a more or less age-independent disease process of its own" (1910, 627). The main arguments for a separate histological position of AD were (1) onset, (2) severity and type of clinical symptoms, and (3) severity of neuropathological change. Kraepelin was too shrewd and Alzheimer too ponderous to take a clear position. So why did this incidental finding and the concept of AD take off?

Five years after Alzheimer's case report, the following had been achieved:

— The presenile, severe form of nonarteriosclerotic dementia had received a name — Alzheimer disease.

— A number of similar cases of presenile dementia with plaques and tangles had been reported by Bonfiglio, Perusini, Sarteschi, Schnitzler, Bielschowsky (1911), Fuller (1907, 1912), Alzheimer himself (1911), and several others.

— Kraepelin and Alzheimer had formed the world's strongest and most renowned international neuroscience research group of that time, and its members had direct access to scientific publishing media in several languages.

— The clinicopathologic paradigm had the greatest scientific appeal when it came to defining diseases. Neuropsychiatry was desperate to catch up with other medical specialties that had already stormed ahead in the days of Morgagni and Virchow. Not many examples lent themselves to this purpose as well as Alzheimer's.

— A number of neuropsychiatric disturbances became treatable once their pathogenetic mechanism, or even etiologies, became more transparent, and were quickly captured by other specialties. This was not true of presenile and senile dementia.

— Alzheimer's case fell into place during an academic discussion among Kraepelin, the towering figure of classificatory optimism, and Hoche and Bonhoeffer, the most prominent exponents of the skeptics. As the scientific community was waiting for the cases to substantiate Kraepelin's classificatory boxes, little further advertising was necessary. Kraepelin could afford a relaxed and considerate attitude. The public knew what to do with cases as appealing as Alzheimer's.

Over the next half-century, the clinical story about AD as a presenile degenerative dementia was retold again and again, but it offered few insights about cognitive impairment (Eiden and Lechner 1950; Hilpert 1926; Leuchtenberg 1942); language and speech disturbances (Schottky 1932; Grünthal 1936); paranoid symptoms and hallucinations (Albert 1964; Fünfgeld 1933); epileptic seizures (Eiden and Lechner 1950; Grünthal 1927, 1932, 1936); and other clinical features of AD. The FIAT report (1947), inaugurated by the allied forces after World War II, listed little of value that had been produced during the Third Reich. The psychiatry section (edited by E. Kretschmer) cites Bostroem's Handbook article on senile and presenile dementia (1939), Stucke's paper on the diagnostic contribution of EEG (1943), Grosch's psychopathological and anatomical case studies (1944), and a tutorial film by Pittrich (Ederle 1947). No original research work on AD is quoted in the neurology section (Hassler et al. 1947).

After Kraepelin's initial description (1910), AD rapidly became a household term that made its way through the small-print paragraphs of textbooks into the canon of neuropsychiatric handbook knowledge. E. Bleuler accepted some of Kraepelin's views and wrote in the first edition of his psychiatry textbook: "Alzheimer's disease, which today cannot be distinguished from Fischer's presbyophrenia, is a dementia with early onset and a clinical picture of a presbyophrenia with confusion, leading to a particularly severe dementia with aphasia, agnostic and apractic symptoms, and death. It may occasionally begin in the forties. The anatomical findings are qualitatively similar to presbyophrenia, but they are quite severe — a general brain degeneration with fibrillary destruction and numerous plaques" (1916, 267).

From then on, AD regularly appeared in most neuropsychiatry textbooks. W. Weygandt (1920, 227) separates AD, with its peculiar histopathological findings, from senile dementia, presbyophrenia, senile paranoia, brain arteriosclerosis, and postapoplectic dementia. O. Bumke (1924, 794) considers AD "an atypical form of senile brain atrophy . . . a severe dementia with comparably early onset (in the fifth or sixth decade) with unspecific prodromal symptoms (vertigo, headache, forgetfulness, fatigue, irritability), rapid progression accompanied by asymbolic, aphasic, apractic, and spastic phenomena."

The common denominator in textbook descriptions of AD is its early onset together with its clinical and neuropathological severity.

Most authors had queries about the relationship to senile dementia/ presbyophrenia, and these difficulties were discussed extensively in the *Neurology and Psychiatry Handbook* articles by Lewandowsky (1912), Spielmeyer (1912), Runge (1930), and Grünthal (1930, 1936). Even though the AD label became very popular within a short period of time, the scientific validity of the concept was still at stake.

The macroscopic appearance of the brain in senile dementia had been described fifty years before Alzheimer's eponymous patient died (Marce 1863). Plaques (Beljahov 1889; Redlich 1898) and even neuro-fibrillary tangles (Bianchi 1906; Fuller 1907) were about to be recognized as substrates of senile dementia, or rather of presbyophrenia. Kahlbaum (1863) had introduced, and Wernicke (1906) revived, the presbyophrenia concept for an amnestic syndrome with confabulation, hyperactivity, euphoria, intact social skills, and personality. O. Fischer (1907) suggested that plaque-like necroses (*drusige Nekrosen*) were the anatomical basis of presbyophrenic dementia and called this disease entity "sphaerotrichia multiplex cerebri," a complicated term that did not gain much publicity. Further histological features of senile and pre-senile dementia were discovered in due course. T. Simchowicz (1914) described the granulovacuolar degeneration in hippocampal pyramidal cells. Divry (1927) identified amyloid in the plaque cores. W. Scholz (1938) saw a plaque-like degeneration of cerebral arteries and capil-laries. This completed the array of light-microscopic findings in senile dementia and AD.

A number of histological features that were diagnostic of other degenerative brain diseases, some of them with presenile onset and dementia, were discovered during the same period—some of them by the same group of people. Alzheimer (1911) found the globoid argento-philic neuronal inclusion bodies in focal neocortical atrophy—the so-called Pick-bodies of so-called Pick disease. Lewy (1912, 1925) detected globoid eosinophilic inclusion bodies in the basal nucleus of Meynert in patients with paralysis agitans—the so-called Lewy bodies of Parkinson and so-called Lewy-body disease.

Creutzfeldt (1920) and Jakob (1921) observed patients with a prese-nile spongiform encephalopathy or spastic pseudosclerosis. Creutzfeldt-Jakob disease and Lewy-body dementia led a quiet life before scientific interest was rekindled fifty years later.

Pick disease caught the headlines with as much success as AD. Sev-eral papers compared both forms of presenile dementia, which could be distinguished both clinically and neuropathologically. Again, the scien-tific community was prepared by J. Cotard's early volume on partial brain atrophy (1868) and by Pick's series of papers (1892, 1901, 1906) and his monograph (1898) on the clinical findings in patients with focal brain lesions. Similar to AD, a number of anecdotal reports followed Alzheimer's description of the histopathological hallmark (Pick's bodies) and the concept gained scientific credibility (e.g., Mingazzini 1913). Gans (1922) suggested the eponym "Pick's atrophy." Onari and Spatz (1926) called it "Pick's disease." Carl Schneider (1927) described its three stages: (1) impaired judgement and behavior; (2) focal symptoms and signs; and (3) severe dementia. Van Bagh (1946) distinguished frontal from temporal lobe atrophy and also described their combinations. This partnership between AD and Pick disease was of mutual benefit because it strengthened both concepts. If there is a differential dissociation between the clinical and focal brain change on one side, and of the histologic hallmarks on the other side, a clinical differential diagnosis with predictive value makes sense, and it is practically useful to accept the existence of these diseases. This split therefore strengthened the case of AD.

The enemy came from within. Alzheimer himself never claimed that AD was a disease in its own right and was well aware of the similarities to senile dementia (1911). A number of quantitative studies on clinicopathologic correlation moved AD dangerously close to senile dementia, which could have led to the extinction of AD — the younger brother swallowed by the much more prevalent senile form of plaque and tangle dementia.

Fischer (1910) reported that significant numbers of plaques and tangles could only be found in the 16 cases of senile dementia he had examined; he did not find them in high numbers in 10 patients with nonorganic psychoses, 45 with progressive paralysis, and 10 normal elderly controls. A closer look by T. Simchowicz (1911, 1914) revealed that there were plaques in the brains of elderly people and that a cut-off could be defined between nondemented elderly who had counts of less then 10 plaques per visual field (1.77 qmm) and demented people who had a count above this threshold. Simchowicz (1911) also tried to establish a "senile index," which was positive in patients with senile dementia because of higher frontal and lower postcentral plaque densities, and negative in presenile dementia because of lower frontal and higher postcentral counts. Simchowicz stated that this plaque count increased with older age and suggested the term "senile plaque." He began to study the relationship between plaque counts in different cortical areas and their associated clinical findings (1914, 1924).

Grünthal (1927) carried out a thorough quantitative clinicoanatomical study and established: (1) the association between focal neuropsychological deficits and focal plaques, tangles, or other pathology; and (2) the correlation between the severity of clinical deficits and the density and extension of plaques and neurofibrillary tangles within a group of patients with senile dementia. The quantitative correlation between clinical deficits and the underlying pathology within a diagnostic group is a powerful argument for a spectrum of clinical and anatomical findings between pathology and normalcy. It does not support a simplistic categorical distinction between separate clinicopathologic disease entities, which would have to be based on qualitative rather than quantitative markers. What other scientists surmised (Simchowicz 1911, 1914, 1924; Spielmeyer 1912) was strengthened by Grünthal's results, and this spectrum view of presenile and senile dementia eventually became the predominant position (Albert 1964; Bronisch 1951).

Because senile dementia was an illogical choice of words, another label was needed. "Alzheimer disease" may not sound like a real winner, but "sphaerotrichis multiplex cerebri" was even less likely. And there was another reason to choose AD: it had to be made clear that this was a true and obvious disease and not just a normal aging process. This fact was much easier to demonstrate using the more severe form of degenerative dementia with early onset.

N. Gellerstedt (1933) studied the brains of fifty elderly individuals with no reported dementia. Using Von Braunmühl's sensitive silver impregnation technique, he found plaques in 84 percent and felt that their density was not closely related to a patient's mental condition. The localization of neurofibrillary tangles appeared to be of greater importance. While they represented a common finding in the allocortex of Gellerstedt's nondemented elderly, they were abundant and spread out all over the isocortex in senile dementia. The implication of Gellerstedt's work was that the differences between senile dementia and normal aging were only gradual. The overstated or simplified reading of his paper was that the presence neither of plaques nor of tangles was of clinical significance in the elderly. It took some time before a (semi)-quantitative correlation between the density of pathological change and the severity of cognitive impairment was reestablished (Blessed et al. 1968; Roth et al. 1966).

Thus, it probably was a clever political decision to extend the concept of AD from the presenile into the senile area instead of surrendering to senile dementia and ending up with no disease at all, but with a senile or presenile aging process that would have been outside the realm of medicine.

References

Albert, E. 1964. Senile Demenz und Alzheimersche Krankheit als Ausdruck des gleichen Krankheitsgeschehens. *Fortschr Neurol Psychiat* 32:625–72.

Alzheimer, A. 1895. Die arteriosklerotische Atrophie des Gehirns. *Allg Z Psychiat* 51:809–11.

———. 1898. Neuere Arbeiten über die Dementia senilis und die auf atheromatöser Gefässerkrankung basierenden Gehirnkrankheiten. *Monatsschr Psychiat Neurol* 3:101–15.

———. 1902. Die Seelenstörungen auf arteriosklerotischer Grundlage. *Allg Zeitschr Psychiat* 59:695–710.

———. 1904. *Histologische Studien zur Differentialdiagnose der progressiven Paralyse*. Habilitationsschrift. München: Ludwig Maximilians Universität.

———. 1906. Über einen eigenartigen schweren Krankheitsprozeß der Hirnrinde. *Neurol Centralbl* 25:1134.

———. 1907. Über eine eigenartige Erkrankung der Hirnrinde. *Allg Zeitschr Psychiat Psych Gerichtl Med* 64:146–48.

———. 1911. Über eigenartige Krankheitsfälle des späteren Alters. *Zeitschr Ges Neurol Psychiat* 4:356–85.

Beljahov. 1889. Pathological changes in the brain in dementia senilis. *J Ment Sci* 35:261–62.

Berrios, G. E. 1990. Alzheimer's disease: A conceptual history. *Internat J Geriat Psychiat* 5:355–65.

Bianchi, L. 1906. *A Textbook of Psychiatry*. London: Balliere & Tyndall. 846.

Bielschowsky, M. 1903. Die Silberimprägnation der Achsenzylinder. *Neurol Centralbl* 21:997.

———. 1911. Zur Kenntnis der Alzheimerschen Krankheit (praesenilen Demenz mit Herdsymptomen). *J Psychol Neurol* 18 (Suppl. 1): 273–92.

Binswanger, O. 1894. Die Abgrenzung der progressiven Paralyse, I–III. *Berl Klin Wochenschr* 49:1103–5, 1137–39, 1180–86.

Blessed, G., B. E. Tomlinson, and M. Roth. 1968. The association between quantitative measures of dementia and of senile change in the cerebral grey matter of elderly subjects. *Brit J Psychiat* 114:797–811.

Bleuler, E. 1916. *Lehrbuch der Psychiatrie*. Berlin: Springer. 250–71.

Blocq, P., and G. Marinesco. 1892. Sur les lesions et la pathogenie de l'epilepsie dite essentielle. *La Semaine Medicale* 12:445–46.

Bonhoeffer, K. 1912. Die Psychosen im Gefolge von akuten Infektionen, Allgemeinerkrankungen und inneren Erkrankungen. In *Handbuch der Psychiatrie*, ed. G. Aschaffenburg, Vol. B, Part 3: 2–120. Leipzig and Wien: Deuticke.

Bronisch, F. W. 1951. *Hirnatrophische Prozesse im mittleren Lebensalter und ihre psychischen Erscheinungsbilder*. Stuttgart: Thieme.

Bumke, O. 1924. *Lehrbuch der Geisteskrankheiten,* 2d ed. Muenchen: Bergmann. 783–805.

Cotard, J. 1868. *L'atrophie partielle du cerveau.* Paris: LeFrancois.

Creutzfeldt, H. G. 1920. Ueber eine eigenartige herdfoermige Erkrankung des Zentralnervensystems. *Zeitschr Ges Neurol Psychiat* 57:1–18.

Divry, P. 1927. Etude histo-chimique des plaques seniles. *J Neurol* 9.

Ederle, W. 1947. Symptomatische Psychosen. In *FIAT Report Psychiatrie,* ed. E. Kretschmer, 18–21.

Eiden, H. F., and H. Lechner. 1950. Ueber psychotische Zustandsbilder bei der Pickschen und Alzheimerschen Krankheit. *Arch Psychiat Nervenkr* 184:393–412.

Fischer, O. 1907. Miliare Nekrosen mit drusigen Wucherungen der Neurofibrillen, eine regeläßige Veränderung der Hirnrinde bei seniler Demenz. *Monatsschr Psychiat Neurol* 24:361–72.

———. 1910. Miliare Nekrosen mit drusigen Wucherungen der Neurofibrillen, eine regelmäßige Veränderung der Hirnrinde bei seniler Demenz. *Mschr Neurol Psychiat* 22:361–72.

———. 1910. Die presbyophrene Demenz, deren anatomische Grundlage und klinische Abgrenzung. *Zeitschr Ges Neurol Psychiat* 3:372–471.

Fluegel, F. E. 1929. Zur Diagnostik der Alzheimerschen Krankheit. *Zeitschr Ges Neurol Psychiat* 120:783–87.

Fünfgeld, E. 1933. Ueber atypische Symptomenkomplexe bei senilen Hirnkrankheiten und ihre Bedeutung für das Schizophrenieproblem. *Monatsschr Psychiat* 211–21.

Fuller, S. C. 1907. A study of the neurofibrils in dementia paralytica, dementia senilis, chronic alcoholism, cerebral lues, and microcephalic idiocy. *Am J Insanity* 63:415–68.

———. 1912. Alzheimer's disease (senium praecox): The report of a case and review of published cases. *J Nerv Ment Dis* 39:440–55, 536–57.

Gans, A. 1922. Betrachtungen über Art und Ausbreitung des krankhaften Prozesses in einem Fall von Pickscher Atrophie des Stirnhirns. *Z Ges Neurol Psychiat* 80:10–28.

Gellerstedt, N. 1933. Zur Kenntnis der Hirnveränderungen bei der normalen Altersinvolution. *Upsala Läkareförenings Förhandlingar* 38:193–408.

Grünthal, E. 1927. Klinisch-anatomisch vergleichende Untersuchungen über den Greisenblödsinn. *Zeitschr Ges Neurol Psychiat* 111:763–818.

———. 1930. Die pathologische Anatomie der senilen Demenz und der Alzheimerschen Krankheit. In *Handbuch der Geisteskrankheiten,* ed. O. Bumke, 11:634–72. Berlin: Springer.

———. 1936. Die präsenilen und senilen Erkrankungen des Gehirns und des

Rückenmarks. In *Handbuch der Neurologie*, ed. O. Bumke and O. Foerster, 11:466–509. Berlin: Springer.

Hassler R., J. Hallervorden, H. Spatz, F. Toebel. 1947. Grosshirnatrophien. In *FIAT Report Neurologie*, ed. G. Schaltenbrand, 2–3.

Hilpert, P. 1926. Zur Klinik und Histopathologie der Alzheimerschen Krankheit. *Arch Psychiat Nervenkr* 76:379–93.

Jakob, A. 1921. Ueber eigenartige Erkrankungen des Zentralnervensystems mit bemerkenswertem anatomischen Befunde(spastische Pseudosklerose-Encephalomyelopathie mit disseminierten Degenerationsherden). *Dtsch Z Nervenheilk* 70:132.

Kahlbaum, K. L. 1863. *Die Gruppirung der psychischen Krankheiten und die Eintheilung der Seelenstoerungen.* Danzig: Kafemann.

Kraepelin, E. 1899. *Psychiatrie: Ein Lehrbuch für Studierende und Ärzte. 6.* Leipzig: Auflage, Barth. 2:348–58.

———. 1910. *Psychiatrie: Ein Lehrbuch für Studierende und Ärzte. 8.* Leipzig: Auflage, Barth. 2:624–32.

Leri, A. 1906. *Le cerveau senile.* Lille: Le Bigot Freres.

Leuchtenberg, P. 1942. Ein klinischer Fall von Alzheimerscher Krankheit mit "akzentuierter" Atrophie der parieto-occipital Region. *Allg Z Psychiat* 121: 97–123.

Lewandowsky, M. 1912. Arteriosklerose und senile Atrophie des Gehirns. In *Handbuch der Neurologie*, ed. M. Lewandowsky, 3:153–54. Berlin: Springer.

Lewy, F. H. 1912. Paralysis agitans. I. Pathologische Anatomie. In *Handbuch der Neurologie*, ed. M. Lewandowsky, 3:920–33. Berlin: Springer.

———. 1923. *Die Lehre vom Tonus und der Bewegung. Zugleich systematische Untersuchung zur Klinik, Physiologie, Pathologie und Pathogenese der Paralysis agitans.* Berlin: Springer.

———. 1925. Primaer und sekundaer involutive Veraenderungen des Gehirns. *Krankheitsforschung* 1 (cited according to Gellerstedt 1933).

Marce, L. V. 1863. Recherches cliniques et anatomo-pathologiques sur la demence senile et sur les differences qui la separent de la paralysie generale. *Gazette Medicale de Paris* 34:433–35, 467–69, 497–502, 631–32, 761–64, 797–98, 831–33, 855–58.

Mingazzini, G. 1913. On aphasia due to atrophy of the cerebral convolutions. *Brain* 36:493–524.

Onari, K., and H. Spatz. 1926. Anatomische Beitraege zur Lehre von der Pickschen umschriebenen Grosshirnrindenatrophie (Picksche Krankheit). *Zeitschr Ges Neurol Psychiat* 101:470–511.

Pick, A. 1892. Ueber die Beziehungen der senilen Hirnatrophie zur Aphasie. *Prag Med Wochenschr* 17:16–167.

——. 1898. *Beiträge zur Pathologie und pathologischen Anatomie des Centralner-
vensystems mit Bemerkungen zur normalen Anatomie desselben.* Berlin: Karger.

——. 1901. Senile Hirnatrophie als Grundlage von Herderscheinungen. *Wien
Klin Wochenschr* 14:403–4.

——. 1906. Über einen Symptomenkomplex im Rahmen der Dementia senilis, bedingt durch stärkere umschriebene Hirnatrophie (gemischte Ap-
raxie). *Monatsschr Psychiat Neurol* 19:97–108.

Redlich, E. 1898. Über miliare Sklerosen der Hirnrinde bei seniler Atrophie.
Jahrb Psychiat Neurol 17:208–16.

Roth, M., B. E. Tomlinson, and G. Blessed. 1966. Correlation between scores
for dementia and counts of 'senile plaques' in cerebral grey matter of elderly
subjects. *Nature* 109–10.

Runge, W. 1930. Die Geistesstoerungen des Greisenalters. I. Die physiolo-
gischen Erscheinungen des Greisenalters. In *Handbuch der Geisteskrankheiten,*
ed. O. Bumke, 8/4:597–666. Berlin: Springer.

Schneider, C. 1927. Über Picksche Krankheit. *Monatsschr Psychiat Neurol* 15:
230–75.

Scholz, W. 1938. Studien zur Pathologie der Hirngefaesse II. Die drusige En-
tartung der Hirnarterien und -capillaren. *Z Ges Neurol Psychiat* 162:694–715.

Schottky, J. 1932. Über präsenile Verblödungen. *Z Ges Neurol Psychiat* 140:333–
97.

Simchowicz, T. 1911. Histopathologische Studien über die senile Demenz.
Nissl-Alzheimers Histol Histopath Arbeiten über die Hirnrinde 4:267–444.

——. 1914. La maladie d'Alzheimer et son rapport avec la demence senile.
Encephale 9:218–31.

——. 1924. Sur la signification des plaques seniles et sur la formule senile de
l'ecorce cerebrale. *Rev Neurol* 31:221–27.

Spielmeyer, W. 1912. Die Psychosen des Rückbildungs-und Greisenalters. In
Handbuch der Psychiatrie, Vol. B/ Part 5, ed. G. Aschaffenburg. Leipzig and
Wien: Deuticke. 85–157.

Van Bagh. 1946. Klinische und anatomische Studien an 30 Fällen von um-
schriebener Atrophie der Großhirnrinde (Picksche Krankheit). *Ann Acad Sci
fennica* 16:1.

Wernicke, C. 1906. *Grundriß der Psychiatrie in klinischen Vorlesungen,* 2d ed.
Leipzig: Thieme.

Weygandt, W. 1920. *Erkennung der Geistesstörungen (Psychiatrische Diagnostik).*
München: Lehmanns. 228.

5

Beyond the Characteristic Plaques and Tangles

Mid-Twentieth Century U.S. Psychiatry and the Fight Against Senility

Jesse F. Ballenger

The conceptual history of Alzheimer disease (AD) is usually discussed within an implicit three-part chronology. There is the classical period, in which the clinical and histopathologic acumen of Alzheimer and Perusini brought the disease into scientific focus (and in which Kraepelin made the inscrutable decision to distinguish between presenile and senile dementia, confounding research for generations). There is the modern period, beginning in the 1970s and continuing to the present, in which technological and conceptual breakthroughs and the pressure of an aging population created explosive interest and progress. Between these two brightly illumined periods lies a stretch of decades in which it is assumed that little scientific interest was taken in the disease and still less progress made — a veritable dark age in the conceptual history of AD.

Of course, this age did not seem nearly so dark at the time. In fact, from the mid-1930s through the 1950s, there was a dramatic surge of interest in senile dementia and AD among U.S. psychiatrists. In the ten years from 1926 to 1935, nine articles concerning senile dementia and/or AD were published in the *American Journal of Psychiatry* and the *Archives of Neurology and Psychiatry*, the two leading professional journals; and in the following decade, thirty-six articles appeared. Though this heightened interest in the dementias of old age was small compared to what would follow in the 1980s, many observers at the time optimistically regarded the 1930s to 1950s as a period of great progress.

More interestingly, although the period brought no new insights into the biological and genetic bases of brain pathology that has been the focus of research since the late 1970s, U.S. psychiatrists in this period forged a distinctly new approach to senile dementia that emphasized psychosocial factors over neuropathology in the etiology of dementia. Dementia was more than the simple and inevitable outcome of a brain that was deteriorating with the processes of aging and/or disease. Dementia was a dialectical process between the brain and the social context in which the aging person was situated. Factors such as premorbid personality structure, emotional trauma, disruptions of family support, and social isolation were regarded as at least as important in explaining dementia as the biological processes that produced plaques and tangles. Similarly, memory loss and other cognitive deficits were, relative to today, less interesting than the emotional and behavioral disturbances that accompany dementia. In short, AD and senile dementia were regarded by most psychiatrists of this period, not as cognitive disorders produced by biological processes within the brain, but as mental illnesses produced by psychodynamic processes occurring between the aging individual and society. So conceived, dementia was not a well-bounded disease entity. It could not be easily differentiated from the entire experience of aging. Psychiatry's way of thinking about senile dementia was deeply connected to the larger project of the emerging field of gerontology—salvaging old age in modern society. Fighting "senility" was the central goal of the first generation of professional gerontologists.

This chapter describes the psychodynamic model of senile dementia constructed by psychiatrists in the United States. By exploring its connections to gerontology, I argue that mid-century U.S. psychiatry's interest in senile dementia should be understood as a crucial part of the broad cultural transformation of old age, without which AD could not have emerged as a major public issue in the 1970s. Thus, this "dark age" in the conceptual history of AD had important connections and continuities with the "renaissance" that would follow.

PSYCHIATRY, THE AGED PATIENT, AND THE CRISIS OF THE STATE MENTAL HOSPITALS

The surge in interest in senile dementia can only be understood in the context of American psychiatry's ambiguous attitude toward aged patients, who were becoming a disproportionately large part of the patient population of the state mental hospitals throughout the first half of the twentieth century. Because psychiatry regarded the aged insane as incurable, their presence in large numbers undermined the therapeutic environment that the state hospitals were supposed to provide. Because the overall population was aging, the problem was regarded by many as an impending crisis—a demographic avalanche that would bury the state hospital as a viable institution and the professional authority of psychiatry along with it.

The problem of aged patients in the state mental hospitals began around the turn of the century with changes in state public policy. Historians Carole Haber and Gerald Grob have shown that through most of the nineteenth century, psychiatrists were able to keep aged patients out of the mental hospitals by arguing that senility did not really constitute insanity; therefore, the senile could be cared for best in the homes of their families, almshouses, or private old age homes. Because almshouse care was the cheapest way of caring for aged patients who had to be institutionalized, local welfare officials also sought to keep the aged out of mental hospitals (Haber 1983, 88–91; Grob 1986).

At the end of the nineteenth century, this situation changed. Both the absolute and proportional number of aged patients admitted to the state hospitals increased dramatically—a trend that continued through the early 1960s (Grob 1983, 182–84, 317). This did not mean that most or even many psychiatrists had concluded that senile dementia should be regarded as a form of insanity suitable for treatment in mental hospitals. Rather, as Grob persuasively argues, the influx of aged patients into the mental hospitals was accounted for by two public policy developments: the decline of the almshouse as a viable public institution, and the decision by states to assume responsibility for all mentally ill persons. As individual states enacted legislation that shifted financial responsibility for the insane to the state governments, local welfare officials reclassified their aged almshouse inmates as insane. Moreover, the care received in mental hospitals was widely perceived as superior to almshouse care, and the social stigma attached to insanity may have been less than that of pauperism, thus making confinement of aged relatives in a mental hospital the preferred choice of most families.

The result of all this was that responsibility for the care of the demented elderly was increasingly thrust upon psychiatry. Though comprehensive and reliable national data are impossible to reconstruct, Grob cited data from Massachusetts and New York that illustrate the magnitude of the change. In 1855, the rate of first admission for male patients over age 60 to Massachusetts mental hospitals was 70.4 per 100,000, and the rate for female patients over age 60 was 60.5 per 100,000; in 1939–41, the rates were 279.5 and 223 per 100,000. In 1919–21, 9.2 percent of first admissions to state hospitals in New York were aged 70 and over; in 1949–51, 26.2 percent were 70 and over. The percentage of the population in New York over age 65 was 4.7 in 1920 and 8.6 percent in 1950 (Grob 1983, 182).

From the 1930s through the 1950s, the professional literature of U.S. psychiatry was filled with dire pronouncements about the burden that aged patients pressed onto psychiatry and the impending crisis of the state hospitals. "Our institutions promise to become in time vast infirmaries with relatively small departments for younger patients with curable disorders," Richard Hutchings cautioned in his 1939 address as president of the American Psychiatric Association (Hutchings 1939, 1). Following up on Hutchings' remarks, the authors of a 1942 study of the senile and arteriosclerotic psychoses noted that the number of persons aged 65 years and over in the U.S. population increased by 35 percent from 1930 to 1940, with a corresponding increase in admissions to mental hospitals. (As shown by Grob, the increase was actually far more than corresponding.) "So pressing is the problem," the authors argued, "that the character of mental hospitals is in danger of again reverting to a functional level of custodial care" (Williams et al. 1942, 712). The prominence of the problem in psychiatry during this period was summed up by former APA president Abraham Myerson in 1944, when he argued that progress in longevity brought with it the "distressing fact that more people . . . outlive their brains." Psychiatry would "have to face this fact, since the real increase in mental diseases comes by the roads of senile dementia with its plaques, and cerebral arteriosclerotic dementia with its more direct cardio-vascular changes" (Myerson 1944, 162).

Psychiatry reacted to this situation in two ways. On the one hand, as the overcrowded state mental hospitals became a public scandal, some psychiatrists redoubled efforts to create alternative policy solutions to the problem of caring for aged patients (Kolb 1956). This was accomplished in the 1960s when the federal government, through provisions in Medicare and Medicaid, assumed responsibility for funding nursing-home care for elderly patients. As a result, many thousands of elderly demented patients were transferred out of the mental hospitals and into nursing homes and various community care arrangements (Grob 1991). On the other hand, as the next two sections of this chapter will discuss, other psychiatrists redoubled efforts to deal with senile dementia within the state hospitals by conceptualizing it as a treatable mental illness.

DAVID ROTHSCHILD AND THE PSYCHODYNAMIC MODEL OF SENILE DEMENTIA

The researchers who devoted increased attention to senile dementia during this period continued to struggle with a number of vexing issues.[1] One concerned the role of arteriosclerosis in senile dementia. Although many researchers made a careful distinction between senile (Alzheimer-type) dementia and cerebral-arteriosclerotic psychoses, the traditional view that arteriosclerotic processes were somehow causative in all cases of dementia in old age continued to appear in the literature. Thus, the diagnosis of arteriosclerosis seems to have been greatly over-used through the 1960s (Beach 1987; Dillmann 1990, 161–63; Haber 1986; Katzman this volume).

Another issue concerned whether to consider senile dementia a physiological or pathological process (i.e., a product of aging or of disease). Tradition favored viewing dementia as an inevitable concomitant of aging, though some disagreed. The issue remains contested (Beach 1987; Haber 1986; Huppert, Brayne, and O'Connor 1994).

Closely related to the issue of aging versus disease was whether AD and senile dementia ought to be categorized as different entities as they had been since Kraepelin created the eponym in 1910 in the eighth edition of his influential textbook. Although AD presented both clinical and pathological signs that were virtually identical to senile dementia, it occurred in persons whose age logically precluded senile changes in the brain. The distinction persisted because it seemed illogical to regard dementia in a person in his or her late forties or early fifties as caused by the normal processes of aging. As research pointing to the clinical and pathological similarities of the two conditions piled up, however, researchers were hard-pressed to maintain the distinction. Proof that the logic of age categories remained compelling is seen in a 1941 article by William McMenemy and Eugene Pollack in which they argued that the distinction between senile and Alzheimer *pre*senile dementia should not be made on the basis of pathology, but on whether "the mental illness commenced at an age when the patient still retained normal vitality, the decline in which is usually evident somewhere between the ages of 60 and 70" (McMenemy and Pollack 1941, 689–90).

A decade earlier, William Malamud and Konstantin Lowenburg (1929) had argued that their own findings and the preponderance of evidence in the literature suggested that AD was not limited to the presenium, although they nonetheless thought that the distinction should be maintained on pragmatic grounds. Since little was actually known about senility, saying that AD was a form of senile dementia would not add anything to the understanding of AD but would blur the meaning of senility by linking it to conditions occurring in earlier ages. In 1936 David Rothschild and Jerome Kasanin argued that practical considerations dictated the opposite: since the pathological pictures were so similar, advances in understanding AD would have the practical benefit of shedding light on the larger problem of senile dementia. "It is evident," they concluded, "that in a broad discussion of Alzheimer's disease one must include also the problems of senility in its normal and pathologic aspects" (Rothschild and Kasanin 1936, 293–94). Although the distinction between AD and senile dementia persisted in official nosology until the mid-1970s, by 1940 it had little meaning. Most researchers of this period acknowledged that AD and senile dementia were, for all practical purposes, the same entity but found no compelling reason to abandon the traditional distinction.[2]

By the mid-1930s, research into senile dementia and AD had established two additional anomalies, both concerning the relationship of pathology to dementia. First, the senile plaques and neurofibrillary tangles that were found in the brains of patients suffering from dementia were also found in the brains of patients suffering from a number of conditions having nothing to do with senility. Second, senile plaques and neurofibrillary tangles had been found at autopsy in the brains of older people who had shown no signs of dementia in life. In grappling with these findings, Massachusetts psychiatrist David Rothschild was ultimately moved to look beyond the deterioration of brain tissue to explain dementia.

In papers published in 1931 and 1936, Rothschild and his colleagues argued that since the pathological structures characteristic of AD and senile dementia had been found in a variety of other conditions, such as spastic paralysis, hyperthyroidism, and multiple sclerosis, these structures were not an expression of any one disease process. Instead, they were an indication of a special type of tissue reaction that might occur in response to a variety of biological factors (Lowenburg and Rothschild

1931; Rothschild and Kasanin 1936). Some researchers pursued this idea, while others sought a single cause for the tissue changes.[3] Rothschild and his colleagues, however, began to explore the relationship between biology and personality.

In their 1936 paper, Rothschild and Kasanin explained the severity of emotional and personality disturbances in AD, which were typically more pronounced than those found in senile dementia, as the attempts of a relatively strong organism to compensate for the oncoming disease. The more dramatic clinical appearance of AD could be understood as "an attempt at rejuvenescence in the face of an abnormal aging process" (1936, 320).[4] When this idea was considered in light of research demonstrating that the brains of some aged persons who had died with normal mentality contained the same pathological structures as those suffering from dementia, the possibility of a strikingly new conception of senile dementia was apparent.

In a flurry of articles published in the major psychiatric journals between 1937 and 1952, Rothschild reported that his own clinical and histological investigations verified a discrepancy, first noted by the German researcher Gellerstedt (1932), between the presence and degree of dementia in the living patient, and the presence and degree of pathological structures found in autopsy. In accounting for this discrepancy, Rothschild rejected an available biological explanation endorsed by another German, A. von Braunmühl (1932), who argued that the pathological structures of senile dementia were actually secondary phenomena of other, undetectable senile changes. It was thus possible to say that "the brain of a senile patient is more severely damaged than that of a patient of normal mentality, even though the demonstrable alterations may be the same in both cases." The problem with von Braunmühl's explanation was that it could be reversed with equal justification: if the real senile changes could not be detected, then it could be argued that the brain of a person of normal mentality was more profoundly damaged than the brain of a severely demented person. Von Braunmühl's theory, Rothschild argued, "is effective only if it is applied in one direction, a direction determined by preconceived ideas as to what tissue damage should be. Therefore, it cannot be accepted as a satisfactory explanation of the[se] troublesome discrepancies" (Rothschild 1937, 777).

Finding a satisfactory explanation moved Rothschild away from what he saw as biological reductionism. "Too exclusive preoccupation with the cerebral pathology," he argued, had "led to a tendency to forget that the changes are occurring in living, mentally functioning persons who may react to a given situation, including an organic one, in various ways" (Rothschild and Sharp 1941, 49). The lack of correlation between clinical and pathological data could best be accounted for by a differing ability among individuals to compensate for organic lesions. An individual's ability to withstand organic damage was decreased both by personality defects and by stress and life crises (Rothschild and Sharp 1941, 53).

Rothschild was not arguing that pathological structures were unimportant. There were "limits beyond which senile lesions will, no doubt, produce a mental disorder in any person." But within a fairly wide range, he argued, they did not lead inevitably to mental illness. Structural alterations were always present, but their significance could only be understood in light of "factors of a more personal nature." Each case, he concluded, required "individual scrutiny, and instead of focusing attention solely on the impersonal tissue process or on more personal influences, the main object should be to estimate the relative importance of these two sets of forces as factors in the origin of the psychosis" (Rothschild and Sharp 1941, 54).

THERAPEUTIC INITIATIVE IN THE STATE HOSPITALS

There was nothing inherently new in Rothschild's work. It clearly reflected the dominance of psychodynamic theory in U.S. psychiatry from the 1920s through the early 1960s (Grob 1983, 1991; Hale 1995), particularly the psychobiologic approach of Adolph Meyer, which conceived of all mental phenomena as a dialectical interplay between biological, social, and psychological forces (Holstein 1996). As Rothschild himself pointed out, his explanation of senile dementia was "in fact, the attitude of modern American psychiatry to mental disorders in general" (Rothschild 1937, 781). Applied to senile dementia, however, this attitude had the effect of challenging the therapeutic nihilism with which psychiatrists habitually viewed older patients. As Elvin O. Semrad put it in a discussion of one of Rothschild's papers published in 1947, "The emphasis on personality factors helped lead me and my associates out of the convenient balm for our frustrations as therapists which preoccupation with the neuropathologic damage and internal medical aspects of these problems allowed" (Rothschild 1947, 127).

In the 1940s and 1950s, there was a surge of interest in therapies that had previously been considered inappropriate for aged patients. This phenomenon reflected both the optimistic avenues that Rothschild's work opened and the desperate empiricism to which psychiatrists were driven by the crisis of the mental hospitals. From 1935 to

1959, thirty-five articles discussing these therapies appeared in the two leading professional psychiatric journals; in the fifteen preceding years, there had only been three. Many of these articles cited Rothschild or related work, and even those that did not, implicitly recognized the changed terrain on which their therapeutic efforts were based. A 1955 article on the use of electroconvulsive therapy on aged patients was typical. Following the usual litany concerning the growing importance of geriatric psychiatry, given the "mounting numbers of patients admitted to the senile wards of mental institutions," the authors noted that "considerable change has taken place in our thinking about the subject" over the previous decade. They then went on to cite Rothschild and other proponents of the psychodynamic model (Ehrenberg and Gullingsrud 1955, 743).

While generally optimistic in tone, which was remarkable given the long-standing psychiatric pessimism regarding senility, this burgeoning literature on treatment reported varying degrees of success, depending on the therapies and goals in question. Electroconvulsive therapy (ECT), aimed at lessening the confusion of senile patients and restoring their ability to function socially, reported the most favorable results. The article quoted above followed 112 patients treated with ECT and reported that 78.5 percent were able to be discharged from the hospital and 55 percent of these were able to remain out for more than a year. Similar levels of success were reported by other studies (Evans 1942, 1943; Susselman et al. 1946; Prout and Hamilton 1952; Wolff 1957). Drug therapies and group and interactive therapies aimed at calming agitation and making senile patients more manageable on the wards also received generally favorable reports (Linden 1953; Ginzberg 1953; Linden and Courtney 1954; Judah et al. 1959). Vitamin and other nutritional therapies, hormones, and drug treatments aimed at preserving or restoring the intellectual capacities of senile patients had much more ambiguous results (Chittick and Stotz 1941; Jetter et al. 1941; Wadsworth et al. 1943; Vernon and McKinlay 1947; J. Haber 1955; Cameron et al. 1957; Cameron 1958).

Increased interest in therapeutic interventions in the care of the senile was accompanied by a heightened interest in developing clinical procedures for evaluating the extent of organic damage in senile dementia. Many psychiatrists stressed the need to differentiate carefully between irreversible organic conditions and dementias that were produced by reversible conditions, such as nutritional insufficiency or drug toxicity. Psychiatrists recognized that hospitalization itself could be a source of dementia because of the disorienting effects of confinement in a strange location, disruption of routine, and the danger of over-medication (Robinson 1942; Avery et al. 1945; Arneson 1958; Titchener et al. 1958). Implicit in the literature was the belief that senile dementia was drastically overdiagnosed. One doctor argued in 1945 that it was common practice in the state hospitals to "accept without staff presentation or review, the diagnosis of psychosis with cerebral arteriosclerosis or senility made on the patient's admission." In the same article, Meyer Solomon argued that this practice often destroyed the morale of the patient and family without foundation. The term "senile dementia" ought to be dropped, he thought, in favor of "geriopsychosis," which would reflect the variability of origins and prognosis in psychotic conditions of the elderly. In any case, psychiatrists would need "to make a careful re-evaluation of our attitudes toward old people and of the too hurried diagnosis and management of their mental disorders" (Avery et al. 1945, 313–14).

It is difficult to evaluate the outburst of therapeutic activity directed at senile patients in the state mental hospitals. Depending on one's point of view, the high success rates reported for much of this therapy might be regarded as evidence either of the correctness of Rothschild's view (the typical view in the 1940s and 50s) or of diagnostic sloppiness (the typical view since the 1960s). Therapeutic efforts may have improved the ability of patients to compensate for organic damage, or they may have been lifting the symptoms of undiagnosed depression that either exacerbated an organic dementia or produced a clinical picture that mimicked senile dementia. Certainly the more rigorous approach to nosology and diagnosis advocated by Martin Roth and his colleagues at Newcastle produced correlations between pathology and dementia that were significantly better than what had been claimed by Rothschild (Roth 1955; Blessed et al. 1968; Tomlinson, Blessed, and Roth 1968, 1970; Katzman and Bick this volume), though these were still far from perfect (Kitwood 1987). In any case, to institutional psychiatrists struggling under the burden of caring for these patients, any therapeutic success, whatever its basis, was clearly welcome.

Regarding the effect of these therapeutic efforts on conditions within the state mental hospitals, one must balance the frequent optimistic pronouncements that the state hospitals were improving with equally frequent pronouncements about their deterioration and the impending crisis. Given the realities of overcrowding, understaffing, and underfunding in many state hospitals, the therapeutic initiatives described in this section were likely to have affected only a relatively small number of patients at state hospitals that were in a position to try them.

Conditions at most state hospitals could hardly be expected to improve until more basic problems of staffing and funding were resolved.

THE PSYCHODYNAMIC MODEL IN PSYCHIATRY AND BEYOND

Although Rothschild's psychodynamic model was clearly dominant among psychiatrists writing on senile dementia through the 1950s, a strict organic approach had never completely disappeared.[5] A handful of articles appeared in the leading psychiatric journals in the 1940s and 50s, explaining dementia on the basis of biological changes alone. Only one, an ambitious study by Meta Neumann and Robert Cohn, addressed Rothschild's theory directly. Neumann and Cohn studied 210 cases of dementia in a state hospital; they asserted firmly that AD and senile dementia were identical, and that the distinction ought to be dropped. They acknowledged the discrepancies cited by Rothschild between the degree of dementia found in the living patient and the degree of pathological damage found at autopsy. Because the overwhelming majority of patients suffering dementia showed large numbers of plaques and tangles at autopsy, however, they concluded that the link should be considered definite. A scattering of anomalous cases was not sufficient grounds for dismissing the evident organic basis of the disease (Neumann and Cohn 1953). This single article perfectly anticipated the position of researchers in the neurosciences who rediscovered senile dementia in the late 1960s. Present-day researchers who are interested in tracing their intellectual lineage have often cited this article as virtually the only meaningful contribution of U.S. psychiatry to understanding senile dementia during this era.[6]

At the time, however, Rothschild's work was far more influential within U.S. psychiatry and beyond. In large part, this was because of his theory's expansiveness: not only did the theory successfully explain the puzzling discrepancies between pathology and clinical dementia but also, it was argued, it could provide insight into the entire experience of aging. Following World War II Rothschild and the psychiatrists who followed him seldom even undertook research into brain pathology. Instead, they increasingly thought of modern social relations as the pathology of senility. The locus of senile mental deterioration was no longer the aging brain; instead, it was a society that stripped elderly people of the roles that had sustained meaning in their lives through mandatory retirement, social isolation, and the disintegration of traditional family ties. Bereft of any meaningful social role, the demented elderly did not so much lose their minds as lose their places in the world.

A typical example was Rothschild's discussion of a 75-year-old man who was admitted to a state hospital because of "memory impairment, mild confusion and marked untidiness of toilet habits of about one year's duration." Rothschild argued that "the striking point in his history was that he had no hobbies and few outside interests, and although he had three presumably intelligent children with whom he lived, they had made no effort to get him interested in any activities after his retirement from work at the age of 69. He would sit for hours at a time just staring into space. It is scarcely surprising that after several years of completely vacuous existence he should regress to an infantile state" (Rothschild 1947, 125).

In generalizing about such cases, Rothschild made it clear that this social pathology was characteristic of modern society. "In our present social set-up, with its loosening of family ties, unsettled living conditions and fast economic pace, there are many hazards for individuals who are growing old," he wrote. "Many of these persons have not had adequate psychological preparation for their inevitable loss of flexibility, restriction of outlets, and loss of friends or relatives; they are individuals who are facing the prospect of retirement from their life-long activities with few mental assets and perhaps meager material resources" (Rothschild 1947, 125).

Other psychiatrists pushed the turn to the social much further than Rothschild. Some attempted to correlate various forms of social pathology with dementia, much as somatically oriented psychiatrists had attempted to correlate brain lesions with a clinical diagnosis of dementia. Their studies showed a positive relationship between admissions to a state hospital with the diagnosis of senile dementia or cerebral arteriosclerosis and factors such as divorce, death of spouse, living alone, recent loss of job, or retirement (Williams et al. 1942; Gruenberg 1954; Busse et al. 1954; Buck 1956).[7]

Others went so far as to argue that brain pathology was little more than a symptom of social pathology. In a 1953 article, Maurice Linden and Douglas Courtney argued that senility, as it was usually thought of, was a "social illusion." They concluded that "senility as an isolable state is largely a cultural artifact and that senile organic deterioration may be consequent on attitudinal alterations" (Linden and Courtney 1953, 912). The authors acknowledged, however, that this hypothesis was difficult to prove. Writing in 1955, David C. Wilson was less circumspect, arguing that the link between social pathology and brain deterioration was simply a matter of waiting for "laboratory proof" to support what was adequately demonstrated by clinical experience — that the "pathology of senility is found not only in the tissues of the body but also in the concepts of the individual and in the attitude of society." Wilson cited the usual hallmarks of pathological social relations in old age: the break-up of the family, mandatory retirement, and isolation. "Factors that narrow the individual's life also influence the occurrence of senility," he asserted. "Lonesomeness, lack of responsibility, and a feeling of not being wanted all increase the restricted view of life which in turn leads to restricted blood flow" (Wilson 1955, 905). Social pathology could even be discerned, it seemed, within the constricted blood vessels of the aging brain.

A popularization of the psychodynamic model explained senility in terms of Freudian repression. In a 1957 feature for the *New York Times Magazine*, David Stonecypher Jr. (although identified as a physician, he did not, it seems, publish on senile dementia in professional journals) noted that "until recently it was widely believed that senility was the result of physical deterioration of the aging brain." But recent studies had shown this to be erroneous. Though other factors may contribute to the appearance of senility, "the *fear* and *frustration* associated with growing old in our society" was itself "adequate to explain the whole picture of senility." The forgetfulness so common in senility was the senile mind's way of protecting itself from painful memories, he argued. "Doctors used to marvel that a man who could not find his way home from the grocery store could still repeat accurately the plays of a football game forty years earlier," Stonecypher noted. But to the psychiatrist armed with the psychodynamic theory of senile dementia, the answer was simple: "The man enjoys remembering the times he was victorious. But the same man, retired from foreman at the plant to become errand boy for his wife, unconsciously finds it so painful to come home that he cannot remember his way" (Stonecypher 1957, 67).

As Stonecypher's example suggests, the psychodynamic model of senility followed the dominant expectations for gender of the period. Despite the fact that by the 1930s it had been documented that the prevalence of senile dementia was significantly higher for women, senility continued to be represented in the professional psychiatric literature as primarily a problem of middle-class men. Typically, discussions of the social production of senility centered around stereotypical male figures and problems—primarily retirement from paid labor and the loss of status and self-esteem it entailed. Stonecypher's popular account made explicit an assumption that was implicit throughout the psychiatric literature: because women's lives were oriented around the home and domesticity, they were sheltered from the worst aspects of the social pathology of senility. "Women get by pretty well," he asserted. "A woman is not deprived of her activities as much as a man, primarily because she maintains her housekeeping responsibilities. Then, too, the woman's interests as she becomes a grandmother are similar to those she had as a mother" (Stonecypher 1957, 27, 67). When women did appear in the psychiatric literature on senile dementia, the precipitating social factor was seen typically as a disruption of domestic life, such as the last child leaving home or the loss of a husband.

By bringing together cultural expectations and anxieties about gender, vexing issues of aging policy, and the horrifying symptoms of dementia (which carried their own deep connections to cultural anxieties about the stability and coherence of the self in post–World War II America), psychodynamic psychiatry made senility a potent political symbol for the emerging field of gerontology. A common argument was that the failure to adequately address the material, social, and psychological needs of the burgeoning aging population would result in a catastrophic increase in senility. "With the number of people who are over 65 increasing significantly each year, our society is today finding itself faced with the problem of keeping a large share of its population from joining the living dead—those whose minds are allowed to die before their bodies do," argued Jerome Kaplan, in advocacy of publicly supported recreation programs for the elderly (Kaplan 1953, 3). Similarly, in a book on the responsibility of churches to provide social opportunities for the elderly, George Gleason compared the elderly to juvenile delinquents: "While there is little tendency for [the isolated elderly] to engage in lawbreaking operations, as juveniles do, their depredations take another form. They tend to fill our general and mental hospitals, and become a burden upon society" (Gleason 1956, 14). The assertion that social and recreational programs lowered the frequency of placement in mental hospitals and other institutions was commonplace in the gerontologic literature of the era, backed up with anecdotal evidence from the professionals who operated these programs. While such programs would be expensive, they would be a bargain when compared to the cost of housing the elderly in mental hospitals and other institutions (Boucher and Tehan 1948; Bowen 1950; Woods 1953).

The eradication of senility (i.e., the expansive, socially produced senility described by American psychiatry) became a rallying point for a diverse array of biomedical and social scientists, policy makers, and advocates who were creating the field of gerontology in the decade after World War II. So construed, the fight against senility involved improving the material circumstances of old age through increasing public and private pensions, abolishing mandatory retirement, and establishing a network of social and recreational services. Perhaps most important, it required replacing the stereotype of senility, which generated hostility toward the elderly and fear of growing old, with positive images of successful aging, which generated the optimistic attitude necessary for the individual and society to meet the challenges of aging.

Geriatrician Martin Gumpert, one of the most energetic and visible proponents of this outlook, argued that the crucial factor was for people to realize that freedom from senility was possible. "If people are asked whether they would like to live for a hundred or a hundred and twenty or a hundred and fifty years, most of them seem horrified. Why?" Gumpert wondered. "They are frightened by the grotesque ugliness, the obscenity, the misery of senility, the hell in which so many beloved ones languish before they die. They look with fear into the mirror that reveals the first symptoms of old age and they would give their souls to arrest its ravages." Gumpert emphatically believed that senility could and would be eradicated. "There are facts to prove it, methods to follow and hopes that can be realized." Man deserved a better fate, "a more serene, more entertaining, more satisfying kind of life," Gumpert concluded. And he would have it. "All the technical means for creating happiness are available today. We need only change the direction of our energy from destruction to reconstruction" (Gumpert 1944, 13–14).

According to several historians, much of this program was accomplished by the end of the 1970s, creating what historian Peter Laslett has called the "emergence of the third age" and others have called the "young old" (Laslett 1991). The material circumstances of old age had markedly improved, significant legal protections had been won against age discrimination in the labor market, negative stereotypes were challenged, and the elderly themselves organized for political advocacy and action on their own behalf (Calhoun 1978; Haber and Gratton 1994).

With these developments, the expansiveness of the psychodynamic concept of senility was no longer acceptable. "Senility" now appeared to be a wastebasket term for a variety of discrete physical and mental disease entities, many of them treatable. "The word 'senile' itself is less a diagnosis than a term of abuse," aging activists like Alex Comfort asserted (Comfort 1976, 47). "Acceptance of senility as a predictable result of getting old perpetuates discrimination against the elderly," argued U.S. Representative Edward Royball, a stalwart congressional voice for the aging. Moreover, "mislabeling all elderly persons as senile also ignores the unique problems of a small but growing minority of elderly who do suffer from a group of diseases called senile dementia.

Those diseases are irreversible and are a growing health problem" (U.S. House of Representatives 1983, 1). Activists for the aging strove at once to attack the myth of senility — that the brain inevitably deteriorated with age — and to win attention and resources to attack the very real problem of AD and related disorders. As later chapters in this volume will show, these goals were vigorously pursued by a powerful coalition of AD caregivers, researchers, and policy makers in the federal government (see chapters by Fox and Bick).

Thus, by the end of the 1970s, if senility had not been eradicated, as an earlier generation of gerontologic activists had dreamed, it had at least been thoroughly disciplined — relegated by biomedical scientists to various discrete, well-defined disease entities that, at least in theory, no longer contaminated the entire experience of aging. Yet despite what clearly seem to be positive developments, the prospect of aging continued to generate anxiety and hostility. Despite the tone of optimism among researchers and activists, AD, as more carefully and rigorously defined and described by contemporary biomedicine, seems to create at least as much public fear and loathing about old age as did the expansive concept of senility out of which it was carved. One could reasonably ask whether, somewhere along the line, Americans had indeed paid for a youthful old age with their souls, as Martin Gumpert had asserted they were willing to do.

Notes

1. The first three paragraphs of this section follow the argument of Thomas Beach (1987) that research on AD has revolved around three issues: the role of arteriosclerosis, the relationship between AD and senile dementia, and whether senile dementia ought to be regarded as a normal part of aging or as a disease entity. Although Beach's framework is useful, forcing the literature of this period into it causes him to miss its most distinctive feature, as the rest of this section will show.

2. For examples of work treating the issue this way, see Lowenburg and Rothschild (1931); Lowenburg and Waggoner (1934); Kasanin and Crank (1933); Gordon (1935); Bay and Weinberg (1941).

3. For a variety of etiologic factors, see Alexander (1934); Alexander and Looney (1938). For single cause, see Sonati (1941).

4. Of course, one might also argue that the difference in clinical pictures between senility and AD lies more in differential expectations of observers for patients at different ages — that is, because expectations for the emotional functioning of an older person are lower than that for a younger, an equally devas-

tating clinical picture might be judged more severe in the case of a younger patient.

5. This generalization is difficult to make because relatively few articles addressed the etiological issue directly. Of the 36 articles appearing in *the American Journal of Psychiatry or the Archives of Neurology and Psychiatry* between 1940 and 1959 that dealt with etiology and classification, 17 can easily be classified as definitively taking one position or the other. Of these, 12 adhere to the psychodynamic approach, 11 of which explicitly cite Rothschild as the authority on the subject. Of the 5 that clearly favor a strict organic explanation, only Neumann and Cohn (1953), as discussed below, engage Rothschild's evidence directly. The remaining 19 articles could not be categorized because their subjects were too narrow — for example, a study ruling out heart disease as a significant factor in the psychoses of the senium could be consistent with either a psychodynamic or organic model. Of these 19 uncategorized articles, 11 were concerned with organic issues, 5 with social issues, and 2 remain sui generis. If these are added in, the picture is much more balanced — 17 articles approaching senile dementia from a psychodynamic angle, 16 from an organic angle.

6. The other article from this period frequently cited is that of British researcher R. D. Newton, who four years before Neumann and Cohn's publication, asserted that senile dementia and AD were the same entity ("The Identity of Alzheimer's Disease and Senile Dementia and their Relationship to Senility," *Journal of Mental Science* 94:225–48, 1948).

7. These studies had the obvious limitation of measuring only admission rates, not prevalence rates. All these factors could feasibly produce more admissions, regardless of whether they actually produced more psychotics. Thus, since they demonstrated that the elderly most likely to be admitted to the state mental hospitals were those whose social situations precluded their being cared for at home, they could be used to support the argument that alternatives to the state mental hospitals should be found to care for the senile aged.

References

Alexander, Leo. 1934. Neurofibrils in Systemic Disease and in Supravital Experiments. *Archives of Neurology and Psychiatry* 32:293.

Alexander, Leo, and Joseph M. Looney. 1938. Histologic Changes in Senile Dementia and Related Conditions. *Archives of Neurology and Psychiatry* 40: 1075.

Arneson, Genevieve. 1958. Hazards in Tranquilizing the Elderly Patient. *American Journal of Psychiatry* 115:163.

Avery, Loren, et al. 1945. Common Factors Precipitating Mental Symptoms in the Aged. *Archives of Neurology and Psychiatry* 54:312.

Bay, Alfred Paul, and Jack Weinberg. 1941. Review of the Symptomology of Alzheimer's Disease. *Archives of Neurology and Psychiatry* 47:862.

Beach, Thomas. 1987. The History of Alzheimer's Disease: Three Debates. *Journal of the History of Medicine and Allied Sciences* 42:327–49.

Blessed, Gary, Bernard E. Tomlinson, and Martin Roth. 1968. The Association Between Quantitative Measures of Dementia and of Senile Change in the Cerebral Gray Matter of Elderly Subjects. *British Journal of Psychiatry* 114: 797–811.

Boucher, Arline Britton, and John Leo Tehan. 1948. No One Under Sixty Need Apply. *Recreation* 42:347.

Bowen, Georgene E. 1950. The Time of Their Lives. *Recreation* 44:375.

Buck, Carol. 1956. Environmental change and Age of Onset of Psychosis in Elderly Patients. *Archives of Neurology and Psychiatry* 75:622.

Busse, Ewald W., et al. 1954. Studies of the Process of Aging: Factors that Influence the Psyche of Elderly Persons. *American Journal of Psychiatry* 110: 897.

Calhoun, Richard B. 1978. *In Search of the New Old: Redefining Old Age in America, 1945–1970.* New York: Elsevier.

Cameron, Ewen. 1958. The Use of Nucleic Acid in Aged Patients with Memory Impairments. *American Journal of Psychiatry* 114:943.

Cameron, Ewen, et al. 1957. Interthecal Administration of Hyaluroniadase: Effects upon the Behavior of Patients Suffering from Senile and Arteriosclerotic Behavior Disorders. *American Journal of Psychiatry* 113:893.

Chittick, Rupert, and Elmer Stotz. 1941. Nicotinic Acid and Ascorbic Acid in Relation to the Care of the Aged. *Diseases of the Nervous System* 2:71.

Comfort, Alex. 1976. *A Good Age.* New York: Simon and Schuster.

Dillmann, Rob. 1990. *Alzheimer's Disease: The Concept of Disease and the Construction of Medical Knowledge.* Amsterdam: Thesis Publishers.

Ehrenberg, Ruth, and Miles O. J. Gullingsrud. 1955. Electroconvulsive Therapy in Elderly Patients. *American Journal of Psychiatry* 111:743.

Evans, Vernon L. 1942. Physical Risks in Convulsive Shock Therapy. *Archives of Neurology and Psychiatry* 48:1017.

———. 1943. Convulsive Shock Therapy in Elderly Patients: Risks and Results. *American Journal of Psychiatry* 99:531.

Gellerstedt, N. 1932. Zur Kenntnis der Hirnveranderungen bei der normalen Altersinvolution. *Upsala Lakaref Forh* 38:193.

Ginzberg, Raphael. 1953. Geriatric Ward Psychiatry: Techniques in the Psychological Management of Elderly Psychotics. *American Journal of Psychiatry* 110:296.

Gleason, George. 1956. *Horizons for Older People.* New York: Macmillan.

Gordon, Alfred. 1935. Pick's or Alzheimer's Disease. *Archives of Neurology and Psychiatry* 24:214.

Grob, Gerald N. 1983. *Mental Illness and American Society, 1875–1940.* Princeton: Princeton University Press.

——. 1986. Explaining Old Age History: The Need for Empiricism. In *Old Age in a Bureaucratic Society: The Elderly, the Experts and the State in American History,* ed. David D. Van Tassel and Peter N. Stearns. Westport, Conn.: Greenwood Press.

——. 1991. *From Asylum to Community: Mental Health Policy in Modern America.* Princeton: Princeton University Press.

Gruenberg, E. M. 1954. Community Conditions and Psychoses of the Elderly. *American Journal of Psychiatry* 110:888.

Gumpert, Martin. 1944. *You Are Younger Than You Think.* New York: Duell, Sloan, and Pearce.

Haber, Carole. 1983. *Beyond Sixty-Five: The Dilemma of Old Age in America's Past.* New York: Cambridge University Press.

——. 1986. Geriatrics: A Specialty in Search of Specialists. In *Old Age in a Bureaucratic Society: The Elderly, the Experts and the State in American History,* ed. David D. Van Tassel and Peter N. Stearns. Westport, Conn.: Greenwood Press.

Haber, Carole, and Brian Gratton. 1994. *Old Age and the Search for Security: An American Social History.* Bloomington: Indiana University Press.

Haber, Joseph. 1955. Stellate Ganglion Infiltration in Organic Psychoses of Later Life. *American Journal of Psychiatry* 111:751.

Hale, Nathan G. 1995. *The Rise and Crisis of Psychoanalysis in the United States: Freud and the Americans, 1917–1985.* New York: Oxford University Press.

Holstein, Martha B. 1996. Negotiating Disease: Senile Dementia and Alzheimer's Disease, 1900–1980. Ph.D. diss., University of Texas Medical Branch at Galveston.

Huppert, Felicia, Carol Brayne, and Daniel W. O'Connor. 1994. *Dementia and Normal Aging.* Cambridge, UK: Cambridge University Press.

Hutchings, Richard W. 1939. President's Address. *American Journal of Psychiatry* 96:1.

Jetter, W. W., et al. 1941. Vitamin Studies in Cerebral Arteriosclerosis. *Diseases of the Nervous System* 2:66.

Judah, Leopold, et al. 1959. Psychiatric Response of Geriatric-Psychiatric Patients to Mellaril. *American Journal of Psychiatry* 115:118.

Kaplan, Jerome. 1953. *A Social Program for Older People.* Minneapolis: University of Minnesota Press.

Kasanin, Jerome, and R. P. Crank, 1933. Alzheimer's Disease. *Annals of Neurology and Psychiatry* 30:1180.

Kitwood, Tom. 1987. Explaining Senile Dementia: The Limits of Neuropathological Research. *Free Associations* 10:117–38.

Kolb, Lawrence. 1956. The Mental Hospitalization of the Aged: Is It Being Overdone? *American Journal of Psychiatry* 112:627.

Laslett, Peter. 1991. *A Fresh Map of Life: The Emergence of the Third Age.* Cambridge: Harvard University Press.

Linden, Maurice. 1953. Group Psychotherapy with Institutionalized Senile Women: Studies in Gerontologic Human Relations. *Archives of Neurology and Psychiatry* 69:400.

Linden, Maurice, and Douglas Courtney. 1953. The Human Life Cycle and Its Interruptions. *American Journal of Psychiatry* 109:906.

———. 1954. Interdisciplinary Research in the Use of Oral Pentylenetetetetrazol (Metrazol) in the Psychoses of Senility and Cerebral Arteriosclerosis. *Archives of Neurology and Psychiatry* 72:385.

Lowenburg, K., and D. Rothschild. 1931. Alzheimer's Disease: Its Occurrence on the Basis of a Variety of Etiologic Factors. *American Journal of Psychiatry* 11:269.

Lowenburg, K., and R. W. Waggoner. 1934. Familial Organic Psychosis (Alzheimer's Type). *Archives of Neurology and Psychiatry* 31:737.

Malamud, William, and Konstantin Lowenburg. 1929. Alzheimer's Disease: A Contribution to its Etiology and Classification. *Archives of Neurology and Psychiatry* 21:805.

McMenemy, William, and Eugene Pollack. 1941. Pre-Senile Disease of the Nervous System: Report of an Unusual Case. *Archives of Neurology and Psychiatry* 45:683.

Myerson, Abraham. 1944. Some Trends in Psychiatry. *American Journal of Psychiatry*, Special Centennial Issue: 161.

Neumann, Meta, and Robert Cohn. 1953. Incidence of Alzheimer's Disease in a Large Mental Hospital: Relation to Senile Psychosis and Psychosis with Cerebral Arteriosclerosis. *Archives of Neurology and Psychiatry* 69:615.

Prout, Curtis, and Donald Hamilton. 1952. Results of Electroshock Therapy in Patients over Sixty Years of Age. *Archives of Neurology and Psychiatry* 67:689.

Robinson, G. Wilse. 1942. The Toxic Delirious Reactions of Old Age. *American Journal of Psychiatry* 99:110.

Roth, M. 1955. The Natural History of Mental Disorders in Old Age. *Journal of Mental Science* 101:281–301.

Rothschild, David. 1937 Pathologic Changes in Senile Psychoses and their Psychobiologic Significance. *American Journal of Psychiatry* 93:757–87.

———. 1947. The Practical Value of Research in the Psychoses of Later Life. *Diseases of the Nervous System* 8:123.

Rothschild, David, and Jerome Kasanin. 1936. Clinicopathologic Study of Alzheimer's Disease: A Contribution to its Etiology and Classification. *Archives of Neurology and Psychiatry* 36:293.

Rothschild, David, and M. L. Sharp. 1941. The Origin of Senile Psychoses: Neuropathologic Factors and Factors of a More Personal Nature. *Diseases of the Nervous System* 2:49–54.

Sonati, Theodore L. L. 1941. Histogenesis of Senile Plaques. *Archives of Neurology and Psychiatry* 46:101.

Stonecypher, David D. 1957. Old Age Need Not Be Old. *New York Times Magazine*, 18 August, 27ff.

Susselman, Samuel, et al. 1946. Electric Shock Therapy of Elderly Patients. *Archives of Neurology and Psychiatry* 56:158, 1946.

Titchener, James, et al. 1958. Psychological Reactions of the Aged in Surgery: The Reaction of Renewal and Depletion. *Archives of Neurology and Psychiatry* 78:63.

Tomlinson, B. E., G. Blessed, and M. Roth. 1968. Observations on the Brains of Non-demented Old People. *Journal of Neurological Science* 7:331–56.

———. 1970. Observations on the Brains of Demented Old People. *Journal of Neurological Science* 11:205–42.

U.S. House of Representatives, Select Committee on Aging. 1983. *Senility: The Last Stereotype: Hearing Before the Select Committee on Aging, House of Representatives, Ninety-eighth Congress, first session, May 18, 1983.* Washington, D.C.: U.S. Government Printing Office.

Von Braunmühl, A. 1932. Kolloidchemische Betrachtungswise seniler und präseniler Gewebsveränderungen. *Ztschr f d ges Nevrol u Psychiat* 142:1.

———. 1934. Versuch um eine kolloidchemische Pathologie des Zentralnervensystems. Das synaertische Syndromcals cerebrale Reaktionsform. *Klin Wchnschr* 13:897.

Vernon, P. E., and M. McKinlay. 1947. Effects of Vitamin and Hormone Treatment on Senile Patients. *Journal of Neurology, Neurosurgery, and Psychiatry* 8:87.

Wadsworth, G. L., et al. 1943. An Evaluation of Treatment for Senile Psychosis with Vitamin B Complex. *American Journal of Psychiatry.* 99:807.

Williams, Harold W., et al. 1942. Studies in Senile and Arteriosclerotic Psychoses: Relative Significance of Extrinsic Factors in their Development. *American Journal of Psychiatry* 98:712.

Wilson, David. 1955. The Pathology of Senility. *American Journal of Psychiatry* 111:902–906.

Wolff, Gunther E. 1957. Results of Four Years Active Therapy for Chronic Mental Patients and the Value of an Individual Maintenance Dose of ECT. *American Journal of Psychiatry* 114:453.

Woods, James H. 1953. *Helping Older People Enjoy Life.* New York: Harper & Brothers.

6

The Rediscovery of Alzheimer Disease During the 1960s and 1970s

Robert Katzman and Katherine L. Bick

The modern era of Alzheimer research began in 1948 with R. D. Newton's argument on the clinical identity of Alzheimer disease (AD) and senile dementia but was not continued until the reports on the ultrastructure of the plaque and tangle by Terry (1963; Terry, Gonatas, and Weiss 1964) and Kidd (1963, 1964) and the classical prospective clinicopathologic study of Blessed, Tomlinson, and Roth reported in 1968. Further impetus was provided in 1976 by the recognition of the public health importance of AD by Katzman and the exciting discovery of the deficit in choline acetyl transferase made independently by Bowen, Davies, and the Perrys.

Before we describe these events, it is important to understand the intellectual disarray about late-life cognitive changes that existed in the 1950s. This disarray was partly due to the failure to establish a clear clinicopathologic relationship between intellectual impairment and either brain weight or abundance of plaques and tangles. In the absence of that connection, the proposal was made that functional psychiatric conditions played a significant role in these disorders of late life. This story is described in the preceding chapter by Jesse Ballenger.

An additional confound in the United States was the emphasis on cerebrovascular events as the major cause of late-life dementia. In 1946 Walter Alvarez, a prominent gastroenterologist at the Mayo Clinic and a prolific writer whose major interest was in patients with psychosomatic symptoms not understood by medicine of his day (or today for that matter), published an extraordinary paper entitled "Cerebral Arteriosclerosis with Small Commonly Unrecognized Apoplexies." Alvarez noted, "One of the commonest diseases of man is a slow petering out toward the end of life, and one of the commonest ways of petering out is that in which the brain is slowly destroyed by the repeated thrombosis of small sclerotic blood vessels." In this article, Alvarez presented detailed clinicopathologic data on seven cases — two of them his own relatives for whom he had lifelong histories. He described this variety of multi-infarct dementia, the lacunar state, more than a decade before C. Miller Fisher's more detailed analysis of this disorder. Alvarez's impact on American medicine was extraordinary. His explanation of most late-life dementing illnesses as due to cerebral arteriosclerosis was almost universally accepted by U.S. physicians and persisted for almost forty years.

That destruction of brain tissue rather than arteriosclerotic plaques in blood vessels is associated with dementia required further evidence, however. J. A. N. Corsellis (1962, 1965) analyzed brains of 300 patients who had died at Runwell, a psychiatric hospital in Wickford, Essex, and in this series, the average age at time of death was 70. He concluded that severe arteriosclerosis of the carotid and vertebral blood vessels was not related to either dementia or parenchymal neuropathology per se. Then, in the prospective clinicopathologic study to be described below, Tomlinson, Blessed, and Roth (1970) found that more than 50 ml. of cerebral tissue had to be infarcted for signs of dementia to have been observed prior to death. Hachinski et al. (1974) later coined the term *multi-infarct* dementia. By the time of the Hachinski publication, clinicians were willing to drop the term *arteriosclerotic dementia.*

The first to argue for the identity of AD with senile dementia was R. D. Newton. His conclusion was based on 150 consecutive autopsies performed at a mental hospital located in Middlesex County, United Kingdom. He argued that although the brains of individuals with dementia showed differences in the number of plaques and tangles, and although individuals presented clinically with a variety of symptoms, the variations in pathological and clinical features were similar in subjects, whether they were older or younger than 65 years at onset.

The modern era in AD research was ushered in by the first successful electron microscopic studies of the AD brain, carried out independently in the United Kingdom by Kidd (1963) and in the United States by Terry (1963). (We have had the opportunity of interviewing both of these pioneers, as well as Blessed, Kay, Roth, Tomlinson, and Wisniewski.) The technology involved in such studies had just advanced to the point where brain pathology could be investigated at the ultrastructural level, although the techniques were still very idiosyncratic and difficult to use.

Both Kidd and Terry had been trained as physicians, but their post-clinical training differed. Kidd was primarily interested in the normal cerebral cortex, had worked with J. Z. Young to study the retina, and learned electron microscopy with David Robertson and George Gray. He then took a post at Maida Vale to work on a senile dementia unit only when he felt that other, perhaps more suitable jobs were not available.

Terry initially began his training as a surgeon but quickly switched to pathology and trained with the leading U.S. neuropathologist, Harry Zimmerman, who had been in the former Alzheimer's laboratory in Munich. Interested in applying the new electron microscopic technology to pathology, Terry spent a year at a cancer research center in Paris learning this technique. After returning to Zimmerman's department at Montefiore Hospital in New York to complete his training, he specialized in neuropathology, developing a major interest in how the brain responded to disease. He accepted a position on the faculty of the Albert Einstein College of Medicine to work with Saul Korey, a neurologist and neurochemist who was dedicated to identifying the biochemical (now, we would say "molecular") basis of neurodegenerative disorders. Terry and Korey sought an approach that would make it possible to study both the ultrastructural and biochemical aspects of fatal neurodegenerative diseases. Terry's first major success with this new approach was the delineation of the lamellar intraneuronal inclusions in Tay-Sachs disease and other lipidoses. Korey died in 1963 of pancreatic carcinoma while his laboratory was isolating and purifying the ganglioside accumulated in the Tay-Sachs brain. He was engaged in trying to identify the chemical structure of this lipid and the enzymatic defect in that disorder. AD was one of many relatively rare neurodegenerative disorders that would be studied.

At both Maida Vale and Albert Einstein in the early 1960s, cerebral biopsies were carried out in the investigation of progressive fatal neurodegenerative diseases both to establish diagnosis and to begin to learn something about the biology of these diseases. Thus, both investigators had available brain biopsy material from AD patients under the age of 65. Neurofibrillary tangles are hardy structures, and both investigators quickly identified the periodic filamentous components of these tangles. Kidd, who published in *Nature* shortly before Terry's article appeared in the *Journal of Neuropathology and Experimental Neurology*, could claim priority; moreover, he correctly interpreted the periodicity of the filamentous structures observed on the electron micrographs of tangles as paired helical filaments, whereas Terry, on the basis of their diameter, believed them to be twisted microtubules. Based on pictures obtained with a tilt-stage electron microscope, Terry's collaborator, Henry Wisniewski later developed a three-dimensional, scaled wire model of these structures that persuaded Terry that Kidd's interpretation of the structure as paired helical filaments was correct (Wisniewski, Narang, and Terry 1976).

Terry was unquestionably the first to identify the straight fibril material constituting the core of the plaque as amyloid. It would be thirty years before advances in molecular biology would permit identification of the material in the paired helical filament as tau protein and the material in the amyloid core of the plaques as the 40–43 amino acid A/β amyloid peptide.

The pioneer articles were truly extraordinary in the detail and accuracy of their findings. It is unfortunate that until 1997 the major biomedical electronic database, MEDLINES, only cited articles written after 1966, so the classic papers of Kidd and Terry, published in 1963 and 1964, were not included. Consequently, many of the findings in these seminal studies in addition to that of the paired helical filaments and amyloid — for example, the Terry paper clearly delineates degenerative changes in synapses, the presence of microglia, disruption of microtubules — were continually being rediscovered. Fortunately, MEDLINES citations have now been extended back to 1963 for many journals, and citations for these classic papers can be easily retrieved.

Shortly after these publications, it became apparent to some of those working in the Terry laboratory (according to Wisniewski) that the brains of very elderly demented individuals also had plaques and tangles with the same ultrastructural features as in the presenile cases. But the issue in regard to the identity of presenile and senile dementias was not settled to everyone's satisfaction by these findings.

The next major step was the prospective clinicopathologic study that was carried out in Newcastle. Blessed, Tomlinson, and Roth demonstrated a strong correlation between quantitative measures of dementia and the number of plaques and tangles or between dementia and the volume of brain destroyed by cerebral infarcts in elderly subjects. Martin Roth, then professor of psychiatry at Newcastle on Tyne, headed a Medical Research Council unit that looked at the relationship between organic and medical disorders and psychiatric disorders. Roth had persuaded his colleague, the pathologist Bernard Tomlinson, to look at the brains of old people who died from mental illnesses. Gary Blessed, a senior registrar in the department, had joined the group primarily to study patients with brain tumors but was asked, additionally, to assess elderly people in the long-stay wards of the local mental hospital and control subjects without mental illness in the general hospital and to obtain postmortems of both mental patients and controls so that Tomlinson could study the brains.

Tomlinson had undertaken quantitative assessment of the lesions in these brains, and to match it, Blessed put together a quantitative test battery that included the ten items of the Roth-Hopkins test related to memory and orientation plus items borrowed from Felix Post's list, including simple tests of concentration like counting forward and backward, five-minute name and address recall (which seemed to be one of the better tests), and items of personal memory. This instrument came to be known as the Modified Roth-Hopkins Test and is now frequently referred to as the Blessed Information-Memory-Concentration Test. Blessed relates that about a year after the assessments were started and his group had obtained 27 cases that had been fully assessed, they were faced with a review visit from the Medical Research Council. "And it was decided to push the results through the university computer and see whether we'd shown any relationship and we found that the correlation between dementia score and Bernard's mean plaque count was about 0.8! . . . We'd hit the jackpot."

A brief report of this initial work, now with 53 cases (24 of which had dementia), was presented by Blessed and Tomlinson at a symposium held by the World Psychiatric Association at the Royal College of Physicians in London on September 28–29, 1965. It was entitled "Psychiatric Disorders in the Aged." Blessed and Tomlinson remark that the "majority of cases of dementia in old age are associated with one of two types of pathological changes in the one brain. . . . One of these is ischaemic cerebral destruction . . . arteriosclerotic dementia. The second type of change is that found in cases of so-called senile dementia, regarded by many as Alzheimer's disease occurring in later life" (1965, 310). Although Michael Kidd and J. A. N. Corsellis also presented at this symposium, the remarks about AD that we have cited elicited little response from the other clinician participants as judged by the paucity of remarks during the formal discussion.

By the time of the 1968 publication of this clinicopathologic study by Blessed, Tomlinson, and Roth, the total number of autopsies had reached 78. In their 1968 analysis, the investigators excluded subjects with significant cerebral infarcts. Twenty-six of these 60 infarct-free patients had a clinical diagnosis of senile dementia; their mean age was 78 years. In this cohort of 60 subjects, the correlation of plaque count to the premorbid dementia score was 0.77. Thus, the pathologic hallmarks of AD were established as the major cause of so-called senile dementia.

The initial impact of the Blessed, Tomlinson, and Roth (1968) study was to impress upon European psychiatrists that some elderly persons may develop AD. However, many clinicians still considered senile dementia to be a distinct entity. In 1969 the first modern symposium on AD was held on November 11–13, in Ciba House in London, with proceedings edited by G. E. W. Wolstenholme and M. O'Connor published in 1970. Roth chaired the symposium. The participants included twenty-three clinicians, pathologists, and scientists from Europe, Japan, and the United States, including Corsellis, Terry, Tomlinson, and Wisniewski.

Although the Blessed, Tomlinson, and Roth (1968) paper had been published a year earlier, only Tomlinson and the participants from the Maudsley referred to its findings. All of the clinicians and pathologists at the meeting accepted the concept that some elderly subjects with dementia had AD and that defining the disease as "presenile" was not correct, but they did not necessarily accept the evidence that AD itself was the most important cause of senile dementia. Ludwig van Bogaert (1970) clearly stated the prevailing clinical view: "Psychiatrists differentiate senile dementia from Alzheimer's disease by specific symptoms which, in each case, overlie the same background of dementia. In spite of lesions of similar quality, the two diseases differ from each other in their intensity and localization. Calendar age is of little importance; what matters in these types of involutional disorder is biological age."

Patrick Sourander and Hakon Sjogren (1970) reported on 68 cases of patients with classical presenile AD and 20 cases of patients with Alzheimer findings who were aged 70 to 79 in an analysis of 318 cases of dementia — thus tacitly accepting the fact that age 65 was arbitrary. However, they contrasted these 20 cases of unquestioned AD in elderly persons to the majority of those aged 70 to 79 who were diagnosed as having senile dementia ("dementia senilis simplex"). The latter were clinically defined on the basis that they lacked the "focal findings" that these authors considered necessary to diagnose typical presenile AD — aphasia, apraxia and agnosia, lack of spontaneity, extrapyramidal features, and seizures. Pathologically, the cases of senile dementia might show some plaques but had "only rare tangles in isocortex."

Quite different results were reported by Tomlinson, Blessed, and Roth in 1970, based on their analysis of the entire series of brains of elderly subjects who had been diagnosed as demented by Blessed, Tomlinson, and Roth (1968) but including, this time, brains with large areas of infarction and other diagnoses that had been excluded from the 1968 paper. Fifty percent of these brains had the histologic features of AD without significant vascular changes; in 17 percent, the dementia appeared to be primarily due to multiple cerebral infarcts; and 18 percent were mixed vascular and AD cases. The remainder had other neuropathologic diagnoses, such as Wernicke encephalopathy, or had nonspecific neuropathologic findings — possibly cases that would now be diagnosed as being among the chromosome 17–related dementias or as due to diffuse Lewy body disease. Thus, this second study established that dementia in the senium could be due to a number of different causes, with AD being the most common.

Clinicopathologic correlations may provide the basis for understanding diseases, but they do not necessarily excite the scientific imagination. Despite the extraordinary impact of this landmark study, very few investigators chose to work on AD at this time. The number of articles on AD had risen from 10 published in 1966 to only 52 in 1976. Interest then increased so that by 1986 there were 826 articles published on AD, and by 1996 there were 2,372. In 1976 additional findings helped to increase interest in AD.

Recognition that the majority of subjects with senile dementia have AD changes AD from a rare to an increasingly common disorder as people live longer. Based on small community studies of elderly persons carried out in the 1950s and 1960s, Katzman (1976) summarized evidence that the prevalence of severe dementia in those over age 65, averaged 4.1 percent, and the prevalence of mild dementia (or "chronic brain syndrome without psychosis") averaged 10.8 percent. In his 1976 editorial in the *Archives of Neurology*, Katzman applied the epidemiologic data together with the findings of Tomlinson that 48 to 58 percent of those with late-life dementia have AD. He estimated that the number of cases of AD in the United States in 1976 was between 880,000 and 1,200,000 and that there were 60,000 to 90,000 deaths per year due to this disease, making AD the fourth or fifth most common cause of death.

Also in 1976 reports on a major cholinergic deficit in AD were surfacing from three independent laboratories in the United Kingdom. Peter Davies, then working in Edinburgh in a research program on schizophrenia although trained as a classical biochemist at Leeds, had always planned to work on human brain chemistry. In the course of the work on schizophrenia, assays for the cholinergic neurotransmitters had already been set up, and AD brain samples were available, in part having been used as disease controls for the schizophrenia samples. The decreases in acetylcholinesterase and choline acetyl transferase in the first AD brains Davies studied were so striking that it seemed incredible that they had not been found before. And of course, they were being found, in what might be called the "golden age" of AD neurochemistry, in Newcastle by Elaine Perry in her association with the Tomlinson, Blessed, and Roth cohort, and in London by David Bowen in Alan Davison's group at Queen Square with material from Corsellis at Runwell Hospital.

Elaine Perry had studied synaptosome preparations with Whittaker at Cambridge and was an accomplished neurochemist when she and her husband, Robert Perry, a neuropathologist, came to Newcastle to join Bernard Tomlinson's department. By this time, the advantages of adding a neurochemical aspect to the meticulous neuropathologic counts of plaques and tangles and their association with the dementia seen in AD were clear to Tomlinson. Elaine's familiarity with the assay systems for the cholinergic neurotransmitter systems made it a natural place to begin to look for neurochemical anomalies in AD. David Drachman's reports of the memory deficits in scopolamine-treated young adults (Drachman and Leavitt 1974) further stimulated looking first at the cholinergic system in the disease. The Perry's work, although published in early 1977, was completed at essentially the same time as that of the others.

David Bowen was born in England, received his Ph.D. in biochemistry at Pittsburgh, and went on to postdoctoral work with Norman Radin at Michigan, where he was "converted to a neurochemist." Two years after he returned to England, he joined Alan Davison's newly formed group at the Institute of Biochemistry at Queen Square. Bowen established a collaborative program with Corsellis so that he was able to obtain human brains within 24 hours of death from patients with a variety of brain diseases, including AD. Bowen's initial neurochemical work indicated that the AD brain had a deficiency in a specific protein, which he later found was dependent not on the disease but on the preagonal state of the patient. A similar problem plagued the finding of the deficiency he found in glutamic acid decarboxylase in the AD brain, which may have led him to downplay the loss in choline acetyltransferase that he also reported, in passing, in his 1976 paper in *Brain* (Bowen et al. 1976).

A matter of concern in regard to these findings was the source of the neocortical choline acetyltransferase. It was known that few cortical neurons were primarily cholinergic. Johnston, McKinney, and Coyle (1979) identified the major source of cortical acetylcholine in rats as a projections system arising from large cholinergic neurons in the ventral globus pallidus area, the nucleus of Meynert. Whitehouse et al. (1982) showed the selective, greater than 75 percent degeneration of the neurons of the nucleus basalis of Meynert in AD patients. The degeneration of this projection system is so profound that it provided the pathological substrate of the cholinergic deficiency in the AD brain.

The idea that a clinical presentation of a global deficit such as is seen in AD may be caused by the loss of specific groups of neurons in the brain was strengthened by the earlier work on Parkinson disease. Hence, the finding of a specific neurotransmitter deficit in the AD brain triggered new studies both on the basic etiology and on the possible therapeutic approaches that could be envisioned. Over the next several years, the failure of precursor replacement therapy—that is, the use of choline or lecithin—caused great disappointment. Physostigmine and related compounds that block the breakdown of acetylcholine were found to have a modest but reproducible effect in improving memory and cognition in AD patients; these drugs are still the major drugs used in AD twenty years later, although an intensive search for new drugs that delay onset or slow down progression is now underway.

Katzman and Terry followed up on the *Archives of Neurology* editorial by writing to the director of the National Institute of Neurological and Communicative Disorders and Stroke (NINCDS), Dr. Donald Tower, a neurochemist initially trained as a neurosurgeon. They suggested that the institute convene a workshop conference on AD to highlight scientific problems that could be studied and to interest skilled investigators in other fields to begin working on the disease. With the excitement that developed from the discovery of the cholinergic deficit in AD, Dr. Tower was sufficiently interested in what had become a new frontier in neuroscience research to enlist Dr. Bick in organizing the conference. He also asked the directors of the National Institute of Mental Health and of the newly established National Institute on Aging to join in sponsoring this conference, the proceedings of which were subsequently published.

By 1979 fledgling AD societies in the United States were brought together by the National Institute on Aging and urged to form a single organization, as will be described by Dr. Patrick Fox in a following chapter.

Alzheimer disease had been rediscovered—once again!

References

Alvarez, W. C. 1946. Cerebral arteriosclerosis with small, commonly unrecognized apoplexies. *Geriatrics* 1:189–216.

Blessed, G., and B. E. Tomlinson. 1965. Senile plaques and intellectual deterioration in old age. In *World Psychiatric Association Symposium: Psychiatric Disorders in the Aged*, 310–21. Manchester, U.K.: Geigy.

Blessed, G., B. E. Tomlinson, and M. Roth. 1968. The association between quantitative measures of dementia and of senile change in the cerebral grey matter of elderly subjects. *Br J Psychiatry* 114:797–811.

Bowen, D. M., and A. N. Davison. 1975. Letter: Extrapyramidal diseases and dementia. *Lancet* 1(7917): 1199–200.

Bowen, D. M., C. B. Smith, P. White, and A. N. Davison. 1976. Neurotransmitter – related enzymes and indices of hypoxia in senile dementia and other abiotrophies. *Brain* 99:59–96.

Corsellis, J. A. N. 1962. *Mental Illness and the Aging Brain*. London: Oxford University Press.

Corsellis, J. A. N. 1965. Cerebral degeneration and the mental disorders of later life. In *World Psychiatric Association Symposium: Psychiatric Disorders in the Aged*, 292–309. Manchester, U.K.: Geigy.

Davies, P., and A. J. R. Maloney. 1976. Selective loss of central cholinergic neurons in Alzheimer's disease. *Lancet* 2:1403.

Drachman, D. A., and J. Leavitt. 1974. Human memory and the cholinergic system. *Arch Neurol* 30:113–21.

Hachinski, V. C., N. A. Lessen, et al. 1974. Multi-infarct dementia: A cause of mental deterioration in the elderly. *Lancet* 2 (July 27): 207–10.

Johnston, M. V., M. McKinney, and J. T. Coyle. 1979. Evidence for a cholinergic projection to neocortex from neurons in the basal forebrain. *Proc Natl Acad Sci USA* 76:5392–96.

Katzman, R. 1976. The prevalence and malignancy of Alzheimer disease: A major killer. *Arch Neurol* 33:217.

Katzman, R., R. D. Terry, and K. L. Bick, eds. 1978. *Alzheimer's Disease: Senile Dementia and Related Disorders, Aging*, vol. 7. New York: Raven Press.

Kidd, M. 1963. Paired helical filaments in electron microscopy in Alzheimer's disease. *Nature* 197:192–93.

———. (1964). Alzheimer's disease: An electron microscopic study. *Brain* 87: 303–20.

Newton, R. D. 1948. The identity of Alzheimer's disease and senile dementia and their relationship in senility. *J Mental Sci*, 94:225–48.

Perry, E. K., R. H. Perry, G. Blessed, and B. E. Tomlinson. 1977. Necropsy evidence of central cholinergic deficits in senile dementia. *Lancet* 1:189.

Perry, E. K., R. H. Perry, P. H. Gibson, G. Blessed, and B. E. Tomlinson. 1977. A cholinergic connection between normal aging and senile dementia in the human hippocampus. *Neurosci Lett* 6:85–89.

Roth, M., B. E. Tomlinson, and G. Blessed. 1966. Correlation between scores for dementia and counts of "senile plaques" in cerebral grey matter of elderly subjects. *Nature* 200:109–10.

Sourander, P., and H. Sjogren. 1970. Clinical implications of Alzheimer's disease. In *Alzheimer Disease and Related Conditions: A Ciba Foundation Symposium*, ed. G. E. W. Wolstenholme and M. O'Connor, 11–32. London: J & A Churchill.

Terry, R. D. 1963. Neurofibrillary tangles in Alzheimer's disease. *J Neuropathol Exp Neurol* 22:629–42.

Terry, R. D., N. K. Gonatas, and M. Weiss. 1964. Ultrastructural studies in Alzheimer's presenile dementia. *Am J Pathol* 44:269–97.

Tomlinson, B. E., G. Blessed, and M. Roth. 1970. Observations on the brains of demented old people. *J Neurol Sci* 11:205–42.

Van Bogaert, L. 1970. Cerebral amyloid angiopathy and Alzheimer's disease. In *Alzheimer Disease and Related Conditions: A Ciba Foundation Symposium*, ed. G. E. W. Wolstenholme and M. O'Connor, 95–104. London: J & A Churchill.

Whitehouse, P. J., D. L. Price, R. G. Struble, A. W. Clark, J. T. Coyle, and M. R. Delon. 1982. Alzheimer's disease and senile dementia: Loss of neurons in the basal forebrain. *Science* 215:1237–39.

Wisniewski, H. M., H. K. Narang, and R. D. Terry. 1976. Neurofibrillary tangles of paired helical filaments. *J Neurol Sci* 27:173–81.

Wolstenholme, G. E. W., and M. O'Connor. 1970. *Alzheimer Disease and Related Conditions: A Ciba Foundation Symposium*. London: J & A Churchill.

7

The History of the Genetics of Alzheimer Disease

Daniel A. Pollen

This chapter reviews the major advances in the genetics of Alzheimer disease (AD), together with several issues that have proved inseparable from the discovery of the genes themselves. For diseases of unknown gene product, gene discovery is often the first step in understanding disease pathogenesis. In the protracted period between gene discovery and treatment, however, the issues of predictive genetic testing create both options and dilemmas for an ever-increasing percentage of the population. Moreover, the discovery of susceptibility genes for late-onset AD has provided opportunities to determine how environmental factors modify gene products and disease progression. I begin with the history of the recognition of genetic factors in AD (Pollen 1996).

Following the 1907 publication of Alois Alzheimer's three-page report on a case of presenile dementia, Kraepelin proposed in 1910 that the presenile form of dementia be designated as "Alzheimer's Disease." By then, Alzheimer had already astutely surmised that atherosclerotic vascular abnormalities were unrelated to the senile processes observed in the brain in late life.

Alzheimer accepted Kraepelin's designation of AD with considerable caution and was never certain whether the presenile disease was simply an unusually severe and premature form of senile dementia. Indeed, he and others at the time thought that there were neuropathological differences in the two forms — with frontal lobe pathology being more severe in senile dementia and with greater devastation of temporal and parietal lobes occurring in presenile dementias. Even the distinctions between senile dementia and normal aging were not yet clear. In 1911 Perusini could find no clear-cut distinction between senile dementia and normal aging — at least as far as the presence, though not the extent, of the senile plaques was concerned (Bick, Amaducci, and Pepeu 1987).

While there is a great risk of oversimplification in summarizing the history that led to the discovery of the first known gene to cause AD, certain landmarks stand out. Between 1927 and 1934, Paul Divry in Belgium defined the "peculiar substance" in the cerebral plaques as "amyloid," a then-obscure class of substances defined by characteristic staining reactions. Contemporaneously, in Germany in 1929, Fredric Strüwe discovered numerous senile plaques in the brains of relatively young patients dying with Down syndrome. Studies of such patients provided the first evidence of a convergent process common to victims of Down syndrome and AD.

By 1932 the first reports that AD might occur on a familial basis came from Germany in independent reports by Shottky and Von Braunmühl. In the United States in 1934, Rothschild documented the higher incidence of AD in females. In England a decade later, this remarkable difference inspired Mayer-Gross's (1944) observation that "a completely unexplained feature of Alzheimer's disease is its prevalence in females."

By 1948 Jervis had discovered that some patients with Down syndrome develop a dementia in their late 30s and 40s that resembles AD. Although R. D. Newton (1948) saw a continuum between presenile dementia, senile dementia, and what he called "normal senility," he nevertheless suspected that obscure genetic factors took hold at vastly distinct stages of life.

In 1958 the French geneticist Jerome Lejeune discovered that Down syndrome was caused by a duplication or extra copy of chromosome 21, hence the new term "trisomy 21." By 1977 Heston in the United States realized that the increased incidence of AD in persons with Down syndrome might be attributable to the extra copy of some gene on chromosome 21.

Early-Onset Alzheimer Disease

The search for the genetic basis of the various forms of early-onset AD took on new momentum in the 1983–84 period. Jim Gusella's 1983 discovery of the linkage of Huntington disease to the short arm of chromosome 4 initiated the use of "reverse genetics" — that is, using DNA markers for linkage analysis to discover the genetic causes of diseases of unknown gene product. Indeed, only one of the AD genes has been discovered on the basis of a putative gene product. That discovery may be traced back to Glenner and Wong, who in 1984 isolated, purified, and sequenced the vascular amyloid peptide. If β-amyloid is a gene product, they suggested that perhaps the genetic defect for both AD and Down syndrome resided on chromosome 21. Within a year, Beyreuther and his colleagues, largely from Cologne, purified and sequenced the peptide found in the senile plaques of patients with AD and Down's syndrome. His team realized that the β-amyloid, protein that they called A4, was actually a small fragment or cleavage product of a much larger precursor protein. By 1987 Jie Kang, then a graduate student, and her colleagues in Cologne had discovered and sequenced the gene for the amyloid precursor protein on chromosome 21.

The way was now clear to test whether cases of AD in several families that had been linked to chromosome 21 were actually due to mutations in the APP gene. At that time, four of the largest known families with familial AD were tested for mutations in the APP gene; of course, none were found.

Fortunately, a group led by Blas Frangione studied Dutch patients with a form of familial amyloid angiopathy that predisposed them to cerebral hemorrhages. Suspecting a mutation in the amyloid gene, Frangione's team discovered a single point mutation in exon 17 of the APP gene. But did this finding have anything to do with AD? After all, the APP gene seemed to have been eliminated as a cause of AD in most of the documented large pedigrees that had been linked to chromosome 21. A brain donation from a victim of an English family linked to chromosome 21 allowed John Hardy's group in London to document that the patient had AD rather than hereditary cerebral hemorrhage with amyloidosis.

On February 21, 1991, Allison Goate and the St. Mary's Hospital team reported the discovery of a mutation that caused a classic form of familial AD. Remarkably, this mutation was on the same APP gene that harbored the Dutch mutation and even on the same exon, albeit at a different position. Since then, a substantial number of single-point and a smaller number of double-point mutations in the APP gene have been discovered. These account for perhaps 1–3 percent of all cases of early-onset familial AD. However, the significance of these discoveries does not lie in the percentage of cases in which these mutations are causal; it is the fact that an abnormality in the metabolism of amyloid can be a proximal cause of at least one form of AD that is significant. Subsequently, models using transgenic mice that overpromote the "long" 42–43 amino acid residues or "long β-amyloid" fragments have been shown to produce many of the neuropathological features of AD. Thus, there is finally a working animal model of AD, and attempts to discover how to arrest the disease process are proceeding apace.

For much of this century, the issue of whether amyloid fragments were a cause or an effect of the AD process has been hotly contested. The discovery of the amyloid gene and the causal mutations for at least one form of AD, as well as the reproduction of key neuropathologic and more recently neuropsychological findings in transgenic mice, have greatly increased confidence that long β-amyloid plays a decisive role in the biochemical cascade leading to the process of cell death in AD. Whether there are other and independent causes of this disease is still unknown.

The breakthrough regarding this issue came in 1995, when Peter St. George-Hyslop and his colleagues in Toronto discovered the presenilin 1 gene on chromosome 14, which probably accounts for the greatest number of cases of familial early-onset AD (Sherrington et al., 1995). Two discoveries led to publications about the presenilin 2 mutations. Within weeks, Hyslop's team (Rogaev et al., 1995) discovered an homologous gene on chromosome 1. Schellenberg's team (Levy-Lahad et al., 1995), had already linked the locus for familial AD in Volga German pedigrees to chromosome 1. Both teams used Hyslop's sequence for the S182 gene to find the homologous gene on chromosome 1; and the results were published in *Nature* and *Science*, respectively, in August 1995. Since then, several groups have convincingly shown that transgenic animals with mutations in the presenilin genes experience excess production of long β-amyloid even before there are any symptoms of disease (Citron et al. 1997).

The issues now hinge on the intermediate steps between the presenilin mutations and the excess production of β-amyloid, and how the excess production of β-amyloid in the brain causes cellular damage. There still remain some kindreds with early-onset AD that are not caused by known mutations on chromosome 21, 14, or 1. Knowledge of the existing genetic defects may, however, suffice to define final common pathways (Lippa et al. 1996)—if these are based on aberrant β-amyloid metabolism. Current interest centers on both extracellular (Barger and Harmon 1997) and intracellular (Yan et al. 1997) mechanisms of β-amyloid toxicity (see also Beyreuther and Masters 1997).

Late-Onset Alzheimer Disease

The early-onset cases of AD probably account for only 5–10 percent of total cases. With the risk essentially doubling every five years between ages 50 to 80, the population at risk for late-onset AD bears a heavy burden. This is especially true for those who develop the disease in their mid-60s to mid-70s when quality of life might otherwise be excellent. The discovery of Alan Roses's group (and the flood of confirming papers) that the apolipoprotein E4 allele increases the risk of late-onset AD by two- to threefold in heterozygotes and up to ninefold by age 80 in homozygotes is the breakthrough that has offered the greatest opportunity to modify the expression of late-onset AD (Roses 1996).

Most workers believe that this susceptibility factor modifies disease risk by interactions with β-amyloid. However, studies of the independent effects of the three major alleles of apoE continue. An understanding of the role of apoE and its relation to β-amyloid metabolism offers one of the greatest hopes for successful intervention in the majority of cases of late-onset AD. There are also unknown familial factors that account for the development of late-onset AD in the same age group, especially for those who develop the disease beyond their late 70s. There are recent reports that a second susceptibility gene for late-onset AD resides on chromosome 12 (Pericak-Vance et al. 1997). Moreover, the HLA-A2 allele on chromosome 6 may accelerate the age of onset of late-onset AD by several years, suggesting that an immune/inflammatory response mechanism may play a small but significant role in the pathogenesis of some types of AD (Payami et al. 1997).

Concepts of Alzheimer Disease

Thus, there are a number of genetic defects that cause AD on an autosomal dominant basis, and there are at least several genetic susceptibility factors that increase risk of AD. If we wish to emphasize the distinctions between the multiple molecular triggers that lead to AD, we might wish to refer to the disparate group as the "Alzheimer diseases." Should there be a final common pathway through which we may eventually intervene to treat, the inclusive term "Alzheimer disease" will remain justified.

Formerly, many workers classified AD as either "familial" or "sporadic," with the latter designation applying most often to elderly victims with no apparent family history. However, with people living longer and with family predisposition and genetic susceptibility factors for late-onset AD becoming increasingly evident, I have chosen to adhere to an "early-onset" versus "late-onset" classification scheme. This dichotomy fits nicely with the genetic dichotomy that those familial cases that occur on an early-onset basis are generally attributable to autosomal dominant, largely fully penetrant genetic defects, whereas the late-onset cases are at least partially attributable to weaker genetic susceptibility factors. This is not to deny that when the sweep of molecular genetics has run its course there may still exist genetically unexplained cases that may then properly be called "sporadic."

PREDICTIVE GENETIC TESTING

The discovery of genetic defects that lead to early-onset AD on a virtually fully penetrant autosomal dominant basis has made it possible for at-risk members of families with known mutations to undertake predictive testing in the asymptomatic phase. Screening tests for the presenilin mutations are also now commercially available for at-risk members of families whose defective genes have not yet been identified. Moreover, when a genetic defect has been identified in a given family, couples have the option for prenatal testing. Of the 30–40 family members at risk for presenilin 1 in two large kindreds that I have followed for over a decade, no one has opted for prenatal testing; only one at-risk member has elected predictive testing. In general, most people simply do not want to know the results of genetic tests until there is treatment for the disease.

PREIMPLANTATION TESTING

The recent successful development of preimplantation testing and *in vitro* fertilization, on the other hand, has created further opportunities and dilemmas for such at-risk family members. The procedure works as follows. Ova are harvested and fertilized by the husband's sperm. At the four-cell stage, one cell is removed for genetic testing. If the mutation in a given family is known, the extracted cell can be tested for the presence or absence of that mutation, using PCR techniques and known primers for the specific mutation. Only embryos that are free of the mutation are then implanted. Thus in theory, no one who carries a known gene for familial AD need reproduce a similarly affected child. The Genetics and IVF Institute in Fairfax, Virginia, is willing to assure prospective parents that the embryo will be free of the mutation — whether or not the at-risk parent knows or wishes to know his or her own genetic status (Schulman et al. 1996). Such techniques were first developed for X-linked disorders, proved applicable for pre-implantation testing in Huntington disease, where the length of the relevant triplet repeat is estimated, and are available for members of families with early-onset AD when the familial defect is known.

There are, however, drawbacks and concerns. The odds of carrying an implanted embryo to term are much less than after a normal pregnancy. Roughly only one out of three pregnancies initiated by in vitro fertilization will reach term, even in healthy young mothers; the numbers are lower in older mothers, especially those with preexisting fertility or gynecological problems. Moreover, the procedure costs $10,000 for each attempted pregnancy. So far, none of the young couples at risk for the presenilin 1 mutation that I have followed have availed themselves of this opportunity, primarily because of the expense of the procedure. These large expenses come at a time when few young families have the economic resources to avail themselves of this opportunity. Yet the cost is low compared to the cost of more than $50,000 per year for nursing-home care of victims that may go on for years — even apart from the untold suffering of victims and their families. Should we encourage governments to provide low interest loans to young couples for preimplantation genetic testing that could be paid back when they are more financially secure?

The Interplay of Environmental Factors in Genetic Risk

At present, there is little evidence that environmental factors play much of a role in the age of onset, the course, or the severity of early-onset familial AD. However, the wide variation in the age of onset of victims with *late*-onset disease — sometimes even within the same family — who may be at special risk by virtue of their apoE genotype, creates opportunities to assess both polygenetic factors and environmental impact. Indeed, there are already studies suggesting that the apoE4 risk may be adversely affected by a high serum total cholesterol and its highly correlated LDL component (Jarvik et el. 1995). Other studies confirm that there may be an interaction between apoE and the risk factors for atherosclerosis in the etiology of AD (Hofman et al. 1997). Moreover, there are a number of studies that suggest that estrogen replacement therapy in women (Henderson et al. 1994; Paganini-Hill and Henderson 1994), prior use of nonsteroidal anti-inflammatory drugs (Breitner 1996), and exposure to tobacco products (presumably the nicotine) (Graves et al. 1991) may decrease the risk of AD.

According to the epidemiological studies of Lindsay Farrer and colleagues (Farrer et al. 1995; Rao et al. 1996), the disproportionate burden of late-onset AD for the female appears to fall on those who inherit one copy of the apoE4 allele. Women who are homozygous for the neutral apoE3 allele have roughly the same increased risk for late-onset AD as age-matched males. Although the recent studies of the decreased risk of AD in women on estrogen replacement therapy are not yet decisive, they offer substantial promise. It would be of great interest to know whether the putative protective effect is greater in women who are heterozygous for apoE4. As the mechanism of action of the various genes becomes better known, we will expect epidemiological clues to play a progressively greater role in the design of rational therapy.

In conclusion, as scientists, we may be justifiably proud of the progress made since Alois Alzheimer's seminal paper in 1907, especially with respect to the importance of genetic factors in the pathogenesis of AD. As physicians who still have little to offer our patients in terms of treatment, however, we must remain humble.

References

Barger, D. W., and A. D. Harmon. 1997. Microglial activation by Alzheimer amyloid precursor protein and modulation by apolipoprotein E. *Nature* 388:878–81.

Beyreuther, K., and C. L. Masters. 1997. The ins and outs of amyloid-β. *Nature* 389:677.

Bick, K., L. Amaducci, and G. Pepeu, eds. 1987. *The Early Story of Alzheimer's Disease*. Padua: Lavonia Press; New York: Raven Press.

Breitner, J. C. S. 1996. The role of anti-inflammatory drugs in the prevention and treatment of Alzheimer's disease. *Annu Rev Med* 47:401–11.

Citron, M., D. Westaway, X. Weiming, G. Carlson, T. Diehl, G. Levesque, K. Johnson-Wood, M. Lee, P. Seubert, A. Davis, D. Kholodenko, R. Motter, R. Sherrington, B. Perry, H. Yao, R. Strome, I. Leiberburg, J. Rommens, S. Kim, D. Schenk, P. Fraser, P. St. George-Hyslop, and D. J. Selkoe. 1997. Mutant presenilins of Alzheimer's disease increase production of 42-residue amyloid β-protein in both transfected cells and transgenic mice. *Nature Medicine* 3(1): 67–72.

Farrer, L. A., L. A. Cupples, C. M. van Duijn, A. Kuirz, R. Zimmer, U. Muller, R. C. Green, V. Clarke, J. Shoffner, and D. C. Wallace. 1995. Apolipoprotein

E genotype in patients with Alzheimer's disease: Implications for the risk of dementia among relatives. *Annals of Neurology* 38(5): 797–808.

Graves, A. B., C. M. van Duijn, V. Chandra, L. Fratiglioni, A. Heyman, A. F. Jorm, E. Kokmen, K. Kondo, J. A. Mortimer, W. Rocca et al. 1991. Alcohol and tobacco consumption as risk factors for Alzheimer's disease: A collaborative re-analysis of case-control studies. *International Journal of Epidemiology* 20(2): S48–57.

Henderson, V. W., A. Paganini-Hill, C. K. Emanuel, M. Dunn, and G. Buckwalter. 1994. Estrogen replacement therapy in older women. *Arch Neurol* 51:896–900.

Hofman, A., A. Ott, M. M. B. Breteler, M. L. Bots, A. J. C. Slooter, F. van Harskamp, C. N. van Duijn, C. Van Broeckhoven, D. E. Grobbee. 1997. Atherosclerosis, apolipoprotein E, and prevalence of dementia and Alzheimer's disease in the Rotterdam Study. *Lancet* 349:151–54.

Jarvik, G. P., E. M. Wijsman, W. A. Kukull, G. D. Schellenberg, C. Yu, and E. B. Larson. 1995. Interactions of apolipoprotein E genotype, total cholesterol level, age, and sex in prediction of Alzheimer's disease: A case-control study. *Neurology* 45:1092–96.

Levy-Lahad, E., W. Wasco, P. Poorkaj, D. M. Romano, J. Oshima, W. H. Pettingell, C. Yu, P. D. Jondro, S. D. Schmidt, K. Wang, A. C. Crowley, Y.-H. Fu, S. Y. Guenette, D. Galas, E. Nemens, E. M. Wijsman, T. D. Bird, G. D. Schellenberg, and R. E. Tanzi. 1995. Candidate gene for the chromosome 1 familial Alzheimer's disease locus. *Science* 269:973–77.

Lippa, C. F., M. A. Saunders, T. W. Smith, J. M. Swearer, D. A. Drachman, B. Chetti, L. Nee, D. Pulaski-Salo, D. Dickson, Y. Robitaille, C. Bergeron, B. Crain, M. D. Benson, M. Farlow, B. T. Hyman, P. St. George-Hyslop, A. D. Roses, and D. A. Pollen. 1996. Familial and sporadic Alzheimer's disease: Neuropathology cannot exclude a final common pathway. *Neurology* 46:406–12.

Mayer-Gross, W. 1944. Recent progress in psychiatry, arteriosclerotic, senile and presenile dementia. *J Mental Science* 90:316–327.

Newton, R. D. 1948. The identity of Alzheimer's disease and senile dementia and their relationship to senility. *J Mental Science* 94:225–49.

Paganini-Hill, A., and V. W. Henderson. 1994. Estrogen deficiency and risk of Alzheimer's disease in women. *Am J Epidemiology* 140(3): 256.

Payami, H., G. D. Schellenberg, S. Zareparsi, J. Kaye, G. J. Sexton, M. A. Head, S. S. Matsuyama, L. F. Jarvik, B. Miller, D. Q. McManus, T. D. Bird, R. Katzman, L. Heston, D. Norman, and G. W. Small. 1997. Evidence for association of HLA-A2 allele with onset age of Alzheimer's disease. *Neurology* 49:512–18.

Pericak-Vance, M. A., M. P. Bass, L. H. Yamaoka, P. C. Gaskell, W. K. Scott, H. A. Terwedow, M. M. Menold, P. M. Conneally, G. W. Small, J. M. Vance, A. M. Saunders, A. D. Roses, and J. L. Haines. 1997. Complete genomic screen in late-onset familial Alzheimer disease: Evidence for a new locus on chromosome 12. *JAMA* 278(15): 1237–41.

Pollen, D. 1996. *Hannah's Heirs: The Quest for the Genetic Origins of Alzheimer's Disease.* Oxford University Press.

Rao, V. S., A. Cupples, C. M. van Duijn, A. Kurz, R. C. Green, H. Chui, R. Duara, S. A. Auerbach, L. Volicer, J. Wells, C. van Broeckhoven, J. H. Growdon, J. L. Haines, and L. A. Farrer. 1996. Evidence for major gene inheritance of Alzheimer disease in families of patients with and without apolipoprotein E 4. *Am J Hum Genet* 59:664–75.

Rogaev, E. I., R. Sherrington, E. A. Rogaeva, G. Levesque, M. Ikeda, Y. Liang, H. Chi, C. Lin, K. Holman, T. Tsuda, L. Mar, S. Sorbi, B. Nacmias, S. Placentini, L. Amaducci, I. Chumakov, D. Cohen, L. Lannfelt, P. E. Fraser, J. M. Rommens, and P. H. St. George-Hyslop. 1995. Familial Alzheimer's disease in kindreds with missense mutations in a gene on chromosome 1 related to the Alzheimer's disease Type 3 gene. *Nature* 376:775–78.

Roses, A. D. 1996. Apolipoprotein E alleles as risk factors in Alzheimer's disease. *Annu Rev Med* 47:387–400.

Schulman, J. D., S. H. Black, A. Handyside, and W. E. Nance. 1966. Preimplantation genetic testing for Huntington disease and certain other dominantly inherited disorders. *Clinical Genetics* 49:57–58.

Sherrington, R., E. I. Rogaev, Y. Liang, E. A. Rogaeva, G. Levesque, M. Ikeda, H. Chi, C. Lin, G. Li, K. Holman, T. Tsuda, L. Mar, J.-F. Foncin, A. C. Bruni, M. P. Montesi, S. Sorbi, I. Rainero, L. Pinessi, L. Nee, I. Chumakov, D. Pollen, A. Brookes, P. Sanseau, R. J. Polinsky, W. Wasco, H. A. R. Da Silva, J. Haines, M. A. Pericak-Vance, R. E. Tanzi, A. D. Roses, P. E. Fraser, J. M. Rommens, and P. H. St. George-Hyslop. 1995. Cloning of a gene bearing missense mutations in early-onset familial Alzheimer's disease. *Nature* 375: 754–60.

Yan, S. D., J. Fu, C. Soto, X. Chen, H. Zhu, F. Al-Mohanna, K. Collison, A. Zhu, E. Stern, T. Saido, M. Tohyamas, S. Ogawa, A. Roher, and D. Stern. 1997. An intracellular protein that binds amyloid-ß peptide and mediates neurotoxicity in Alzheimer's disease. *Nature* 389:689–95.

PART III

Alzheimer Disease as a Social and Cultural Entity

Social Construction. These two words succinctly evoke an intellectual battle that has raged over the meanings and boundaries of nature, society, and science in the modern world. Although the intellectual approaches to this problem are in fact quite diverse, the tendency of the combatants to engage in caricature makes it possible to speak as though there were two clearly defined and inevitably conflicting camps. On one side stand positivistic scientists and their allies, who assert that knowledge derived through scientific procedures and validated by the scientific community is pure knowledge, untainted by the social environment that surrounds it, and should thus be regarded as the authoritative account of nature. On the other side stand relativistic historians and social theorists, who assert that science is a social process like any other and that the knowledge it produces is always tainted by the ideological imperatives of the scientific community and should thus be regarded as no more authoritative than any other account of nature. Though most scholars recognize that these are caricatures, after two decades of what has been called "the science wars," in which these caricatures have too often been the central terms of debate, it has become difficult to approach these issues in any other way.

We suggest, along with a growing number of scholars, that it is time to abandon the starkly drawn battle lines of the "science wars" to create a middle ground where insights coming from many directions can provide a more satisfying account of what scientific concepts tell us about the natural world, our society, and ourselves. The chapters in this section will suggest ways in which constructivist studies can contribute to a better understanding of the concept of Alzheimer disease (AD).

The essential difference between scientific studies and constructivist studies of science lies in their respective objects of inquiry. While the scientist follows a series of elaborate social, intellectual, and technological procedures in order to make some aspect of the natural world a fit object for investigation, the constructivist takes those procedures as the very object of inquiry. While the scientist works to erect walls between the prejudices of the social world and the field of scientific observation, the constructivist analyzes the means by which these walls have been erected, questions whether they are as solid as the scientist believes, and watches carefully as the scientist moves between the supposed sanctity of those walls and the larger society. Sociologist Bruno Latour distinguishes between "ready-made science" and "science in action." Where the scientist presents science as a "ready-made" finished product, making the steps taken along the way appear to follow an inevitable logic, the constructivist scholar presents science "in action," showing how each step along the way was problematic and fraught with contingency (Latour 1987).

But a critical perspective need not be an inherently hostile one. Most constructivist work evinces respect for scientific work on its own terms but seeks a more satisfying account of that work than is typically offered by the scientist. Constructivist accounts have seldom set out to impugn the integrity of scientists or to question the validity of scientific knowledge as scientific knowledge. They recognize that scientists must primarily be concerned with science, not with its social construction. Researchers are trying to create valid scientific knowledge and ultimately to find useful treatments for AD — a task that understandably precludes intensive inquiries concerning the philosophy and sociology of scientific knowledge. Nonetheless, constructivist approaches can contribute much to an understanding of the way the concept of AD has evolved and how it is situated in a broader social and cultural context. This more nuanced account can, in turn, help to decide the sorts of knowledge that should be pursued in the future. Thus, while critical approaches to scientific knowledge about AD should not be regarded as inherently hostile to the goals of scientists, the insights they contribute should provide an important critical perspective on the agenda for future research.

Constructivist accounts can further the understanding of the concept of AD in at least three ways. First and most obviously, constructivist accounts can help us to better understand the process of creating knowledge about AD and, more fundamentally, how it is we have come to talk about disease at all when confronting this puzzling condition. Rob Dillmann's chapter illustrates this sort of contribution. Trained in both clinical medicine and the philosophy of medicine, Dillmann describes the epistemological difficulties inherent in the concept of disease in general and AD in particular, and cautions against the "rationalist fallacy" of mistaking ideas for reality. Concepts of disease are more than simple observations and descriptions of an ontological entity; they are rational constructions that link together the relevant and exclude the irrelevant from an overwhelmingly complex constellation of potential evidence in order to create knowledge that can be used by clinicians and researchers. Dillmann examines the original concept of AD by Alzheimer and Kraepelin, the conceptual unification of AD and senile dementia in the 1960s, and the development of the cholinergic hypothesis in the late 1970s, showing how each of these conceptualizations required an element of metaphysical conjecture in order to construct a workable and useful concept of AD. These metaphysical conjectures are not to be deplored, Dillmann asserts; for they have served a crucial heuristic strategy for organizing research. But they also carry important consequences that should not go unexamined if we are to understand fully the limits and potential of our knowledge about AD.

Second, constructivist accounts can enrich our understanding by drawing attention to the wider social and cultural context in which scientific knowledge is created. Martha Holstein shows that scientific concepts of AD have always been embedded in a broader cultural framework. The relationship between aging, senile dementia, and AD has been a thorny conceptual problem from Alois Alzheimer's time to our own. Holstein shows that researchers have always engaged that problem from within the framework of dominant cultural attitudes and social expectations toward aging. Though the evidence in favor of differentiating between AD and senile dementia was highly equivocal, this became the accepted view by the 1920s, in large part because it was consistent with broadly held ideas about the effects of aging. Approaching the problem from a cultural framework that expected some degree of mental deterioration in old age, physicians interpreted dementing symptoms in a 70-year-old much differently than similar symptoms in a 50-year-old. The former was only an accentuation of changes that were expected with aging, while the latter was clearly abnormal. Such assumptions, Holstein shows, have been at the center of psychiatric concepts of dementia throughout the twentieth century.

Finally, constructivist accounts of the concept of AD can remind us that concepts of AD are not timelessly relevant and true, but are useful and true only in particular cultural contexts, for particular social and intellectual purposes, and according to a particular set of socially constituted authorities. These contexts can be thought of as local rather than national or global, as Jaber F. Gubrium shows in his chapter. Gubrium describes how AD was conceptualized in the particular context of caregiver support groups in the 1980s. Gubrium is interested in the way these groups used narratives of their own experience as caregivers to construct useful and satisfying concepts of the inner worlds of both the person suffering from AD and the caregiver. In so doing, these groups helped define and expand a cultural space for a new disease entity by constructing its concrete, everyday reality. Concepts of the disease as articulated by professionals were not always relevant for this purpose; indeed, it was occasionally asserted in these groups that professionals understood little about the ordinary experience of the disease. While scientific concepts of AD learned through encounters with professionals and in the public culture of AD were a resource for caregivers' narratives, they hardly dominated them. To a large extent, the local culture of each group constituted its own authority, an authority rooted in the experience of each caregiver as constructed through personal stories of everyday experience with the disease. Gubrium's work thus shows that to understand the concept of AD, we need to look beyond the discourses of biomedicine — an insight that will be the focus of the next section of this book, which concerns the perspective of patients and caregivers.

Reference

Latour, B. 1987. *Science in Action: How to Follow Scientists and Engineers Through Society.* Cambridge: Harvard University Press.

8

Alzheimer Disease

Epistemological Lessons from History?

Rob J. M. Dillmann

In analyzing the history of Alzheimer disease (AD), two approaches can be taken. First, one can focus on the consecutive *events* and the *agents* that brought them about. This is important in order to know what happened and who was involved. In this general approach two focuses can be distinguished. The first is a focus on the mainstream, the flow of history, which always looks better — and logical — with hindsight. The second focus is on (necessary) conditions, contingencies, and what I usually call "socio-logical" processes. Although this chapter does not consist of a description of consecutive events, at some points it will be clear that I use the second focus regarding the history of AD. In this sense, my view could be described as moderately "constructivist" (see Latour 1987, 1988).

The second approach does not primarily concern events and agents, but instead concerns *concepts, ideas, and hypotheses*. As such, this approach is at odds with most of the contemporary constructivist analyses of science, which deem concepts to be secondary to the socio-logical processes that work in history. In this chapter, however, concepts, ideas, and hypotheses will be central — especially the concept of disease. Many of the misunderstandings, loops, and mishaps in the history of AD cannot be understood without knowledge of the ways in which clinicians and researchers tried, through the concept of disease, to impose some order on the empirical observations they made. In this approach it is not enough to focus on particular theories concerning, for instance, the pathogenesis of AD. One should especially focus one's attention to the concept of AD as the central category by which patients and disease processes are identified by researchers.

In this chapter I analyze the characteristics of the concept of AD, distinguishing among its three main types. These types coincide quite well with particular periods. The first is the Kraepelinian concept of neuropsychiatric disease, which permeates the early concept of AD. The second is the syndromal concept, introduced in the 1970s and 1980s, in which psychiatric diagnosis tried to free itself from a narrow somatic interpretation of psychiatric disorders. The third is the concept of disease used within the context of the "cholinergic hypothesis." These analyses outline the advantages of using "Alzheimer disease" as a concept, as well as the risks and disadvantages.

The history of AD is complex in many ways. It combines several clinical, scientific, social, and epistemological problems into one particular story. As such, it is an illustration of all the difficulties involved in the acquisition of biomedical knowledge (i.e., knowledge concerning individuals, diseases, and the possibilities for intervention in the disease processes). Which problems and difficulties can be distinguished? The first problem is the delineation of the biological processes underlying a psychiatric disorder. As such, AD was born in the middle of the "mind-brain problem." Second, AD had to be distinguished from the processes of aging. Concepts such as senile psychosis, which preceded AD and senile dementia, indicate that this process was not easy. Third, AD encompasses, as do most diseases, an enormous number of empirical observations based on many different tools of observation. These tools range from "simple" observations of the behavior of patients, to PET and MRI scans, to DNA-markers — and all that lies in between. How can all these findings be integrated into one plausible pathogenetic concept?

I believe that there are several epistemological points that must be identified. The first is a phenomenon that can be observed quite often and might be called "the rationalist fallacy": the tendency to take ideas for realities. A metaphysical element is present in most scientific conjectures, and it is no different in AD research. This is not something to be condemned, but it is something to be reckoned with. In AD research, this phenomenon has played a role at several moments in history: when Alzheimer was coloring his specimen to "show" the metabolic processes; when "focal symptoms" were considered to be pivotal in the clinical distinction; when AD was coined as a "cholinergic disease."

The second point concerns the complex task of integrating the whole complex of AD-related knowledge into an intelligible whole. In this process, the concept of "Alzheimer disease" — that is, the conjecture that there exists a disease that can be known and investigated in its own right — has been critical. In this respect, the general use of the term *Alzheimer disease* can be interpreted as a so-called ontological concept of disease, implying that disease exists as a natural entity. It can be maintained, however, that the use of this term served as an important and useful heuristic strategy with, unfortunately, important side effects. The potential influence of these side effects can be assessed more clearly if we shed some light on concepts of disease in general.

CONCEPTS OF DISEASE

The obvious is rarely questioned. This is also true for one of the core concepts of medicine, the concept of disease, which is a useful, but not very reliable tool for patients, doctors, and researchers from different disciplines. It is used in various contexts, as illustrated by the concept of AD. It is therefore useful to distinguish at least a few different meanings of the concept of disease. Two questions are useful in guiding this discussion: On what grounds do we usually distinguish between healthy persons and diseased persons, or normal and diseased biochemical processes? And, provided we can distinguish between the two, on what grounds do we conjecture that the changes ("disease process") that cause the symptoms in one patient are identical to those in another patient? Labeling a person as "having a disease" that is the same as that of another person supposes both epistemological problems to have been solved.

The distinction between disease as a concept, a theoretical conjecture, and an object or a natural entity, is essential. Although the common everyday use of the term *disease* suggests that we can speak about it and manipulate it as if it were a natural entity (such as the everyday use of concepts such as "time" or "gravitational force"), in effect what we are doing is taking an idea or Kantian categorization into reality. This was what happened to Alzheimer as he was peering through his Zeiss microscope to identify the pathological processes in his histologic specimen.

A second distinction that is useful in this respect is between two general approaches to the causes of disease: generalism and externalism (Fried and Agassi 1983). The externalist view holds that all diseases can be distinguished on the basis of an identifiable cause. The generalist view is that disease is interwoven into an organism struggling to regain equilibrium, and that therefore it cannot be identified clearly. The recurrent debate in the field of genetics is a good example. Some diseases can be clearly associated with particular mutations in one gene, whereas others seem to be the result of complex interactions between genes, gene products, and external pathogens such as viruses or toxins. The genetics of AD is a more specific example of these two views.

The most generally applicable definition of disease as a concept can be found in Engelhardt's work (1981). The general background of his view is that diseases cannot be encountered as natural phenomena that are subject to taxonomy, like plants and animals. His approach underlines the normative elements in definitions of disease and is neatly summarized in this quotation:

> Diseases are, in fact not only multifactorial, but multidimensional, involving genetic, physiological, and sociological components. The presence of the various components does not merely entail a superimposition of modifying variables upon these basic structures. Rather it implies that diseases have a basically relational, not a subject (i.e., substance)-predicate (i.e., accident) nature. That is, there is not necessarily a bearer for every disease, a substrate for each type of disease. . . . The result is a multidimensional concept of disease with each dimension — genetic, infectious, metabolic, psychological, and social — containing a nexus of causes bounded by their appropriate, usually different, nomological structures. (Engelhardt 1981, 37–38)

This multidimensional approach to disease leaves open, however, the problem of creating sufficient observational reliability within a particular dimension — such as the realm of clinical symptoms. This came about in psychiatry along quite different lines, which will be discussed below.

Nevertheless, Engelhardt's description makes clear that several steps are involved in addressing disease. The first is to distinguish between a *thing* and a *concept.* Clearly, disease is a concept or conjecture that guides the general way of reasoning in the biomedical sciences (i.e., that phenomena demonstrated by groups of people have identical and identifiable causes).

The second is to realize that several types of disease concepts can be distinguished. Engelhardt's is one of them. Another example is the concept developed by Boorse (1977), which implies that disease is to be understood as a statistical deviation from an empirically established "species design."

The third step is to define the level of specific pathogenetic theories of particular diseases. At this level, the distinction between generalist and externalist theories can be made as a general distinction among pathogenetic theories. This is also the level of the distinction between infectious, genetic, environmental, and other diseases.

These distinctions must be kept in mind in addressing AD, which can be understood as a collection of historical concepts. In addition, there have been many rival pathogenetic theories. In addressing the concepts that were dominant during particular periods, all of these distinctions are relevant and must be kept in mind.

THE KRAEPELINIAN CONCEPT OF ALZHEIMER DISEASE

It is generally agreed that AD was mentioned for the first time at a meeting of psychiatrists and neuropathologists in Tübingen on November 3 and 4, 1906. Alzheimer reported a case study of a patient with some remarkable findings. His patient, a 51-year-old woman, showed "early clinical symptoms which deviated from the common ones and could not be classified under any well-known clinical pattern. The anatomical patterns were also different from those of the usual disease processes" (Alzheimer 1907; translation in Bick 1987).

The first symptoms consisted of strong jealousy; the patient accused her husband of having several affairs. Shortly thereafter, she experienced disturbances in her ability to memorize and to recall events. During her stay in a mental institution, she became totally helpless and disoriented in time and place. Furthermore, she suffered from delirium and auditory hallucinations, focal symptoms, and disturbances in perception. During autopsy, changes considered to be specific were found, especially when Bielschowsky silver stain was used on brain tissue:

> Inside an apparently normal looking cell, one or more single fibers could be observed that became prominent through their striking thickness and specific impregnability. At a more advanced stage, many fibrils arranged parallel showed the same changes. Then they accumulated, forming dense bundles and gradually advanced to the surface of the cell. Eventually the nucleus and cytoplasm disappeared, and only a tangled bundle of fibrils indicated the site where once the neuron had been located. As these fibrils can be stained with dyes different from the normal neurofibrils, a chemical transformation of the fibril substance must have taken place. This might be the reason why the fibrils survived the destruction of the cell. It seems that the transformation of the fibrils goes hand in hand with the storage of an as-yet-not-closely examined pathological product of the metabolism in the neuron. (Alzheimer 1907)

The history of AD starts with these lines. Several conditions for this "takeoff" are worth mentioning, however. The first is the presence of institutionalized care, which incorporated systematic assessment and follow-up of the patients. This process began with Kraepelin's clinic in Heidelberg (see Berrios and Hauser 1988) and enabled Kraepelin to develop his system of clinical classification, which included links with the course and outcomes of patients. Although the first reported patient was cared for by Sioli, the teacher whom Alzheimer worked under in Frankfurt until 1902, it is quite clear that the systematic approach in Kraepelin's clinic favored the delineation of new disease entities. This is particularly true for Perusini's publication, which was used (in its un-published form) by Kraepelin for his "canonical" statement concerning the existence of AD in the eighth edition of his *Psychiatrie* (Kraepelin 1909/1910, 624–28; Perusini 1910).

The second relevant condition was the presence of histology as a reliable instrument for observation. In the second half of the nineteenth century, German industry demonstrated a remarkable growth that stim-ulated German science. Zeiss's development of the apochromatic mi-croscope and the development of a large number of synthetic dyes sup-ported the founding of histology.

The third condition is the conceptualization of psychiatric disease such as that developed by Kraepelin. This condition requires more de-tailed attention.

Kraepelin's Concept of Psychiatric Disease

The concept of AD has a clear historical context. In this context, three problems were essential: (1) the relationship between psychiatric symptoms and disease processes in the brain (i.e., the mind-brain dis-tinction); (2) the identification of disease entities or clinical symptom patterns; and (3) the identification of the tissue processes responsible for the disease.

Kraepelin's viewpoints concerning psychiatric disease clearly changed during the sixty years of his career. Furthermore, they are by no means as "reductionistic" or "Linnean" as has often been suggested. Initially, Kraepelin adhered to Griesinger's symptomatologic viewpoint (without accepting Griesinger's "Einheitspsychose"). He subsequently shifted from a symptomatologic approach to a clinical approach, in which the actual clinical symptom complex as well as the etiology, course, and outcome of mental disease were pivotal for the establish-ment of "Krankheitseinheiten" (Kraepelin 1896). Finally, at the end of his career, he denounced the concept of "Krankheitseinheiten" and suggested that mental disease was expressed in three main clinical forms ("die Erscheinungsformen des Irreseins") (Kraepelin 1920).

The 1896 Kraepelinian concept of disease had several features that were quite relevant for understanding both the establishment of AD and the nosological confusion that would characterize its history in the twentieth century.

1. Kraepelin understood the relationship between mind and brain in the sense of parallelism. Although the precise relationship between the functions of the brain and psychic functions is not known, Kraepelin presumed it was "law-like." In 1887 he compared the nature of the object of psychiatry with the two faces of Janus (Kraepelin 1887, 4).

2. The existence of mental disease provided the best opportunity to study the parallelism between mind and brain. Establishing discrete, well-defined disease entities was crucial.

3. Kraepelin emphasized that the explanation of mental disease had to be found in the brain and its functions, which were to be approached by neuropathology, physiology, and (experimental) psychology. Nevertheless, Kraepelin kept using the term "mental disease" (*Geisteskrankheit*).

4. Given the absence of empirical knowledge of brain pathology, Kraepelin emphasized that the delineation of mental disease should be attempted clinically. He felt that clinical observation was the only way to establish clinical pictures (*Krankheitsbilder*) and to relate psychic and physical disturbances to each other (Kraepelin 1883, 12; 1896, 5).

In 1887 Kraepelin introduced important additional criteria for the establishment of mental disease: etiology, course, and outcome (including autopsy).

Kraepelin and Alzheimer Disease

Kraepelin coined the term "Alzheimer's disease" in 1910, based on the four cases used in Perusini's 1910 publication. Perusini's paper included the case used by Alzheimer in his 1907 publication (Kraepelin 1910, 624–28). The cases were mentioned under the heading *Altersblödsinn*, best translated as 'senile dementia,' but were also assigned a somewhat special position. Kraepelin considered the clinical phenomena demonstrated in these cases to be quite different from those of senile dementia and suggested that they were related to the presenile diseases.

Alzheimer himself was not so sure. The case he presented in 1911 did not show neurofibrillary tangles, and the plaques (*miliaire Herdchen*,

Drusen) were interpreted as a concomitant change, rather than the cause of the dementia. His conclusion was based on the observation that the changes could be very small, even in patients with severe disturbances, while the plaques themselves displace, not infiltrate, the brain tissues. His final conclusion dismissed the hypothesis of the separate existence of "Alzheimer disease" completely:

> There is then no tenable reason to consider these cases as caused by a specific disease process. *They are senile psychoses, atypical forms of senile dementia.* Nevertheless they do assume a certain separate position, so that one has to know of their existence as one has to know of Lissauer's paralysis, in order to avoid misdiagnosis. (Alzheimer 1911, 378; translation by Förstl and Levy 1991)

These statements were the start of a controversy that lasted about seventy years and focused on two questions. First, is AD identical with, or a type of, senile dementia? Second, is senile dementia a disease, or is it the result of "senile involution" or "plain aging"?

Kraepelin's proclamation of Alzheimer disease seems peculiar. Alzheimer, one of the neuropathologists Kraepelin convinced to work in the laboratories of his clinic and himself a prestigious researcher (especially because of his work on general paralysis, published in 1904), was not able to distinguish the histologic picture of the aforementioned cases from the picture of senile dementia. Still, Kraepelin declares the existence of AD. This declaration is very obvious, not hidden somewhere in the thousands of pages of the eighth edition of his textbook. "Alzheimer's disease" appears in the table of contents, which was in fact Kraepelin's classification system. Kraepelin's arguments supporting AD as a separate entity are interesting. First, he cites the age of the patients. Second, he notes the peculiar clinical picture: language disturbances, "fits" and spastic movements (focal signs), and severe dementia.

Age was generally considered to be a parameter in disease classifications. Each period of life had its own diseases and/or disease manifestations. Kraepelin acknowledged age as a predisposition for different types of disease, and mental disease in elderly people was mentioned as a different category in his textbooks (Kraepelin 1896, 1898, 1910). If AD had been accepted as a form of senile dementia, it would have violated the age-specific categorization of the disorder — that is, senile dementia would have to be known as a disease that could affect nonsenile persons under the age of 65. By designating AD as a separate disease, the question of whether senile dementia is a disease entity to be distinguished from aging was avoided. Thus, it is likely that the specific position of AD in Kraepelin's textbook was inspired by convenience.

The second argument Kraepelin offered concerned the specific clinical picture. This argument was consistent with the early Kraepelinian viewpoint concerning the delineation of mental disease, which emphasized a clinical approach and the search for essential signs. The patient in question was reported to illustrate a clinical picture that had not been observed previously, including the existence of "focal signs." Moreover, Kraepelin was informed about the course (rapidly progressive) and the outcome of the condition (death, with peculiar changes observed in autopsy). The combination of clinical and neuropathological changes that occurred in the course of the disease perhaps convinced Kraepelin that it was possible to delineate this condition without being led astray.[1]

Disease and Aging

From the beginning, the history of AD has been pervaded by debates regarding the difference between aging and senile dementia on one hand, and between senile dementia and AD on the other. In 1910 Simchowicz—a co-worker of Alzheimer and Nissl—argued that the distinction between aging (*das normale Senium*) and disease (*Dementia senilis*) is not possible on clear clinical or pathological grounds. The presumed abnormality is thus transferred to the pathological stimulation of a normal process. In that way, both the "normal" physiological processes of aging (*normal* is used in a statistical sense to mean something that happens to most people) and the "pathological" pivot are safeguarded (Simchowicz 1911, 425). Simchowicz's nosologic viewpoint as well as his opinions on aging and senile dementia are similar to those of Fischer, working in the laboratory of Pick in Prague (Fischer 1907, 1910).[2]

Nevertheless, we have two problems: (1) The aging process itself demands a different operationalization of normality. What is a normal or "physiological" involutionary process? (2) The classical medical question concerning the difference between normality and pathology remains. Where does Simchowicz draw the line between "physiological" and "pathological" aging? At what level is the speeding up of the aging process pathological? Simchowicz tried to transfer the unanswerable question of first-order normality (aging is not disease) to the domain of second-order normality (accelerated aging is pathology). But he did not answer the question in the second-order domain.

The main line of the argument is remarkably clear. AD is considered to be an atypical form of senile dementia. In combination with Kraepelin's remarks referring to senile dementia, the ambiguous relationship with normal aging becomes clear: "In the most serious cases, the psychological alterations of old age result in the disease patterns of dementia. The main feature of this disease consists of a gradually developing particular psychological weakness, in which perception and memory impairments appear as the most characteristic symptoms. The perception of external impressions becomes more error-prone and slowed" (Kraepelin 1910, 594; translation in Bick et al. 1987).

It is illuminating to consider a contemporary example of the discussion — a discussion between Evans and Katzman concerning the relationship between AD and aging published in CIBA Foundation Symposium 134. Evans suggests that the concept of disease, as used in medicine, can be unhelpful when used to distinguish between normal aging and disease. It fosters a dichotomous way of dealing with problems that could better be replaced by a model emphasizing interaction between intrinsic and extrinsic factors. Since aging processes are at the moment out of scientific reach, the study of "age-associated phenomena" should be performed without preconceived notions about their origins. Evans thus suggests that aging research be reframed in an empirical context without an a priori distinction between aging phenomena and disease phenomena (Evans 1988). Katzman, an AD pioneer, reacts like this:

> Let me challenge your view that the traditional distinction between the concepts of "disease" and "normal aging" is misguided. I have spent a number of years trying to persuade people that Alzheimer's Disease is a disease, and not simply what used to be called "senility" or "Senile dementia": and there has been marvelous progress in research. In my view, this is because people now consider Alzheimer's as a disease. Clearly, environmental factors contribute, but I have been unable to establish that any change after the disease begins, related to any obvious environmental factor, has anything to do with the course of Alzheimer's. It seems to be biologically driven. (Katzman, in Evans 1988, 47)

Katzman seems to defend the position Kraepelin took in 1910 — that AD is a particular disease, that it is not identical with aging or senile dementia. Evans, however, takes the position of Alzheimer — that AD is not a separate entity but is a phenomenon (or a cluster of phenomena) that can be observed in a (large) minority of elderly people.

The aging of all living beings is, in fact, an anthropological theme that finds a particular form in research, diagnosis, and treatment (or support) of patients with a diagnosis of AD. The relationship between aging and AD is complicated and varied: (1) The incidence of AD is exponentially related to the age of the population (Katzman 1988a). As life expectancy increases, the number of AD patients increases to the extent that it has been called a "major killer" (Katzman 1976). (2) Most of the phenomena that can be observed in AD can also be observed in the very old, and their number increases with age. (3) The neuropathological diagnosis of AD is age-dependent (Khachaturian 1985). (4) According to some authors, the difference between "normal" aging and AD is arbitrary (Katzman, Terry, and Bick 1978; Evans 1988; Roth, Tomlinson, and Blessed 1967; Roth 1986).

The combination of the concepts of aging and disease in research apparently contributes to a confusing situation. However, some of the issues can be clarified. It must be kept in mind that there are several causes for the differences observed between young and old contemporaries that could be mistakenly interpreted as phenomena of aging: (a) Differential survival: those who reach high ages may be different from those who die earlier. The group that survives to grow old may represent a positive selection of the original cohort. Therefore, there is a chance that older and younger people differ because the older people are relatively more "fit." (b) Cohort effects: differences between young and old could be caused by differences in the circumstances of their lives, such as education, habits, environmental changes, and other sociocultural characteristics. (c) Differential challenge: older people are confronted with different and relatively more severe challenges. These might account for differences from younger people (Evans 1988).

All people change and become old as time passes. The changes are obvious and compromise all bodily functions and structures. They are general, gradual, irreversible, and usually unfavorable. Thus, it seems as if aging has both descriptive and normative components.

The descriptive component suggests that we start looking for the biological mechanisms that cause the phenomena described as aging. We must, however, be cautious here. Where and when do the differences we observe between people become known as "aging"? When we compare younger and older people, or compare ourselves with our memories and pictures, the observed differences are also related to another difference: the amount of time between the first and second observation.

If aging consists of differences in the body expressed in relation to time, we should use the term "mechanisms of change" rather than "mechanisms of aging" (difference in relation to time is change). The measurement of change and the evaluation of these changes combine to become the phenomenon of "aging." Thus, there is no need to refer to mechanisms that "cause aging," because aging is what we use to characterize differences in the first place. The research that addressed mechanisms that are responsible for these differences can be investigated and may be explained, but not as mechanisms that are responsible for aging. They can be viewed as mechanisms that are responsible for changes in people, changes that are summarized as "aging."

What conclusions can be drawn from this? The concept of disease is a useful tool to demarcate a particular domain of observation. The remainder belongs to the domain of aging. In the previous section, however, we hypothesized that the meanings inherent in the concept of aging do not include a descriptive component. The central point was that aging refers to changes in organisms — that is, differences that occur in the course of time. The concept of disease also addresses differences in organisms. In this case, however, the accent is on the differences between different people at a particular moment of observation. Thus, aging is *diachronic*, and disease is *synchronic*.

The people observed to be in the upper tail of the empirical distribution are taken to be instances of AD. Yet, they ended up in this range through a gradual process in time. Heston's data indicate that people can be divided according to the behavior of this process in time — that is, its moment of onset (Heston et al. 1981) We do not know whether the process differs too. It does seem that an earlier age of expression is associated with accelerated progression. Should we understand these differences as "differences in aging?" If we use *aging* in the sense of the time scale, we ought to say that people who demonstrate these phenomena ("aging changes") earlier in life, are aging prematurely. If we compare the changes they exhibit with those of the general population, we might say that the aging process is more intensive. These changes could be understood as "changes of disease" if we pointed out that these people will, to a very large extent, express Alzheimer's changes, whereas most of the others will not. We may conjecture, for instance, that these differences are related to a particular genetic constitution.

In fact, both viewpoints share the observation that changes in organisms over time ("aging") occur in the group of people that is evaluated as being different and the group that is considered to be normal. Thus, biological processes result in changes within organisms; the probability that an organism will exhibit a particular range of these changes might be increased by a particular genetic constitution.

The conclusion is that aging and disease are conceptually different. *Aging* refers to differences that develop over time. *Disease* refers to differences in states of organisms that are considered to be the result of a particular biological mechanism. Another conceptualization provides a new picture. A particular biological background — a combination of genetic makeup, forthcoming biological mechanisms, and environmental strains upon these mechanisms — can influence the function that expresses the relationship between differences in observation and time. One could demarcate such a background as "disease." Yet the process of changing in time is still present in this particular group of people: one can age and end up in the category of AD.[3]

The "age-dependency" of AD is true in an empirical sense: the incidence of AD is related to the age of people. But that observation does not warrant the statement that AD *depends* on age. Age is an instrument by which we compare people; it does not belong in the realm of biological causes. AD phenomena differ quantitatively from other phenomena observed in the elderly. There might, however, be distinctive biological causes that influence the moment of occurrence and the amount of these changes.

THE NEO-KRAEPELINIAN CONCEPT OF ALZHEIMER DISEASE

The question of whether AD (or senile dementia) was a disease or was caused by aging was accompanied for decades by great difficulties in the process of clinical diagnosis. As indicated before, this had something to do with the Kraepelinian concept of "focal signs." Kraepelin used them as an indication of a decreased distance between the parallels of mind and brain. Therefore, they could serve as the pivot of clinical diagnosis. The only problem was that they had not been defined clearly. In AD (and often in senile dementia as well), aphasia and apoplectiform attacks were considered to be clear diagnostic signs.[4] At this point, the difference between the clinical descriptions of AD, senile dementia, and vascular dementia became increasingly unclear.

The lack of distinction between AD and senile dementia again became an issue in the 1960s. Tissot's viewpoint is the most clear example of the confusion in this respect. He indicated that cases of senile dementia could end up "Alzheimerized" (Tissot 1967). These problems could only be solved by the introduction of more refined and systematic approaches to the clinical diagnosis of psychiatric disorders in the elderly. Its main proponent was Roth (1955), who in 1970 concluded that:

Traditionally the distinction between Alzheimer's Disease and Senile dementia was a clear one. It rested on the occurrence in Alzheimer's Disease
of focal phenomena: the Parietal lobe group of features, the characteristic
mixture of apraxia, agnosia, aphasia, spatial disorientation and so on. In
Senile dementia, on the other hand, a simple amnestic dementia was held
to be the principal ingredient of the clinical picture. . . . The German
workers have recently called this distinction into question. Lauter and
Meyer claim to have demonstrated focal phenomena in the senile cases. In
the light of these is the distinction (between Alzheimer's Disease and Senile
dementia) valid clinically or pathologically, or are we left with age criteria
alone? (Roth 1970)

It took some more years before the clinical distinction between AD
and senile dementia was dismissed completely. Instead, the terms "senile dementia of the Alzheimer Type (SDAT)" for patients in the senium, and "Alzheimer disease" for patients in the presenium, were rec-
ommended. These recommendations were issued by the members of a
workshop conference on AD, senile dementia, and related disorders,
and were published in 1978 (Katzman, Terry, and Bick 1978, 579–85).[5]
The nosological viewpoint that resulted from the conference was par-
simonious: "Although the clinical and pathological manifestations of
these disorders are almost identical in the senium and the presenium,
different but as yet unknown etiologic factors might be operative in,
for example, a 50-year-old as compared to an 80-year-old" (Katzman,
Terry, and Bick 1978, 579).

In addition to the unclear difference between AD and senile dementia, confusion was stimulated by the notion that aging and senility were
somehow connected to arteriosclerosis. This is illustrated by the fact
that until 1930, senile dementia was diagnosed at about three times the
rate of vascular dementia; from 1945 to 1958, the opposite was true
(Constantinidis, Garrone, and de Ajuriaguerra 1962). Major textbooks
on psychiatry held the view that "organic psychosis" after the age of 50
should be regarded as cerebral arteriosclerosis. These accounts of senile
psychosis, senile dementia, or vascular dementia were accompanied by
popular myths and mystifications. In 1972 Friedlander wrote an article
about Woodrow Wilson's disease entitled "How Cerebral Arteriosclerosis Has Altered World Politics"(Friedlander 1972). It is therefore
hardly a surprise that a recent U.S. president was acknowledged to have
AD—again, a sign of the times.

For the explanation of the nosological and clinical confusion between AD, senile dementia, and cerebral arteriosclerosis, the structure

of Kraepelin's concept of disease, the concept of focal signs, and the casuistic diagnostic approach in psychiatry in those days are relevant. The ambiguity of Kraepelin's concept of disease, comprising both the clinical and the neuropathological realm, is in fact at the root of the debates that lasted until the end of the 1970s.

In the previous section we described the attempts to distinguish AD and senile dementia from aging. We observed that a temporary solution to this problem was found in a pragmatic criterion concerning the neuropathological changes in the brain. The situation concerning clinical diagnosis shows a similar problem. The Kraepelinian approach failed because: (1) the clinical categories were difficult to distinguish from each other; (2) the definitions of these categories comprised both neuropathological and clinical phenomena; (3) there was too much reliance upon focal signs; and (4) there was insufficient correlation between clinical and neuropathological phenomena.

During the 1970s some consensus was achieved concerning nosologic definitions and a diagnostic system of classification in psychiatry (*DSM-III*). The focal sign and the Kraepelinian concept of disease (the "royal way to diagnosis") were replaced by the consensus and empirical corroboration of the *DSM-III* (the "republican highway to diagnosis").

Since 1960 much attention in psychiatry has been directed toward the "reliability" and "validity" of medical diagnosis. The criticism on psychiatry — as expressed in Szasz's "Myth of Mental Illness," for instance — was one of the stimulating forces behind this reconsideration of psychiatric nosology (Szasz 1960). It especially stimulated the question of "validity": What do psychiatrists call a "psychiatric disease" or "disorder?" The famous Rosenhan paper (1973) made Szasz's criticism even more tangible, and it caused a shock that echoed for quite some time (Weiner 1975; Spitzer 1975; Crown 1975; Millon 1975; Farber 1975; Rosenhan 1975).

In 1972 Feighner and his colleagues published a paper that introduced the use of explicit criteria to psychiatric diagnosis (Feighner et al. 1972). The authors stressed the importance of diagnosis for the prediction of course and outcome, planning of treatment, and communication between healthcare professionals. They also defended the use of formal diagnostic criteria to provide insight into the question of whether patients who were dealt with in different disciplines and viewed from different research objectives were comparable.[6]

A whole program of "validation" was suggested: (1) clinical description of the disorder, (2) laboratory studies, (3) delimitation from other disorders, (4) follow-up study, and (5) family study. The designation "neo-Kraepelinian" is indeed quite adequate. The crucial and most interesting step is the first one: "describe the disorder." It consists of an elaboration of a single striking clinical feature or a combination of features thought to be related. The laboratory findings, "when consistent with a defined clinical picture . . . permit a more refined classification" (Feighner et al. 1972, 57). Patients with similar clinical and/or laboratory findings may nevertheless suffer from different diseases. This problem should be solved by the use of exclusion criteria. Borderline cases should be excluded as well so that the "index group may be as homogeneous as possible" (57). The patients thus identified should be subjected to follow-up and family studies in order to obtain knowledge concerning prognosis and (possible) patterns of inheritance.

Feighner's proposal for "Organic Brain Syndrome" follows:

> "Organic Brain Syndrome." This diagnosis is made when either criterion A or criterion B is present.
> A. Two of the following manifestations must be present. (In the presence of muteness the diagnosis must be deferred.)
> (1) Impairment of orientation.
> (2) Impairment of memory.
> (3) Deterioration of other intellectual functions.
> B. This diagnosis is also made if the patient has at least one manifestation (A) in addition to a known probable cause for organic brain syndrome."
> (Feighner et al. 1972)

Although similar in content to the *DSM-II* definition of 1968, this definition differs from it in some important aspects. First, the diagnostic criteria are formulated very clearly, and the concept "two of the following" is introduced. Exclusion criteria are not used in the Feighner paper, and the meaning of the diagnostic terms is not clearly defined. These changes were made in the transfer to the *DSM-III* definition (1980). In the subsequent transition from *DSM-III* to *DSM-III-R* (1987), the concept of "organic brain syndrome" is changed to "organic mental syndrome." In the *DSM-IV* of 1994, the syndrome concept is left behind, and the general category of dementia (with specific subdivisions) is reintroduced. The apparent inconsistency in the concept of "organic mental syndrome" was one of the reasons for this change. The diagnosis of AD remained a diagnosis of exclusion (of other causes of dementia); the emphasis on the chronic progressive course of the DSM-III-R did not return in *DSM-IV.*

The changes brought about by Feighner's approach were clearly inspired by the proposals made by Hempel, a philosopher of science. In Hempel's 1961 "Introduction to Problems of Taxonomy," he tries to develop a general approach to (psychiatric) taxonomy, based on philosophy of science. He suggests that each (sub)class may be regarded as an extension of a concept (such as primate, mental illness, etc.). He asserts that the subjects to be classified are individual cases, which are assigned to the various classes according to the kinds of mental disorders: "[T]he specification of a classificatory system requires a corresponding set of classificatory concepts: Each class provided for in the system is the extension of one of these concepts . . . the establishment of a suitable system of classification in a given domain of investigation may be considered as a special kind of scientific concept formation" (Hempel 1961, 5). Hempel's lecture was a major topic in a work conference on "Problems in Field Studies in Mental Disorders" held in 1959 under the auspices of the American Psychopathological Association.

Using *DSM-III*, the identification of a person as a member of a class presupposes the existence of a particular set of operational criteria that must be met. The criteria in *DSM-III* are partly the result of empirical investigation and partly the result of consensus concerning the most important characteristics of mental diseases. Since knowledge concerning the etiologic and pathogenetic backgrounds of most of these diseases is lacking, it is impossible to know whether the current classes are meaningful, except for their roots in psychiatric tradition and the empirical associations that are reflected in them.

The fact that the DSM is also meant to be used in clinical psychiatry introduces a second problem. If the classes are narrowly defined, a psychiatrist will not always be able to identify a patient as a member of any class. Even if he or she succeeds, the relevant aspects of this particular patient might not be expressed in the class definition — which, after all, only expresses what patients have in common, not their differences. Hence, the class to which a patient belongs might not give useful information concerning the interventions and therapy the physician might suggest or impose. In other words, the physician is not able to connect general psychiatric knowledge to the patient without resorting to considerations beyond those that enable him to assign a person to a particular class. Each patient has two images: on one hand, there is the person with his or her own characteristics, goals, and life history; on the other hand, this person is a (partial) illustration of one class of a system of classification (i.e., a case). As far as medical knowledge is concerned, the specifics of a person's diseased state cannot be taken into account. The definition of a concept of disease is based on consensus among physicians concerning the characteristics of persons assumed to be having the same disease. The n-th case is viewed in light of this collection of previous cases — or, more precisely, in light of what are thought to be characteristic features of these cases. The particular n-th case is bound to show (small) differences from this picture; these differences are not taken into account by reformulating this picture as a class.

The precise status of the diseased person is apparently unclear. A particular patient is always viewed as particular from the viewpoint of general knowledge; a particular person identified as a bearer of a disease is always viewed as an illustration of existing general knowledge concerning this disease. On the other hand, some diseased persons show variations from the general view and slip from known territory into an unknown variation of it. At that moment, they cease to be a particular illustration of a general category, or even scientific law, and become terra incognito. This terra incognito is always found at the end of a classification system and at the beginning of clinical practice.

Specific Pathogenetic Theories: "Cholinergics"

The "cholinergic hypothesis" has been a major domain of research into the pathogenesis and therapy of AD since 1976. In 1978 the term "cholinergic hypothesis" was introduced by Perry and co-workers (Perry et al. 1978). At the end of the 1970s, it was found that the levels of Choline acetyltransferase (ChAt) were lowered in the brains of patients with AD (Davies and Maloney 1976). Furthermore, it was found that reduced levels of ChAt activity were found in the cortex of animals with a destruction of the basal forebrain (Coyle, Price, and Delong 1983) This suggested that this area of the brain, in which the Nucleus Basalis of Meynert is localized, might be involved in the pathogenesis of patients with AD (Whitehouse et al. 1981; 1982). This last link was in part based on the observation that cholinergic drugs such as physostigmine were able to produce memory disturbances in healthy individuals that were similar to those observed in elderly people (Deutsch 1971; Drachman and Leavitt 1974). In this process of modeling the pathogenesis of AD, the example of Parkinson disease was quite important.

On the basis of this particular hypothesis, a large number of pharmacological intervention studies have been performed, resulting in the registration of tacrine, donepezil, and rivastigmine (all cholinesterase inhibitors) in several countries. Several other cholinesterase inhibitors are currently being investigated (quilostigmine, zifrosilone, etc.). Research into the pathogenesis of AD as a "cholinergic disease" has shifted toward the genes involved in the development of AD, including the pathogenesis of amyloid A4 and its relationship to apolipoprotein E (Masters et al. 1994; Roses, Weisgraber, and Christen 1996).

The cholinergic hypothesis did not influence current nosologic demarcations. AD is still AD and is not designated as a disease of "cholinergic neurotransmission from forebrain to cortex." Diagnostic procedures were not influenced by the cholinergic hypothesis: diagnosis remained clinical, and its confirmation remained neuropathological (using the presence of plaques as a criterion). The recent finding that lectin binding analysis of CSF AChE could provide a diagnostic test for AD with 80 percent sensitivity and 97 percent specificity is quite interesting in this respect (Saez-Valero et al. 1997). Cholinergic therapy is not used as a test for the clinical diagnosis; there are no subdivisions of patients who do and who do not respond to drug therapy.

In short, the cholinergic hypothesis was not denominated as "disease." It had to tie together too many elements of knowledge from very different epistemological fields. Its principal problem was its focus on neurochemistry and neuropharmacology, fields of knowledge that could be correlated with the clinical and neuropathologic fields without eliminating the remaining contingency.

The fact that the status of "disease" could not be obtained does not prevent the concept of disease from playing a particular role in research connected to the cholinergic hypothesis. First, it appears that the unification of research results from several fields of knowledge into one particular disease concept is a major goal. All kinds of changes need to be causally connected: plaques; tangles and granulovacuolar degeneration; AChE and ChAt changes; losses of neurons in the NBM; the presence of cholinergic markers in plaques; the effects of cholinomimetic drugs; the improvement of the clinical picture of patients with AD. The cholinergic hypothesis succeeded in connecting quite a few of these changes.

Secondly, it seems that the concept of disease is active in an implicit way. The changes researchers perceive, usually differences between patients with AD and those considered to be normal ("controls"), are interpreted as the result of disease — that is, a process that can be described as an existing object.

Thus, the concept of disease has two important functions. It serves as a guideline for expanding current knowledge. It serves as a conceptual impetus — that is, changes that put us on the path to more knowledge are assumed a priori to be the results of disease, sometimes even the results of a specific disease. Disease plays an important but equivocal and "poetic" (creative, constructive) role. It is accepted as a "given" in order to investigate changes as if they expressed "disease." Yet it is not a given, because no one is sure whether AD is two or even more diseases—or even no disease at all.

The theatrical aspects of the cholinergic hypothesis become more apparent when we remember that it was literally carved out of the existing elements of knowledge pertaining to AD. Thus its goal was to unify existing results of research, a process that would transform these results into evidence of the disease. In order to reach the goal, things had to be left out; indeed, the cholinergic hypothesis left out quite a bit—for example, all disturbances in other neurotransmitter systems, a whole range of clinical phenomena that were not related to memory, and many neuropathological findings such as the tangles and the granulovacuolar changes.

As an attempt to unify a range of elements of knowledge, the cholinergic hypothesis was not completely successful. It seems as if the lack of clear clinical success was the most important setback for the hypothesis. This finding provides some insight into the constraints in medicine on the successful demarcation of a disease or a particular conceptualization of disease: clinical relevance. The hypothesis needed to yield therapeutic success or at least clinically relevant nosologic demarcations. The importance of clinical therapeutic relevance makes biomedicine unique in comparison to other branches of science. The existence of a neurobiologic fact is sufficiently warranted when it is backed by particular laboratory procedures. The existence of a disease is always linked to its relevance for the clinician and for the patient suffering from the phenomena distinguished as "disease." In a laboratory, where an object is the result of controlled circumstances, possibilities are narrowed down until the situation is sufficiently under control to yield a publication in a relevant journal. The step from there to the clinical domain is indeed large.

Although cholinergic drugs have yielded hopeful results in strictly controlled (laboratory) settings, they are not yet a clear match for the far-reaching and devastating changes in patients with AD. The changes induced by tacrine and other acetylcholinesterase inhibitors can be observed on a clinical level. They are still only marginally relevant compared to the range of changes in patients and the unremitting progressive course of the disease.

CONCLUSION: THE CONCEPT OF DISEASE

The concept of disease has played an important role in the history of AD. This is clearly illustrated by Kraepelin's approach to psychiatric disease. His conviction that symptom complex, course, and neuropathological findings were the central elements of any definition of disease clearly influenced his decision to coin the term *Alzheimer disease* — despite the openly expressed doubts of Alzheimer. More specifically, the concept of focal signs would play a crucial role in the problems of discriminating between AD, senile dementia, and vascular dementia. If his emphasis had been different, AD would have been named "Fischer disease." Kraepelin's conviction that the relationship between mind and brain should be understood as a "parallelism," in combination with the viewpoint that the distance between the two was diminished in mental disease, was the basis for the central position of the focal sign. This central position was replaced in the 1970s by memory deficits, largely because of the central role played by the cholinergic hypothesis at that time.

The cholinergic hypothesis was an important tool in bridging the "barrier between mind and brain." It provided important insights into the relationship between particular neuropathological phenomena and clinical symptoms. It was, however, not strong enough to change AD into a "cholinergic disease." The concept of disease was nevertheless quite important in the process of unifying the research results into one particular pathogenetic theory. The fact that the clinical relevance of many of the acetylcholinesterase inhibitors was very modest was, of course, detrimental to the central position of the cholinergic hypothesis. In this sense, the test of clinical relevance plays an important role in obtaining a definite status for a disease concept.

The class concept of disease, illustrated in the *DSM-III* and *DSM-IV*, has other implications. First, the definition of the class concept is based on the accumulated experience and consensus among psychiatrists and other clinicians at a particular point in time. This implies that there is not homogeneity among the persons belonging to the class: heterogeneity is the rule. Second, it is very likely that persons can be categorized into several classes. The question of comorbidity is, therefore, primarily a matter of codescriptivity. There are several implications of codescriptivity. It is an artifact based on imperfect class concepts, or it is an indication of two pathogenetic events or two different expressions of the same event. The choice among the class definitions in *DSM-III* and *DSM-IV* (using the approach of x phenomena present out of n phenomena defined) blurs the edges of the collection of individuals ascribed to the class. Last, because the choice for a class concept leads to a group of homogeneous individuals, many individuals cannot be classified. Since these aspects might not be confined to the group of persons ascribed to the class, heterogeneity is the rule.

The demarcation of diseased biological processes does not have a clear ontological basis. In the case of AD, the distinction between normal and diseased individuals is the result of the use of a set of arbitrary neuropathological and clinical criteria. Although the distinction is arbitrary, it is not useless: it has been used to separate a particular group of people from the encompassing group showing aging changes. This limits the domain of research and might facilitate the development of solutions for AD. There is, however, also a risk: since AD is a reality *claim*, it is impossible to tell what AD really *is*. Any conjecture that implies such an ontological statement runs the risk of closing a scientific question or debate in a premature stage.

The demarcation of AD is intimately connected with the question of whether it is different from aging. The distinction between aging and disease is based on a conceptual ambiguity. The concept of aging lacks a descriptive component: age is an instrument by which we discern differences between people. The state of an organism at a particular moment is compared to its state at another moment. This use of the term *age* — which refers to differences in time — is instrumental; we use it as a yardstick. The changes (or differences) that can be observed might be explained, but can we explain them as "processes or mechanisms of aging"? In fact, we cannot. Aging is not a mechanism; it is a way of comparing people. Why should we introduce the yardstick by which we *perceive* changes as the *cause* of these changes? If we could explain all the relevant biological processes or characteristics of aging, aging would then become an empty category. It might, of course, be possible that these changes in time move someone into another category — the category of disease. This category is used to compare people with others, preferably of the same age. Even if one ended up in this category, one would still age. Hence, the question of whether AD is different from aging is misguided. Both refer to processes that occur during the course of time.

AD addresses a particular range of observed phenomena. Patients with AD age, but they might do it differently than other persons. This difference might be conceptualized as a biological process. In other words, aging can be understood as changes in time, and AD as referring to differences between people at a particular moment that result from a different way of changing in time. In a general sense, AD is a subset of the changes identified by the usage of the concept of aging. This subset is the result of a normative decision to evaluate a particular area of the range as "abnormal." Moreover, it is connected with the particular claim that the changes are caused by an identifiable process of disease.

These observations indicate that the concept of disease is particularly useful as a conceptual tool that performs several functions at the same time. Interpreting disease as a natural entity — the rationalist fallacy — is often a major obstacle for conceptual innovations and the formation of new pathogenetic theories. The functions of the concept of disease are summarized as follows:

a. Disease is a particular way of organizing knowledge.
b. This organization of knowledge comes about in medical research by the collaboration of research subjects, techniques, and concepts.
c. The combination of technique and specimen yields a domain of observation. Such a domain is transformed into an epistemological field by the utilization of concepts, including specific concepts of diseases (such as genetic, infectious, autoimmune, etc.).
d. Research concerning disease usually consists of more than one epistemological field. The concept of disease exemplifies the assumption that these fields can be unified. Sometimes this unification is due to the assumption that disease (as a natural entity) is reflected in knowledge of disease. Although it is useful to create an epistemological point of stability to orient one's research, it must be emphasized that this unification is provisional.
e. Within each epistemological field, the concept of disease serves to demarcate particular areas as areas of disease — thus defining both disease and normality.
f. The viewpoint that disease is the result of a conceptual demarcation is irreconcilable with the viewpoint that we might have knowledge of disease. What we have is fragmented knowledge, which is often the result of generalizations concerning individuals who are diseased in a clinical sense. These fragments are connected and viewed as knowledge of disease.
g. Functions of the concept of disease, such as demarcation and unification, are supported by the assumption that disease exists as a natural entity of which we have knowledge. The assumption that disease is a natural object might be understood as a useful conceptual maneuver.

h. The claim that knowledge of disease refers to a natural object — "disease" — provides the crucial connection between general medical knowledge and the individual to whom this knowledge refers.

Notes

1. Moreover, Kraepelin had suggested the idea of a presenile form of dementia as early as 1898 (in the form of presenile delusional insanity, a group of patients showing many of the characteristics of dementia praecox) (Kraepelin 1898). The same clinical picture (*die präsenile Beeintrachtigungswahn*) is discussed in 1910 in the category of the "*Rückbildungspsychosen.*" AD, however, was mentioned in the section discussing senile mental disease (*das senile Irresein*). Apparently, AD was somewhere in between. It was considered to be a presenile disease in its own right and was discussed in the section of the senile diseases. Kraepelin's proclamation is slightly ambiguous.

2. Interestingly AD — certainly in its modern conceptualization — looks more like Fischer's disease than it looks like AD. Fischer worked in the laboratory of Pick in Prague, and had published on senile dementia in 1907 and 1910. In his work, the distinction between disease (senile dementia) and aging was pivotal. He considered an extra pathological process or factor necessary to explain senile dementia, and distinguished it quite clearly from the regular again process. For instance, in 1907 Fischer postulated a fungal origin of senile dementia, and in 1910 he suggested an as yet unknown pathological process that was responsible for all the changes observed in the brains of patients with senile dementia (1910, 391). He proposed that this disease be called "Spaerotrichia cerebri multiplex." Fischer tried to avoid the necessity of assuming a grasded difference between normalityu and pathology by stressing that the existence of plaques as such is enough to proclaim the existence of disease. In this case patients show the clinical picture of "presbyophenie" as formulated by Wernicke (highly graded dementia, memory and cognitive disturbances and confabulations (Fischer 1910). Fischer does not use clinical criteria to demarcate and disease: the presence of plaques is sufficient. Fischer's choice to designate plaques (or *Drusen*) as the primary element of his disease clearly has some advantages from the nosological viewpoint. An identifiable morphological structure in the brain — generally absent in healthy persons — is considered to be pathological. This clearly demasrcates dementia from normal aging.

3. Evans concluded that the concept of disease has accumulated implications that are not helpful in clinical practice in research into aging; the most important is the difference between "normal aging" and "disease" (Evans 1988). As far as research is concerned, our conclusion is that the concept of aging is at least as (un)helpful as the concept of disease. One of the characteristic problems

of the concept of disease in the context of aging research is that the latter addresses changes observed over periods of years and decades. Such a time span is hard to cover using the concept of disease. In the case of clinical practice and in the context of biomedical research, it cannot be maintained that the concept of disease is a mere obstacle. It just refers to an approach that is different from aging.

4. At this point an interesting parallel with Pick disease is present. Pick conjectured that senile dementia was a disease with general atrophy of the brain and focal disturbances accompanied by cerebral atrophy in the left "lobus sphenoidalis" (the temporal lobe) (Pick 1892). As such, this concept of senile dementia was quite similar to the "classical parietal lobe syndrome of Alzheimer" coined by Roth (Roth and Morissey 1951).

5. The Workshop Conference was convened by the National Institute of Neurological and Communicative Disorders and Stroke, the National Institute of Aging, and the National Institute of Mental Health, all in the United States. The impetus for this conference was provided by epidemiologic data indicating a rising prevalence of AD and SDAT and a growing concern regarding the burden these disorders placed on healthcare systems. Since the recommendations were presented to the editing committee of the American Psychiatric Association (Katzman, Terry, and Bick 1978), it is likely that the nosologic recommendations in question influenced the content of *DSM-III* (published in 1980).

6. In the period 1972–82 this publication was cited about 1,650 times, and the criteria mentioned in it were frequently used to assign diagnoses to patients in research samples (See Blashfield 1984, 37–47). The conclusion seems warranted that the publication had considerable influence. The group of "neo-Kraepelinian" psychiatrists — the term stems from Klerman — was largely responsible for the initial promotion of the paper. Four of the authors belonged to this group.

References

American Psychiatric Association. 1968. *Diagnostic and Statistical Manual of Mental Disorders, 2d ed. (DSM-II)*. Washington, D.C.

——. 1980. *Diagnostic and Statistical Manual of Mental Disorders, 3rd ed. (DSM III)*. Washington, D.C.

——. 1987. *Diagnostic and Statistical Manual of Mental Disorders, 3rd rev. ed. (DSM-III-R)*. Washington, D.C.

——. 1994. *Diagnostic and Statistical Manual of Mental Disorders, 4th ed. (DSM-IV)*. Washington, D.C.

Alzheimer, A. 1907. Über eine eigenartige Erkrankung der Hirnrinde. *Allg Zschr f Psychiatr Psychisch-Gerichtl Mediz* 64:146–48A.

———. 1911. Über eigenartige Krankheitsfallen des späteren Alters. *Zeitschr fdg Neurol u Psychiatr* 4:356–85.

———. 1913. 25 Jahre Psychiatrie. *Arch f Psychiatrie u Nervenkrankh* 52:853–66.

Berrios, G. E., and R. Hauser. 1988. The Early Development of Kraepelin's Ideas on Classification: A Conceptual History. *Psychological Medicine* 18:813–21.

Bick, Katherine, et al. 1987. *The Early Story of Alzheimer's Disease*. Padova, Italy: Liviana Press.

Blashfield, R. K. 1984. *The Classification of Psychopathology*. New York: Plenum Press.

Blessed G., G. Tomlinson, and M. Roth. 1968. The Association Between Quantitative Measures of Dementia and of Senile Changes in the Cerebral Grey Matter of Elderly Subjects. *Brit J Psychiatr* 114:797–811.

Boorse, C. 1977. Health as a Theoretical Concept. *Philosophy of Science* 44:542–73.

Constantinidis, J., G. Garrone, and J. de Ajuriaguerra. 1962. L'Hérédite des Démences de l'âge avancé. *Encéphale* 51:301–44.

Coyle, J. T., D. L. Price, and M. R. Delong. 1983. Alzheimer's Disease: A Disorder of Cholinergic Innervation. *Science* 219:1184–90.

Crown, S. 1975. On Being Sane in Insane Places: A Comment from England. *J of Abnormal Psychology* 84(5): 453–55.

Davies, P., and A. J. F. Maloney. 1976. Selective Loss of Cholinergic Neurons in Alzheimer's Disease. *Lancet* 2:1403.

Deutsch, J. E. 1971. The Cholinergic Synapse and the Site of Memory. *Science* 174:88–94.

Drachman, D. A., and J. Leavitt. 1974. Human Memory and the Cholinergic System: A Relationship to Aging? *Arch Neurol* 30:113–21.

Engelhardt, H. T. 1981. The Concepts of Health and Disease. In *Concepts of Health and Disease*, ed. A. L. Caplan, H. T. Engelhardt, and J. J. McCartney. Reading, Mass.: Addison-Wesley.

Evans, J. G. 1988. Ageing and Disease. In *Research and the Aging Population* (Ciba Foundation Symposium 134), 38–57. Chichester, UK: Wiley.

Farber, I. E. 1975. Sane and Insane: Constructions and Misconstructions. *J of Abnormal Psychology* 84(6): 589–620.

Feighner, J. P., E. Robins, S. B. Guze, et al. 1972. Diagnostic Criteria for Use in Psychiatric Research. *Arch Gen Psychiatr* 26:57–63.

Fischer, O. 1907. Miliare Nekrosen mit drusigen Wucherungen der Neurofibrillen, eine regelmässige Veränderung der Hirnrinde bei seniler Demenz. *Monatschr Psychiatr u Neurol* 22:361–72.

———. 1910. Die Presbyophrene Demenz, deren anatomische Grundlage und klinische Abgrenzung. *Zeitschr fdg Neurologie u Psychiatr* 371–471.

Förstl, H., and R. Levy. 1991. Translation of Alzheimer, A., On a Certain Peculiar Disease of Old Age, 1907. *History of Psychiatry* 2:71–101.

Fried, Y., and J. Agassi. 1983. *Psychiatry as Medicine: Contemporary Psychotherapies.* The Hague/Boston/Lancaster: Martinus Nijhoff/Kluwer.

Friedlander, W. J. 1972. Cerebral Arteriosclerosis. *Stroke* 3:467–73.

Hempel, C. G. 1961. Introduction to the Problems of Taxonomy. In *Field Studies in the Mental Disorders*, ed. J. Zubin. New York: Grune & Stratton.

Heston, L. L., A. Mastri, V. E. Anserson, and J. White. 1981. Dementia of the Alzheimer Type: Clinical Genetics, Natural History and Associated Conditions. *Arch Gen Psychiatr* 38:1085–90.

Katzman, R. 1976. The Prevalence and Malignancy of Alzheimer's Disease: A Major Killer. *Arch Neurol* 33:217–18.

———. 1988. Alzheimer's Disease as an Age-Dependent Disorder. In *Research and the Aging Population* (Ciba Foundation Symposium 134), 69–85. Chichester, UK: Wiley.

Katzman R., and R. D. Terry, eds. 1983. *The Neurology of Aging.* Contemporary Neurology Series. Philadelphia: Davis.

Katzman, R., R. D. Terry, and K. L. Bick. 1978. Recommendations of the Nosology, Epidemiology, and Etiology and Pathophysiology of the Workshop-Conference on Alzheimer's Disease-Senile Dementia and Related Disorders. In *Alzheimer's Disease: Senile Dementia and Related Disorders*, Vol. 7 of *Aging*, ed. R. Katzman, R. D. Terry, K. L. Bick. New York: Raven Press.

Khachaturian, Z. S. 1985. Diagnosis of Alzheimer's Disease. *Arch Neurol* 42: 1097–105.

Kraepelin, E. 1883. *Compendium der Psychiatrie.* Leipzig: Fischer Verlag.

———. 1887. *Die Richtungen der Psychiatrischen Forschung. Vortrag gehalten bei Übernahme des Lehramtes an der Kaiserlichen Universitat Dorpat.* Leipzig: FCW Vogel.

———. 1896. *Psychiatrie, 5th ed.* Leipzig: Barth.

———. 1898. *Psychiatrie, 6th ed.* Leipzig: Barth.

———. 1909/1910. *Psychiatrie, 8th ed.* Leipzig: Barth.

———. 1920. Die Erscheinungsformen des Irreseins. *Zeitschr fdg Neurol u Psychiatr* 62:1–29.

Latour, B. 1987. *Science in Action.* Oxford: Open University Press.

———. 1988. The Politics of Explanation: An Alternative. In *Knowledge and Reflexivity: New Frontiers in the Sociology of Science*, ed. S. Woolgar, 155–76. London: Sage.

Masters, C. L., K. Beyreuther, M. Trillet, Y. Christen, eds. 1994. *Amyloid Protein Precursor in Development, Aging and Alzheimer's Disease.* Berlin: Springer.

Millon, T. 1975. Reflections on Rosenhan's "On being sane in insane places." *J Abnormal Psychology* 84(5): 456–61.

Perry, E. K., B. E. Tomlinson, G. Blessed, K. Bergmann, H. Gibson, and R. H. Perry. 1978. Correlation of Cholinergic Abnormalities with Senile Plaques and Mental Test Scores in Senile Dementia. *Brit Med J* 2:1457–59.

Perusini, G. 1910. Über klinisch und histologisch eigenartige psychische Erkrankungen des späteren Lebensalters. In *Histolog u Histopathologische Arbeiten*, ed. F. Nissl and A. Alzheimer, 3:297–351. Jena: Fischer Verlag.

Pick, A. 1892. Über Beziehungen der senilen Hirnatrophie zur Aphasie. *Prag Mediz Wochenschr* 17:165–67.

Rosenhan, D. L. 1973. On Being Sane in Insane Places. *Science* 179:250–58.

———. 1975. The contextual nature of psychiatric diagnosis. *J Abnormal Psychol* 84:462–74.

Roses, A. D., K. H. Weisgraber, and Y. Christen, eds. 1996. *Apolipoprotein E and Alzheimer's Disease*. Berlin: Springer.

Roth M. 1955. The Natural History of Mental Disorder in Old Age. *J Ment Sci* 101:281–301.

———. 1970. Contribution to Discussion Concerning Paper of Sourander and Sjögren, "The concept of Alzheimer's Disease and its clinical implications." In *Alzheimer's Disease and Related Conditions*, ed. G. E. W. Wolstenholme and M. O'Connor, 33. London: Churchill Livingstone.

———. 1986. The Association of Clinical and Neurological Findings and Its Bearing on the Classification and Aetiology of Alzheimer's Disease. *Brit Med Bull* 42(1): 42–50.

Roth, M., and M. B. Morissey. 1952. Problems in the Diagnosis and Classification of Mental Disorder in Old Age; with a Study of Case Material. *J Ment Sci* 98:66–80.

Roth, M., and D. H. Myers. 1969. The Diagnosis of Dementia. *Brit J of Hosp Medic* 2:705–17.

Roth, M., and B. E. Tomlinson. 1966. Correlation Between Scores for Dementia and Counts of "Senile Plaques" in Cerebral Grey Matter of Elderly Subjects. *Nature* 209:109–10.

Roth, M., B. E. Tomlinson, and G. Blessed. 1967. The Relationship Between Quantitative Measures of Dementia and of Degenerative Changes in the Cerebral Grey Matter of Elderly Subjects. *Proc R Soc Med* 60:254–60.

Saez-Valero, J., G. Sberna, C. A. McLean, et al. 1997. Glycosylation of Acetylcholinesterase as Diagnostic Marker for Alzheimer's Disease. *Lancet* 350:20.

Simchowicz, T. 1911. Histologischen Studien über die senile Demenz. In *Histologische und Histopathologische Arbeiten über die Grosshirnrinde*, ed. F. Nissl and A. Alzheimer, 4:267–444. Jena: Fischer Verlag.

Spitzer, R. L. 1975. On Pseudoscience in Science, Logic in Remission, and Psychiatric Diagnosis: A Critique of Rosenhan's "On being sane in insane places." *J of Abnormal Psychology* 84(5): 442–52.

Szasz, T. S. 1960. The Myth of Mental Illness. *American Psychologist* 15:113–18.

Tissot, R. 1967. Various aspects of the speech of degenerative dementia in old age. *Acta Neurol Psychiatr Belg* 67(11): 911–23.

Tomlinson, B. E., G. Blessed, and M. Roth. 1968. Observations on the Brains of Non-demented Old People. *J Neurol Sci* 7:331–56.

———. 1970. Observations on the Brains of Demented Old People. *J Neurol Sci* 11:205–42.

Weiner, B. 1975. "On being sane in insane places": A Process (Attributional) Analysis and Critique. *J of Abnormal Psychology* 84(5): 433–41.

Whitehouse, P. J., D. L. Price, A. W. Clark, J. T. Coyle, and M. R. DeLong. 1981. Alzheimer's Disease: Evidence for Selective Loss of Cholinergic Neurons in the Nucleus Basalis. *Ann Neurol* 10:122–26.

Whitehouse, P. J., D. L. Price, R. G. Struble, A. W. Clark, J. T. Coyle, and M. R. Delong. 1982. Alzheimer's Disease: Loss of Neurons in the Basal Forebrain. *Science* 215:1237–39.

9

Aging, Culture, and the Framing of Alzheimer Disease

Martha Holstein

Alzheimer disease (AD) has assumed almost mythic proportions in American society. This disease affects over four million people and has stimulated the expenditure of substantial public and private resources in the search for the key to its complex and probably multiple etiologies, its threat to fundamental sources of human identity, and its affect on others in addition to the patient. In spite of these expenditures, AD is a refractory disorder that is unlikely to be "cured" any time in the near future. Instead, scientific investigators now have a more modest goal — to delay the onset of symptoms by five years. Sociologists, anthropologists, psychologists, and others are interested in how this disorder (or disorders) is perceived, how different perceptions shape responses to the patient, and how psychological factors contribute to symptom formation.

This vast research enterprise and the enormous public consciousness about AD's devastation are surprisingly recent. Senile Dementia of the Alzheimer type (SDAT) or Dementia of the Alzheimer Type (DAT), terms commonly employed to distinguish an Alzheimer-type dementia from other dementias, became firmly established as a disease category approximately twenty years ago. Before the mid-70s, most physicians considered AD, a disease that affected individuals in their forties and fifties and occasionally even younger, to be quite rare. Older people with symptoms and brain pathologies comparable to those of younger patients were diagnosed with senile dementia, senility, senile psychoses, or organic brain syndrome. This mixture of diagnostic labels revealed how poorly developed the science (or art) of differential diagnosis was with respect to mental conditions that affect older people. It also reflected the customary view that mental decline in old age is common and essentially untreatable.

Today, neither senility as a diagnostic label nor the idea that mental decline may be an inevitable feature of growing old is acceptable. The dominant discourse about AD holds that dementia of the Alzheimer type (DAT) is a disease without age boundaries that is qualitatively and quantitatively different from "normal" aging — except that age represents the single most important risk factor for its onset. It seeks, in Gubrium's (1986) words, "unity in diversity." The causes of AD are located deep within our DNA.

These transitions in the concept of AD graphically illustrate how negotiation processes establish that certain physical and/or mental conditions deserve the disease label — a decision that often cannot be singularly explained by scientific discovery. For example, while most physicians in the United States accepted AD as a diagnostic label by 1920, the relatively few recognized cases of AD lacked definitive neuropathological signs and commonly accepted behavioral symptoms. The familiar plaques and tangles appeared in other diseases and conditions; postmortem neuropathologic examination could rarely separate younger from older patients, although the brains of younger patients seemed to be more severely diseased. While this lack of specificity necessarily limited the definitiveness of conclusions about the exact nature of AD, it did not preclude investigators from deciding that AD was *not* senile dementia (SD). The few dissenting voices (Newton 1948; Neumann and Cohn 1953) — including that of Dr. Alzheimer in a 1911 paper — had no audience for many years.

Thus, Drs. Fuller, Southard, and their contemporaries adopted the diagnostic label "Alzheimer disease," tentatively proposed by the famed nosologist Emil Kraepelin to differentiate it from the familiar condition known as senile dementia. SD was too encumbered to meet the needs of the time. Its very name announced that it was a condition of old age. Conventional conceptions about disease and health were based on age norms. The belief that mental decline in old age is an expected part of an overall pattern of decline meant that what was clearly "abnormal" at 50 might be quite "normal" at 70. Thus, physicians were uncertain if SD was a disease or "normal," though perhaps extreme, physiological aging.

Assumptions, beliefs, and uncertainties about involutionary processes and the accompanying mental and physical changes were captured in nosology and created a relatively closed conceptual account. This system left little room for younger patients like Frau Auguste D., Dr. Alzheimer's 51-year-old patient, whose age and condition initiated the flurry of attention. Rarely requiring articulation, these views were embedded in medical history, education, and popular attitudes. They filtered perceptions and influenced even the most careful work. Given the state of research on aging at the time, these assumptions faced few challenges.

In contrast, the new diagnostic label "Alzheimer disease" was un-hampered by medical and lay views about mental illness, senility, senile dementia, and cultural meanings of old age; as such, it presented a chance for scientific investigation and perhaps remediation. Physicians logically determined that AD, which could only be viewed as patholog-ical, was a presenile disease related to, but different from, SD. This solution did not compel physicians to resolve their perplexities about normalcy and pathology in old age, but it did allow them to retain assumptions about disease classification and time-honored etiologic views about SD. Thus, despite admitted uncertainty, medical opinion in the United States in 1920 almost universally supported a dual under-standing of SD and AD. In this view, AD was a rare disorder affecting individuals in the presenium; its etiological link to processes associated with early or atypical involution was assumed without being explained.

In the remainder of this chapter, I focus on how factors internal and external to science influenced the conceptualization of AD as different from SD for much of this century. In particular, I consider how shifting medical and cultural perceptions of old age and ways of classifying men-tal disease supported this distinction and later its reversal. These factors are important because they helped constitute the conceptual world of investigators, which, in turn, filtered their experiences. Conceptual worlds are critical; they bring some observations, interpretive possi-bilities, and options into focus while obscuring others. They establish horizons of possibility. How any issue is framed is, therefore, always a choice; it can be framed otherwise. "Evidence conforms to conceptions just as often as conceptions conform to evidence . . . analogously to social structures, every age has its own dominant conceptions as well as remnants of past ones and rudiments of those in the future" (Fleck 1985 [1935], 28).

The conceptual framework of physicians who studied postmortem neuropathology in the early twentieth century helps explain why their original uncertainty evolved into a firm belief system that separated SD from AD for over fifty years. Today, other conceptual frameworks shape thinking and conclusions about DAT, and newer and different frame-works hover on the horizon. These too are negotiated positions that dovetail with prevailing professional views about aging and old age, other critical social and professional forces, and changing scientific discoveries.

THE CONCEPTUAL WORLD: CULTURE, AGING, AND DEMENTIA

Writers have been writing about old age for as long as there have been written words. As historian Carole Haber pointed out, "No scheme ever omitted old age as a separate and distinct segment of the life cycle" (1983, 49). American notions about old age have varied. By the late nineteenth century, however, old age had become associated with an almost unrelenting pattern of decay in which the line between the nor-mal and the pathological was quite indistinct. Contemporary historians of old age and aging disagree about why Americans held such negative views of aging in the late nineteenth and early twentieth centuries, but the result was widely shared cultural biases against the elderly. Studies such as one by George Miller Beard (1881) portrayed old age (which, incidentally, started roughly at the age of 45) as the "inevitable casualty in the great 'race of life'" (Cole 1991, 164); inventiveness and creativity dissipated. In a similar vein, William Krause (1900), an upstate New York neurologist, asserted that senility, decline, and decay were syn-onymous to the medical mind:

> The sturdy frame, once the personification of grace and strength now resembles the mighty oak of the forest, slowly decaying at the center until, only the bark remaining, it topples over from its own sheer weight. . . . The furrowed brow, the wrinkled face, the stooped frame and shuffling gait all are omens of that dissolution that comes without pain, without dis-ease. The nerve currents from the spent storage centers become gradually weaker until the flash of the final spark and the circuit is broken. (648)

In his valedictory address at the Johns Hopkins University School of Medicine in February 1905, no less a figure than the renowned physi-cian William Osler argued that men over the age of 40 were com-paratively useless and those over 60 absolutely useless (Cole 1991, 170–71). To some practitioners, old age was often depicted as a medical problem in toto. Thus, one physician advised older people: "Go into medical training, as it were, for the remainder of the battle of life, like a pugilist for the coming fight, for there will soon come to him the need for all the reserve power of his system, hemotogenic, neuronogenic, thyrogenic, peptogenic, metabolic, phagocytic, etc. The doctor, as the dock to the ocean voyaging ships, should be often sought for needed repair in order that further voyaging may be safer" (Hughes 1909, 67).

Using the words *senile dementia* and *senility* interchangeably to describe mental deterioration in old age, physicians rarely distinguished between simple forgetfulness and its more malignant form. I. J. Nascher, a physician known as the "father" of modern geriatrics, for example, described a 76-year-old woman's behavioral changes as her hearing, memory, and reasoning power became impaired as a "garrulous dement." An aged merchant, once a dominant personality, became a "pliant nonentity" (Nascher 1911, 52, 54). He made these observations despite his general view that old age itself was not a pathological condition but rather a distinct physiological stage of life (Achenbaum 1995). A decade later, famed psychiatrists Smith Ely Jelliffe and William Alanson White (1923) described a "normal" old age in terms of certain inevitabilities — memory loss, inability to recognize others, marked egotism, occasional irritability, and interference. Alfred Scott Warthin (1929) remarked that central nervous system involution meant:

> loss of memory, failing powers of observation, attention and concentration, slowness of all mental reactions, lessened ability to initiate ideas, increasing errors of judgment, loss of effectivity, irritability, retrograde amnesia, pseudo-reminiscence, automatism, aphasia, psychical fatigue, and weakness, daytime sleeping and nocturnal insomnia, melancholia, changes and perversions in personal habits, illusions and delusions, loss of orientation, and ultimately the fully developed stage of 'second childhood' and senile dementia (106).

Theoretical support for a decline-and-loss paradigm flowed easily from the application of the laws of conservation of energy and entropy (thermodynamics) to organic phenomena (Rabinbach 1990): if the body behaved like a machine, then like a machine, it would wear down. According to a popular metaphor, each body had a limited fund of vitality. Once depleted, the body had few reserves; these losses led to the physical and mental transformations associated with old age (Haber 1983).

These descriptions indicate why "normalcy" was such a slippery concept, why it had significance far beyond the medical encounter, and why age norms were so influential in shaping thinking. Ideas about normalcy helped form social expectations and social responses to old age. In most instances, American physicians adopted the position taken some years earlier by the great experimental physiologist Claude Bernard — that the line between the normal and the pathological was one of degree. Imagine, however, where this line would be drawn if the literature repeatedly described old age in Nascher's or Warthin's terms. Physicians also tended to generalize from their patients' characteristics to the entire population. Finding mutual support among their peers and from the period's medical literature, they formed impressions about the expected mental and physical changes that might accompany old age. If most older people they encountered had reduced lung capacity, for example, or displayed significant memory loss, they would assume that these conditions were normal. Notions about normality constituted a shared understanding among most physicians and older people and their families; as such, they did not demand any external verification. Whether old age itself was pathological may have been unclear; it seemed patently obvious, however, that it was riddled with medically adverse conditions for which palliation rather than cure was the highest hope.

This tendency to think of "normal" aging in essentially negative terms continued well beyond mid-twentieth century (Ferraro 1959; Eros 1959; Jones and Kaplan 1956; Palmer, Braceland, and Hastings 1943). No sharp lines, no mini-mental status exams, no differential diagnosis divided "normal" senility from senile dementia. Where to draw that line "must often be an arbitrary one" (Rothschild 1956, 308). Noted British neurologist Macdonald Critchely (1939) shared the uncertainty of his American colleagues. He commented that the "frontiers between healthy and abnormal old age — between senescence and senility — [are] so ill-defined as to be scarcely recognizable." Often it "becomes merely a matter of personal opinion whether a particular symptom or physical sign is to be regarded as normal or pathological" (Critchely 1939, 488).

Normal or pathological? A disease or part of the aging process? These oppositional and irresolvable categories provided the conceptual counterpoint for thinking about AD. If AD could be understood as being different from SD — that is, as a clearly pathological condition affecting people under 65 that may or may not be related to processes of aging, then it could be detached from all the uncertainty that surrounded dementia and aging. It did not demand resolution of what seemed so unclear. In a psychiatric world dominated by the search for the organic underpinnings of mental disease, this new condition would also serve the professional needs of psychiatrists. AD was a disorder in which signs and symptoms could be linked to neuropathology. As such, it met the prevailing requirement for defining a condition as a disease —

that is, it was organically based and located in identifiable and ever smaller components of the body (for a detailed description of this argument, see Holstein 1996).

As research on aging took shape in the middle third of the twentieth century, this inherited frame of reference limited the problems that research on aging would address. For example, while physicians did not treat SD lightly, it was not central to an emerging research agenda. In the popular culture, advice books that instructed people in the maintenance of good health (Haber 1983) had little to say about SD. Popularly, the notion that senility was "just old age" apparently prevailed and contributed to a general therapeutic and research nihilism. In these circumstances, American physicians had little incentive (and even fewer resources) to conduct research on the mental conditions that affected older patients. While biologists like Elie Metchnikoff dreamed of a time when "normal" or "physiological" aging would replace what he saw as "utterly pathological" (Achenbaum 1995), old age and its diseases remained among "the most obscure subjects in the field of biology" (Rothschild and Kasanin 1936, 318). Something would have to change before questions about old age became sufficiently compelling for investigators to break free from the conceptual limits imposed by traditional views of aging.

NOSOLOGY AND ETIOLOGY

These views provided the underpinnings for nosologic categories for mental and other diseases. Age was an important framework for thinking about disease. I. J. Nascher, for example, had adapted the familiar stages of life metaphor when he suggested that age was a convenient and visible marker of many of life's events, including specific physiological norms. Age also served as an important basis for classifying mental illness and so helped shape what investigators selected for notice (Beach 1987; Bick 1994). Thus, William Krause (1900) wrote: "Disorders of the nervous system show selective inclination in regard to *age*, *sex*, and *season* [emphasis in the original] to a greater degree than any other class of diseases. . . . It can be proven conclusively that certain neural disorders accompany and are a part of the different epochs in the life history of an individual and are not probable or even possible at different and remote periods" (641, 643).

If certain diseases occurred at certain ages, then diagnosis by exclusion became an important tool. Alzheimer adopted this exclusionary exercise when he initially expressed doubts that Frau Auguste D. could have SD. While her condition resembled SD, it could not be the same because it occurred at an inappropriately early age. By labeling the disorder *senile* dementia, earlier nosologists emphasized the time of life at which the condition occurred and not its form. This label also contained an implicit etiology — that is, the very processes of growing old "caused" the dementia.

From the beginning, this association of old age, SD, and involutional changes in the brain would raise perplexing questions. One result was a semantic and practical challenge that inevitably influenced the concept of AD. What diagnosis should physicians affix on younger patients who exhibited patterns of symptoms and neuropathologies that were comparable but not identical to those of their older patients with SD? They were unable to solve the semantic problem by adopting the solution that is current today — that is, the position that their younger patients did not have SD, but rather that their older patients had AD. As a result, they encountered a gray area in which it is hard to decide whether similarities or differences should weigh most heavily (Fleck 1985 [1935]). They chose to focus on differences. The age assumptions that supported nosology permitted physicians to solve the problem of nonspecificity without requiring a single disease classification. They generally described AD as an early, accelerated, or atypical form of senility without explaining those terms. Adopting a position that highlighted diversity over unity, they also emphasized the greater severity and other unique features of the early-onset disease form.

The foregrounding of differences also kept options open for varied explanatory accounts. Pathological signs, however similar, might have different causes. By discovering *a* cause, they believed that they might not have discovered *all* causes. Thus, similar neuropathological and even behavioral changes in older and younger patients did not necessarily imply a comparable etiology. Confusion surrounding the diagnosis of mental disorders in old age reinforced the wisdom of this move. In addition to providing few clues to understanding the disorder, the term *senile dementia* was used so broadly that it was hard to know what a specific diagnostic label might connote. There was little agreement on symptomatology and even less agreement about etiology. In part because of this diagnostic agnosticism (see Chapter 6 on the Rothschild period for other reasons), the belief that neuropathology singularly *caused* behavioral changes was challenged for a time in midcentury. The seeming plethora of mental ills that affected older people, often loosely called organic brain syndrome, confused efforts to understand AD and its etiology. Without a clear diagnosis, studies that attempted to correlate pathology and symptoms were bound to be inconclusive. Given all the uncertainties, it seemed best to keep what appeared relatively clear — AD in younger patients — separate from the diagnostic perplexity evidenced by SD.

One further aspect of the physician's conceptual world reinforced their interpretation of the cases they encountered and sought to classify. Most physicians held time-honored, though not universally accepted, ideas about what caused SD. Since many of these etiological factors could only be found in aging persons, it would be difficult to assume that AD had the same causes as SD. Signaling the continued belief that senile dementia's etiology originated in the aging process, psychiatrist William Pickett (1904) wrote that "senile dementia is that mental impairment which is a direct result of cerebral deterioration *from old age*" (81, emphasis added). He did not indicate whether he believed this deterioration inevitably accompanied old age, nor did he identify specific factors associated with old age as being responsible for the cerebral deterioration. While generally supporting the etiologic connection between the processes of aging and SD, and not having a commonly accepted explanation of those processes, physicians had wide scope for adapting traditional, or offering new, explanatory frameworks. Even investigators like E. E. Southard, Harvard's Bullard Professor of Neuropathology, who were most committed to the newest research strategies, often made empirical leaps when their research did not demonstrate clinicopathologic correlations.

University of Pennsylvania professor Charles Burr (1907), for example, suggested that senile dementia in persons without diseased arteries "is sometimes caused by a failure of the excretory organs of the body to fulfill properly their functions" or, if not that, perhaps the cause lay in some "perturbation of function of the ductless glands" (234). E. E. Southard (1910) asserted that "the hypothesis is very near that some part of the mental picture must be related to these defects of the long-distance receptors. . . . These may be the cause, not the effect, of cerebral atrophy" (687). Almost thirty years later, Arthur Noyes (1939) observed in a popular psychiatry textbook that "there is much to suggest that the tissue deterioration [that occurs during the senile period] is due to an innate inadequacy in durability of neurons. Why senile psychoses occur in some persons and not in others is still unknown" (290).

In pursuing etiological explanations, the next generation of research (though not necessarily researchers) focused more specifically on three anatomical observations: brain atrophy; cerebral arteriosclerosis; and specific changes in the brain, such as senile plaques and neurofibrillary tangles. Primarily interested in establishing clinicopathologic correlations, they easily returned to older, more speculative hypotheses when newer research techniques did not exhibit specific correlations. They could not, however, resolve a basic dilemma: Were the illnesses experienced by older people caused by age or by disease? In particular, was SD caused by age or by disease? This question persists.

MOVING TOWARD A CHANGED CONCEPTUAL FRAMEWORK

Systematic medical and biological research on the processes of aging began to fracture the link among perceptions of old age, common etiological assumptions, and the tendency to classify disease on the basis of age. By 1930 demographic changes heightened awareness about aging. With funding from the Macy Foundation, Edmund V. Cowdry convened a conference on aging in Woods Hole, Massachusetts, in 1937. From that meeting emerged *Problems of Ageing* (1939), the first multidisciplinary text on aging and an important milestone in understanding old age. Some common questions that physicians asked about old age included: What changes in aging are individual? Which may be regarded with reasonable certainty as inevitable? What are the conditions superimposed on them? Should arteriosclerosis be regarded as "normal" or as a result of wear and tear, or may it be dependent mostly upon disease processes that can be prevented? (Malamud 1941, 49, 39). To answer such questions, investigators studied what they called "normal" aging as the foundation for understanding abnormal aging (Lewis 1946; Rudd 1959).

Opening a 1957 conference on the Process of Aging in the Nervous System, Pearce Bailey, the Director of the National Institute on Neurological Diseases and Blindness remarked: "I suspect that much of our current information about the process of aging in the nervous system has accumulated by incidental observation and had not been deliberately sought. Perhaps the nature of the process should be explored much more thoroughly in the future than it has been in the past" (Bailey 1959, viii).

Investigators were concerned about structural alterations in the aging nervous system — baseline data for studying abnormal changes. By the 1950s, animal models of cellular and other changes, basic studies of the central nervous system, specific studies of cerebral blood flow and oxygen consumption, studies of intelligence and memory, and investigations of EEG patterns and the aging brain were produced in growing numbers.

Such research only gradually modified understandings. Longitudinal studies of age-related changes required complex research designs and organization that were still new to medicine and the social sciences. Much research in this early period reflected individual ventures (Achenbaum 1995), which made studies that accounted for the simultaneous changes in all organ systems and in the older person's social world particularly difficult. Such research would also demand long-term financing and the commitment of research time. In addition to these practical problems, many physicians still shared society's pervasively negative attitudes toward old age.

Some researchers, including Nascher, and some social reformers began to challenge prevailing assumptions that decline in old age was both inevitable and lodged in internal changes. Nascher, for example, undertook a study of poverty in old age to buttress his belief that pathological conditions in the elderly were multicausal. Once the problems associated with old age were analyzed contextually—for example, by critiquing a society that failed to give older people a sense of security, observers could argue that it was no wonder that "ultimately social responsibility is lost and replaced by childish selfishness, a natural result of the instinct of self-preservation and unappreciated age" (Reed and Stern 1942, 254). As gerontology and geriatrics emerged more visibly as fields of study, more attention was devoted to the social sources of physical and mental problems associated with old age. While often continuing to describe "normal" senescence as dogmatic, inflexible, and intolerant of environmental changes, the new generation of researchers and clinicians predicted that change could occur if social and economic conditions were ameliorated. What physicians once considered inevitable and generated by internal cellular or other changes (which "bad" living accelerated), seemed to become more susceptible to remediation through social action.

While there was no agreement about models of aging—that is, whether one adopted a model conceptualized in terms of disease or in terms of "normal" change processes, there was some growing optimism that old age was subject to amelioration if only one understood it enough. Ironically, social reformers such as Abraham Rubloff generally adopted the profoundly negative views of aging that dominated society as the platform on which to build reform efforts. While these views served noble ends—improving the conditions of the elderly—the means to effect change were less certain. In addition, as advocates worked to transform these negative images of aging, the foundation that supported public programs also seemed to evaporate.

By the 1950s efforts to define more precisely the mental disorders that occurred in later life accelerated. In a highly regarded study, the British psychiatrist Martin Roth (1955) defined senile psychosis as a condition with a history of gradual and continually progressive failure in common activities of everyday life. In describing the clinical picture, he emphasized failures of memory and intellect and disorganization of personality without known causes such as infection, neoplasm, chronic intoxication, or cerebrovascular disease. He further argued that affective psychoses, late paraphrenia, and acute confusion were distinct from the two main causes of progressive dementia in old age — senile and arteriosclerotic psychoses. This research, which gave physicians some basic tools with which to distinguish progressive dementia of senile or arteriosclerotic origin from affective disorders, did not, however, quickly transform the work of clinical geriatric psychiatrists. The diagnostic label "senile dementia" continued in wide and loose usage (Goldman 1978; Wells 1978). As late as 1978, commentators remarked that "organic brain syndrome," as used in *DSM-II*, was a poorly defined, catchall diagnosis; however, it was still commonly used in state mental hospitals where physicians rarely sought to diagnose older patients differentially (Seltzer and Sherwin 1978, 21).

The broad definitional boundaries for organic brain disease meant that some writers considered SD as a dementing process in old age that was associated with the histological changes of AD; while at the same time, other writers considered it only a clinical syndrome without those pathological changes (Tomlinson, Blessed, and Roth 1970). Furthermore, physicians often classified older people with slight deviations from the normal as having SD, and as a result, there was much overdiagnosis (Wells 1972). Thus, classification continued to prove troublesome.

Investigators recognized the overlap between physical and psychiatric disorders in their older patients and the frequent melding of "functional" and organic disorders. They understood the need for greater diagnostic rigor without achieving it. At a 1970 symposium sponsored by the Ciba Foundation, the British psychiatrist B. F. Tomlinson queried a presenter by saying, "We must know whether the term senile dementia is being used to refer to a clinical syndrome without any assumed pathological connotations, or to describe dementia in old age with the pathological hallmarks of Alzheimer's disease. If we don't get this agreed now, confusion will reign throughout our seminar" (Tomlinson 1970, 33).

Nevertheless, by the mid-70s early longitudinal studies about mental functioning in old age stimulated popular as well as professional interest. Physician-researchers had become *public* advocates for a changed conception about old age, to be followed by a new understanding of AD. Robert Butler (1975) had a prepared audience when he affirmed that "intellectual abilities declined not as a consequence of the mysterious process of aging but *rather as the result of specific diseases*. Therefore, senility is not an inevitable outcome of aging" (899; emphasis added).

The interpretation of such studies served to narrow the gray area between normalcy and pathology. The corollary belief that what once was attributed to aging per se was now to be sought in medical disease, sociocultural effects, and personality factors was becoming an article of faith for many biogerontologists and other aging advocates. Changes of this sort supported what would become a dramatic reversal in the conceptualization of AD.

This work culminated in the establishment of the National Institute on Aging (NIA) in 1974 and facilitated resistance to "ageism," a term coined by Robert Butler in 1965. These moves sought to reposition the aged and present counterimages to former stereotypes. In this atmosphere, contemporary views about AD developed. Changing views about aging were only one aspect of the conceptual shift that facilitated the rethinking. It was only subsequent to these changes that an active campaign began to eliminate the word *senility* from the medical vocabulary. It has proved more difficult to remove it from popular thinking. Contemporary views of AD have both contributed to and benefited from this reconceptualization of aging and old age.

ESTABLISHING A UNIFIED DEFINITION

Anglo-American researchers unified SD and AD very quickly into an explicit disease category known variously as Senile Dementia of the Alzheimer type (SDAT), Dementia of the Alzheimer Type (DAT), or simply Alzheimer disease (AD) (see Fox 1989 and Chapter 12 in this volume for a fuller discussion of this period). Declaring that "aging is not a disease," they argued that the manifestations of biological aging were quite different than the common chronic diseases of the aged. AD, in this view, was explicitly *not* an extreme form of "normal" aging. This dichotomy prevails in gerontology, geriatrics, and, more generally, in the medical sciences (Blumenthal 1993). Gubrium (1986) thus notes that by the late 1970s the "facts of aging" on the one hand, and the "facts of disease" on the other, were taken as givens, requiring no further analysis. Questions about disease versus age were "swept aside, unimportant for those who work on the concrete facts — the data of disease"

(207, 209). In this model, a distinct border divides normal aging and disease; one is not the other. AD is a unified entity in a singular category, separate from aging (Gubrium 1986, 52).

T. Franklin Williams, then director of the National Institute on Aging, captured this view: "The advantage of trying to make a distinction between aging and disease is . . . that if one can identify a change in older people which is not universal or inevitable, there must be extrinsic causes and these may be preventable or modifiable. If they are inevitable, on the other hand, that is 'aging'" (1988, 48). In this view, aging itself results in few pathological conditions. Instead, there are many diseases that particularly beset older people.

Diseases imply the intrusion of an extrinsic or exogenous factor or factors that had been or would be identified. The recent focus on genetics enlarges this notion by shifting attention to intrinsic, molecular-level "causes." For investigators, it seems probable that these factors will prove to be the cause or causes of the qualitative differences that separate AD from normal or biological aging. AD thus resembles many forms of cancer—while it is more common in older than in younger people and so is age-dependent, it is not "caused" by "normal" age-related changes. These changes only make the person more receptive to the disease process. Tacitly, both early twentieth-century researchers and their modern counterparts saw AD in ontological terms; the disease existed apart from its embodiment in actual illnesses. In this way, it was easy to lose sight of the features of the disease—especially many behavioral factors that were linked to, but not necessarily directly caused by, the neuropathological changes.

Although there are still dissenting voices (Blumenthal 1993; Huppert, Brayne, and O'Connor 1994; Goodwin 1991), the dominant position today is that SDAT is a disease in which exogenous and endogenous events cause pathological changes in the brain. These changes, in turn, result in the signs that render a tentative diagnosis of AD probable. Without denying its age-dependent characteristics, key leaders have insisted that AD represents more than a continuous distribution of physiopathologic variables in association with specific risk factors.

The perceived "givenness" of this disease model, and the particular consequences that flowed from it, are significant. Medicine, as a social enterprise, has developed what Goodwin (1991) called "an ideology of senility." It is a model that understands AD in classic disease terms—with a specific etiology, visible signs and symptoms, concrete structural alterations in the brain, and causing discomfort and suffering (Caplan 1981). It confirms the ontologically required split between health and disease — or, in the language that prevailed earlier in the century, between the normal and the pathological. A corollary belief is that the most effective response to a disease understood in this way is through basic research designed to reveal its specific etiology, an important step in the pursuit of interventions and, ultimately, cure.

It matters that a condition is called a disease. This acknowledgment generally implies action: a commitment to medical intervention and research to determine both cause and cure. It influences public attitudes and public policy, especially as the public investment in science and medical care accelerated in the twentieth century. In the past half-century or more, it has also come to mean coverage by health insurance and granting privileges to the person with the disease that are unavailable to the well (Reznek 1987; Engelhardt 1981). It can shape the patient's self-image and the family's expectations and behaviors. Other and in some ways equally important stakes, such as funding and research careers, were pragmatic. The development of a disease model was essential for obtaining resources for new research. Thus, this view contributed to the construction of careers, the instruction of students, and the politicization of AD.

This model also fit well with the expectations of a society that had recently identified ageism as a prevailing social problem (Butler 1969) and challenged assumptions that had attributed to age conditions with the potential for remediation. It was important that AD became a disease defined by biological variables — which is, with few exceptions, the modern conception of AD. This age versus disease discussion assumes particular prominence when there are so many stakes involved in addition to the altruistic goal of reducing pain and suffering. Earlier in the century, one must assume that physicians shared the altruistic goals of medicine but were less troubled by the uncertainty of the disease versus aging distinction since few interventions were possible and the ravages of old age were assumed; moreover, no research money was at stake. Whatever the remaining problems, the "diseasing" of AD is entrenched today.

No single factor can explain the new preparedness to think differently. Instead, several factors prepared researchers to see one way and no other (Fleck 1985 [1935], 64). Factors endemic to both medicine and science joined cultural perceptions about old age as a shifting subtext that modified the intellectual horizon within which researchers worked. For example, how physicians categorized symptoms influenced how they perceived similarities and differences between SD and AD. This cognitive activity was contextual, value laden, and conditioned by culture and history (Fleck 1985 [1935]).

While researchers were not yet prepared to focus on similarities between AD and SD, at some point roughly in the 1930s, it no longer seemed inevitable that the etiology of AD was rooted in a premature senility. The first shift, then, was simply, but importantly, the gradual etiologic distancing of AD from the poorly understood "processes of aging." Other causes began to appear more likely. That "senile" plaques became neuritic plaques implied a subtle shift in thinking. This move expanded etiologic possibilities without immediately resulting in changed ideas about either AD or SD. As the century advanced, new factors — advancements in technical capacities such as statistics and microscopy, basic understandings of the neurosciences, the evolution of diagnostic techniques, the improvement in epidemiological and genetic research, and the development of specialty residency programs — further structured perceptual shifts about SD and AD. Later, the emergence of "big science" and the politicization of individual diseases through citizen action also influenced thinking.

CONCLUSION

The account I have just offered tells us something important about the negotiation of disease. If, as many believed, SD was rooted in the aging process itself, then investigators generally could interpret it in three ways. They could consider the mental changes associated with old age in its entirety as pathological; or, in contrast, they could view SD as a "normal" concomitant of aging. They could also adopt a continuum model in which the normal and the pathological blurred into one another. For the first half of the twentieth century, the view that aging processes were strongly, if not causally, implicated in the clinical manifestations of SD came the closest to medical understandings. Since social and individual expectations anticipated decline in old age, and since one implicit way of thinking about a disease was that it limited what was considered normal functioning, then SD would not be considered a disease. Even if statistical norms had been available, they could not have determined whether the behaviors associated with SD should be accepted as "normal" in old age. That is fundamentally a value question.

One could, theoretically, continue to believe that biologic and pathologic aging exist along a continuum — a quantitative distinction — and still consider SD a disease. For this shift to occur, a change in expectations about what was acceptable and what was unacceptable in old age would be required; this change would alter the norms. A pathological condition would violate norms of acceptable functioning in old age. It would also generally be linked to a quantitative distinction in brain pathology. A continuum model can be either behavioral or organic in its focus, but one will usually reinforce the other.

For most of this century, behavior patterns that had been normalized by cultural expectations were rarely interpreted as a disease. Commonly held notions about old age and the relationship of normal old age to pathology formed the cultural matrix within which symptoms of dementia were understood. More specifically, the culture of medicine reinforced more general cultural values through its classification of mental disorders on the basis of age and through its etiological views about both AD and SD.

Even more specifically, in part because their environment harbored so many uncertainties, most investigators tended to emphasize differences rather than similarities between the disorders. This choice preserved options for varied explanatory accounts. Pathological signs, however similar, might have different causes. Influenced by these views, physicians found it easier to see a "disease," in the ontological sense, in a young person. They accepted a disease label even if it were difficult to explain why brain pathologies discovered in these younger people were so similar to changes that occurred in old age. For an older person, they were more likely to face a troubling uncertainty — was the evident intensification of changes that occurred in "normal" aging, even when the symptoms and neuropathology were quite similar to those in a younger person, a disease or normal aging? Could the "same" condition be a disease in the younger person and "normal" in the older person? This dilemma was rarely stated explicitly; however, its source is discoverable in physicians' musings about the indistinct line between the normal and the pathological in old age. Disease is indeed a slippery concept.

The relatively loose classification of mental disorders in old age also left wide areas of uncertainty. As a result, investigators had considerable room for speculation and for developing innovative ideas about SD. For example, if the boundaries between normal old age and SD were almost imperceptible, psychiatrists such as Rothschild could easily identify one or several external life events that pushed the individual across this gray line. In the same way, if the distinctions between various mental disorders of the senium were vague, researchers could test out different treatment modalities and obtain positive results. Or they could assert, as did

Rothschild (see Chapter 6), that there were no, or at best only rough, correlations between brain pathology and symptoms in senile psychoses. That result would be expected if the clinical diagnosis were relatively inconclusive. When combined with the other uncertainties, this agnosticism with regard to differential diagnosis left a gap that encouraged the thinking that flourished from the 1930s onward.

Physicians in the first two-thirds of the twentieth century did not treat questions about normalcy versus pathology, or aging versus disease, lightly as they sought to understand early-onset and late-onset dementia. Attitudes toward old age and the clinical changes that seemed manifest in this period of life served to highlight age as an almost insurmountable barrier to a common understanding of SD and AD, thereby shaping their perceptions. It was not because they could not conceive of AD as an early or atypical senility, as one contemporary writer suggests; after all, they did just that for at least twenty years after Alzheimer's first published paper (Fox 1989). While never making clear what they meant by the terms "atypical" or "early senility," they assumed that the condition might have different causes than the senility of late life that would, in time, be revealed. After all, senility was little more than a rough and ready category for many changes that occurred in old age.

Shifting views about AD and SD thus cannot be explained solely by the processes of scientific discovery. One encounters a text or text analogue—in this case, the brute data of brain pathology and memory loss, confusion, and other symptoms of dementia, which must be interpreted. Our interpretative horizon is not unlimited. It starts with prejudgments and is regularly revised to accommodate new information or historical shifts. In his presidential address to the American Psychiatric Association forty years ago, Kenneth Appel alerted his audience to this feature of research: "We are not outside observers of external neutral facts or things. Facts are constructions, aspirations of the exploring process which are built up and organized by consensual thought" (1954, 12).

For the neurologists and psychiatrists who studied dementia, many changes, both internal and external to medicine and science, separately and together, molded the gestalt that became their interpretive horizon. These changes informed judgments at the same time that new work helped modify previously held positions. As a medical anthropologist recently observed, "Once medicine tries to explain, manipulate, or order some biological reality, a process of contextualization takes place in which the dynamic relationship of biology with cultural values and the social order has to be considered. At each stage, biomedical conceptualizations were important, but they did not form in isolation. Social forces and interactive decisionmaking among key investigators shaped biological convictions" (Lock and Gordon 1988, 7).

Medical researchers negotiated disease categories within implicit boundaries shaped by culture, professional norms, technological possibilities, and intellectual context (Bechtel and Richardson 1993; Rosenberg and Golden 1992). In the case of AD and SD, different ways of explaining previously known phenomena slowly changed the way people thought about these disorders; as their horizons shifted and conceptual links loosened, new possibilities opened. These possibilities had been present, in some sense, from the very beginning. Dr. Solomon Fuller wrestled with uncertainty with each postmortem and then concluded that he had "found" a case of AD. Today, different genes are implicated in some cases of DAT; more might be found some day. Certainly genetics, which seems to represent the hope for remediation, is the dominant area of research (as other chapters in this volume suggest). Research on dementia is a major enterprise fueled by resources from both public and private sources.

How we think about any particular condition is important for another reason: it inevitably influences how we respond to patients who have the disorder and how they might think of themselves. For example, physicians who care for people with dementia describe their patients as "terrified." Terror itself is a cultural creation. In cultures where AD has not been politicized and staked out as an important area for research and funding, cultural conceptions of the condition (which may not even be labeled as AD) make it likely that it can be integrated into everyday life as just one of those "things" that happen to many older people. In Sawako Ariyoshi's (1987) novel *The Twilight Years*, as the old man Shigezo deepens into profound forgetfulness and incapacity, his daughter-in-law, Akiko, takes over his care. The primary problem that Ariyoshi addresses is not Shigezo's terror (he is actually rather calm as he deepens into his dementia); rather it is Akiko's slow transformation of her own busy life to care for her once ornery and even abusive father-in-law. Terror is simply not a part of the conversation.

Who is better served—Shigezo or the newly diagnosed patient at a major medical center? Have we done a disservice to patients and their families by the particular cultural construction of AD that is dominant in American society today? What does this construction suggest about American values, belief systems, and notions about old age? If culture shapes perceptions and understandings of disease, so does disease tell us something important about culture. Perhaps reflection about these interactions and their power is a worthy task for the twenty-first century.

References

Achenbaum, W. A. 1995. *Crossing Frontiers: Gerontology Emerges as a Science.* New York: Cambridge University Press.

Appel, K. 1954. Presidential Address: The Present Challenge of Psychiatry. *American Journal of Psychiatry* 111:1–12.

Ariyoshi, S. 1987 [1972]. *The Twilight Years.* Trans. Mildred Tahara. Tokyo: Kodansha International.

Bailey, Pearce. 1957. Foreword: Significance of the Process of Aging in the Nervous System. In *The Process of Aging in the Nervous System*, ed. James Biren and William Windle, vii–viii. Springfield, Ill.: Charles C. Thomas.

Beach, T. 1987. The History of Alzheimer's Disease: Three Debates. *Journal of the History of Medicine and Allied Sciences* 42:327–49.

Bechtel, W., and R. Richardson. 1993. *Discovering Complexity: Decomposition and Localization as Strategies in Scientific Research.* Princeton: Princeton University Press.

Blumenthal, H. (1993). The Aging-Disease Dichotomy Is Alive, But Is It Well? *Journal of the American Geriatrics Society* 41:1272.

Bick, K. 1994. The Early Story of Alzheimer's Disease. In *Alzheimer's Disease*, ed. R. R. Katzman and K. Bick, 1–8. New York: Raven Press.

Burr, C. 1907. Insanity in the Aged. *International Clinics* 17:231–41.

Butler, R. 1969. Age-ism: Another Form of Bigotry. *Gerontologist* 9:243–46.

———. 1975. Psychiatry and the Elderly: An Overview. *American Journal of Psychiatry* 132:893–900.

Caplan, A. 1981. The Unnaturalness of Aging: A Sickness Unto Death. In *Concepts of Health and Disease: Interdisciplinary Perspectives*, ed. Arthur Caplan, H. Tristram Engelhardt, and John McCartney, 733. Reading, Mass.: Addison Wesley.

Cole, T. 1991. *The Journey of Life: A Cultural History of Aging In America.* New York: Cambridge University Press.

Cowdry, E. 1939. *Problems in Ageing.* Baltimore: Williams and Wilkins.

Critchley, M. 1939. Ageing of the Nervous System. In *Problems of Ageing: Biological and Medical Aspects*, ed. E. V. Cowdry. Baltmore: Williams and Wilkins.

Engelhardt, H. T. 1981. The Disease of Masturbation: Values and the Concept of Disease. In *Concepts of Health and Disease: Interdisciplinary Perspectives*, ed. A. Caplan, T. Engelhardt, and J. McCartney, 267–80. Reading, Mass.: Addison Wesley.

Eros, G. 1959. The Aging Process — Physiological and Pathological. *Diseases of the Nervous System* 20(Suppl.): 112–18.

Ferraro, A. 1931. The Origin and Formation of Senile Plaques. *Archives of Neurology and Psychiatry* 25:1042–62.

———. 1959. Senile Psychosis. In *American Handbook of Psychiatry*, 2:1019–45. New York: Basic Books.

Fleck, L. 1985 [1935]. *Genesis and Development of a Scientific Fact*, ed. T. Tenn and R. Merton, trans. F. Bradless and T. Tenn. Chicago: University of Chicago Press.

———. 1986. Some Specific Features of the Medical Way of Thinking. In *Cognition and Fact: Materials on Ludwik Fleck*, ed. Robert S. Cohen and Thomas Schnelle. Dordrecht: D. Reidel.

Fox, P. 1989. From Senility to Alzheimer's Disease: The Rise of the Alzheimer's Disease Movement. *The Milbank Quarterly* 67:58–102.

Goldman, R. 1978. The Social Impact of the Organic Dementias of the Aged. In *Dementia: A Biomedical Approach*, ed. Kalidas Nandy, 2–17. New York/Amsterdam: Elsevier/North Holland Biomedical Press.

Goodwin, J. 1991. Geriatric Ideology: The Myth of the Myth of Senility. *Journal of the American Geriatrics Society* 39:627–31.

Gubrium, J. 1986. *Old Timers and Alzheimer's Disease: The Descriptive Organization of Senility.* Greenwich, Conn.: JAI Press.

Haber, C. 1983. *Beyond Sixty-five: The Dilemma of Old Age in America's Past.* New York: Cambridge University.

Holstein, M. 1996. Negotiating Disease: Senile Dementia and Alzheimer's Disease, 1900–1980. Ph.D. diss. University of Texas Medical Branch, Galveston.

Hughes, C. 1909. Normal Senility and Dementia Senilis. The Therapeutic Staying of Old Age. *Alienist and Neurologist* 30:63–76.

Huppert, F., C. Brayne, and D. O'Connor, D. 1994. *Dementia and Normal Aging.* Cambridge, UK: Cambridge University Press.

Jellife, S. E., and W. A. White. 1923. *Diseases of the Nervous System: A Text-Book of Neurology and Psychiatry.* Philadelphia and New York: Lea and Febiger.

Jones, H., and O. Kaplan. 1956. Psychological Aspects of Mental Disorders in Later Life. In *Mental Disorders of Later Life*, ed. O. Kaplan, 98–156. Stanford: Stanford University Press.

Krause, W. 1900. The Influence of Age Upon the Production of Nervous Disease. *Alienist and Neurologist* 21:642–52.

Lewis, A. 1946. Ageing and Senility: A Major Problem of Psychiatry. *Journal of Mental Science* 92:150–70.

Lock, M., and D. Gordon, eds. 1988. *Biomedicine Examined.* Dordrecht: Kluwer Academic Publishers.

Malamud, W. 1941. Mental Disorders in the Aged: Arteriosclerotic and Senile

Psychoses. *Public Health Service Reports*, Suppl. 168. Washington, D.C.: United States Public Health Service.

Nascher, I. J. 1911. Senile Mentality. *International Clinics*, 21st ser., 4:48–59.

Neumann, M., and R. Cohn. 1953. Incidence of Alzheimer's Disease in a Large Mental Hospital: Relation to Senile Psychosis with Cerebral Arteriosclerosis. *Archives of Neurology and Psychiatry* 69:615–36.

Newton, R. D. 1948. The Identity of Alzheimer's Disease and Senile Dementia and their Relationship to Senility. *Journal of Mental Science* 94:225–49.

Noyes, A. 1939. *Modern Clinical Psychiatry*, 2d ed. Philadelphia and London: W. B. Saunders.

Palmer, H., F. Braceland, and D. Hastings. 1943. Somatopsychic Disorders of Old Age. *American Journal of Psychiatry* 99:856–63.

Pickett, W. 1904. Senile Dementia: A Clinical Study of Two Hundred Cases with Particular Regard to Types of the Disease. *Journal of Nervous and Mental Disease* 31:81–88.

Rabinbach, A. 1990. *The Human Motor: Energy, Fatigue, and the Origins of Modernity*. Berkeley: University of California Press.

Reed, G. M., and K. Stern. 1942. The Treatment, Pathology, and Prevention of Mental Disorders in the Aged. *Canadian Medical Association Journal* 46:249–54.

Reznek, L. 1987. *The Nature of Disease*. London: Routledge and Kegan Paul.

Rosenberg, C., and J. Golden. 1992. Framing Disease: Illness, Society, and History. In *Framing Disease: Studies in Cultural History*, ed. C. Rosenberg and J. Golden, xiii–xxvi. New Brunswick, N.J.: Rutgers University Press.

Roth, M. 1955. Natural History of Mental Disorders in Old Age. *Journal of Mental Science* 101:281–301.

Rothschild, D. 1956. Senile Psychoses and Psychoses with Cerebral Arteriosclerosis. In *Mental Disorders of Later Life*, 2d ed., ed. Oscar Kaplan, 289–33. Stanford: Stanford University Press.

Rothschild, D., and J. Kasanin. 1936. A Clinicopathologic Study of Alzheimer's Disease: Relationship to Senile Conditions. *Archives of Neurology and Psychiatry* 36:293–321.

Rudd, T. 1959. Preventing Senile Dementia: The Need for a New Approach. *Journal of the American Geriatrics Society* 7:322–26.

Seltzer, B., and I. Sherwin. 1978. Organic Brain Syndrome: An Empirical Study and Critical Review. *American Journal of Psychiatry* 135:13–21.

Southard, E. E. 1910. Anatomical Findings in Senile Dementia: A Diagnostic Study Bearing Especially on the Group of Cerebral Atrophies. *American Journal of Insanity* 66:673–707.

Tomlinson, B. E. 1970. General Discussion. In *Alzheimer's Disease and Related Conditions*, ed. R. Katzman, R. Terry, and K. L. Bick. New York: Raven Press.

Tomlinson, B. E., G. Blessed, and M. Roth. 1970. Observations on the Brains of Demented Older People. *Journal of the Neurological Sciences* 11:205–42.

Warthin, A. S. 1929. *Old Age, the Major Involution: The Physiology and Pathology of the Aging Process.* New York: Paul B. Hoeber, Inc.

Wells, C. (1972). Dementia Reconsidered. *Archives of General Psychiatry* 26: 385–88.

———. (1978). Chronic Brain Disease: An Overview. *American Journal of Psychiatry* 135:1–12.

Williams, T. Franklin. Discussion: Ageing and Disease. In *Research and the Ageing Population*, ed. David Evered and Julie Whelan, 48. Chichester, Great Britain: John Wiley and Sons.

10

Narrative Practice and the Inner Worlds of the Alzheimer Disease Experience

Jaber F. Gubrium

Alzheimer disease has been formally recognized as a diagnostic category for nearly a century, dating back to the case history of a 51-year-old female patient, Auguste D., presented by physician Alois Alzheimer at a meeting of German psychiatrists in 1906. The case was "peculiar" because signs of dementia were being exhibited at an unusually young age. This so-called presenile dementia took the name of its discoverer and became known as "Alzheimer disease," or AD. Decades later nosologic developments established AD as a dementia of "the Alzheimer type," which virtually eliminated the age distinction and further designated AD as one of several other forms of dementia (Wells 1977).

As a matter of routine diagnostic practice, however, AD is of more recent vintage. Until the 1970s, AD was not much of a working diagnosis. My own ethnographic fieldwork in U.S. nursing homes at the time indicated that organic brain syndrome (OBS) and cerebral vascular accident (CVA) were the recorded diagnoses for elderly patients with debilitating dementia symptoms. Rarely if ever was AD listed on patient records (Gubrium 1997 [1975]). As an illness category used by family members, dementia sufferers, and the public at large, AD was effectively born in the late 1970s along with the founding of what was then called the Alzheimer's Disease and Related Disorders Association, or ADRDA

(now the Alzheimer's Association). The rapid growth in public awareness of the disease was accompanied by huge increases in funding for
research and service provision. As Philip Stafford put it, "Clearly, something has happened to carve out cultural space for a disease which, prior
to 1970, was practically unheard of" (1992, 168).

This chapter deals with this cultural space as it was ordinarily articulated in the narratives of service providers, family members, and significant others of those afflicted with AD in the 1980s. It was the period in
which the future of AD was being formed at the level of everyday life. In
accordance with the "two victims" theme of the disease movement, the
chapter considers how folk understandings were used to construct two
inner worlds—the disintegrating mind of the disease sufferer, and the
developing thoughts and feelings of the caregiver.

THE NARRATIVE MATERIAL

For over three years in the early 1980s, I conducted fieldwork in
local chapters of the ADRDA in two North American cities. At the same
time I participated in, and systematically observed, the proceedings of
various support groups for caregivers. Some of the support groups were
formally sponsored by the ADRDA; others were either hospital-based
or had other institutional affiliations. In one of the cities, fieldwork was
also conducted in a day-care center for dementia sufferers (Gubrium
1986a). The analysis in this chapter centers on some of the social processes at work in the support groups based on the theme that cultural
understandings resonate with experience through storytelling.

The illustrations presented are drawn from narrative material collected in four support groups; they represent a small part of the larger
study from which the findings are derived—which, in turn, is a fraction
of what has become a network of over 2,000 support groups nationwide.
Participants in the groups were usually the spouses, adult children, or
other close relatives of dementia sufferers. Most were elderly themselves. Spouses tended to be in their 70s and 80s; adult children were
typically in their 50s or 60s. A few significant others, such as long-time
friends and neighbors, participated, and they too were up in age. On
rare occasions a grandchild who had taken on the responsibility for
caring for a demented grandparent would attend. While most participants cared for their demented relative at home, a few continued to
attend after the relative was placed in a nursing home. This continued
attendance was attributed to a desire to help others in their former
circumstances, a continued need for support from the group, or the

assumption of the role of group facilitator. Although most participants were women, some husbands and adult sons did attend, and many exhibited great enthusiasm for the understanding they received.

All groups were moderated by a facilitator, either a veteran caregiver or a volunteer service professional, usually a nurse or a social worker. The facilitator's function was to facilitate ongoing talk and interaction in the groups. Some felt it important to simply "keep things going" but otherwise remained in the background. Others were didactic, conveying the latest information about progress in treatment or care and occasionally inviting speakers to address the group on topics of interest. Some assertively but sympathetically cajoled participants to think seriously about their circumstances and the future.

Support group meetings articulated the disease's cultural space in a variety of ways. They served as a readily available source of information about national and regional developments. Talk of recent and possible "breakthroughs" in research and treatment was commonplace; facilitators and savvy participants made it a point to convey new information. Oddly enough, such new information might be combined with, or followed by, self-help discussions aimed at encouraging people to "go it alone" — that is, without the well-meant but useless interference of researchers and professionals. It was occasionally said that professionals knew little about the ordinary character of an affliction that had no cure. Pessimism was expressed about the possibility of a cure for what otherwise sounded much like the condition of the aging mind, which was once simply called "senility." Items from the disease's broader public culture were also discussed, such as media and video portrayals of the disease experience. Both ordinary and celebrity portraits were often presented. Rita Hayworth's and Ronald Reagan's stories are notable in this regard. Support group narratives combined these resources with the biographical particulars of their storytellers' personal lives, thereby presenting local cultural renderings that were both general and particular to folk understandings of the disease experience.

Narrative material was collected in two ways. Some groups agreed to have the proceedings tape-recorded; after transcription, the recordings provided detailed narrative material for analysis. Other groups preferred that I participate and unobtrusively take notes if I wished. In these instances, process notes were taken — that is, the general flow of conversations and the sequence of speakers were briefly documented and soon afterward reconstructed in greater detail. As rapport developed, some of the groups that had initially consented only to participant observation invited me to record the proceedings. For example, one participant asked, "Wouldn't it be much easier on you to just tape the meeting?" Needless to say, I agreed. The names of all persons and places were subsequently coded and appear here as pseudonyms.

NARRATIVE PRACTICE

My approach to the everyday activity of storytelling or narrative practice as it relates to personal experience, especially the identities of those concerned, has broad sociological significance. Ordinary talk and social interaction is of great importance to the examination of the structure and organization of inner worlds.

The "everyday" and the "ordinary" are no longer considered to be the poor and ignorant country cousins of what is otherwise professionally or scientifically known about personal experience (see Coulter 1989; Pollner 1987). Rather, such ordinary activities as storytelling are now, in many respects, considered to be the first and foundational elements of that knowledge (cf. Lyotard 1984). The personal story, in particular, is presently commanding considerable research attention. Early texts are being reread for their heuristic value (Allport 1942; Dollard 1935; Murray 1938; Shaw 1930, 1931; Thomas and Znaniecki 1927 [1918–20]), while narrative analysis has emerged as a significant method of procedure (see Cortazzi 1993; Dégh 1995; Denzin 1989; Hinchman and Hinchman 1997; Linde 1993; Richardson 1990; Riessman 1990, 1993).

Increasingly, we are learning to recognize that experience comes to us in the form of stories and that narrative practice is a key feature of knowledge about our various worlds — including, in this case, the inner worlds of the AD experience (Gubrium and Holstein 1998).

Personal stories range from brief accounts of daily events to blow-by-blow renderings of a lifetime of experience. Personal stories never stand on their own, however; they are always stories told, heard, and responded to in the context of the countless occasions for storytelling. In other words, stories are part and parcel of everyday life. They are reflexively linked with the actions and auspices of storytelling, which in the contemporary world are more multi-sited than ever (Gubrium and Holstein 1994, 1997). As Ludwig Wittgenstein (1953) reminded us time and again in conceptualizing language games, stories not only tell of experience, but they are a "form of life" in their own right.

Schools, clinics, counseling centers, correctional facilities, hospitals, support groups, and self-help organizations provide narrative opportunities for conveying personal experiences, including stories about private spaces we regularly claim to be our very own, such as our minds and selves. The local cultures of these institutions are an important part of the resources used by participants to convey to themselves and to others who they are, what they were, and what they will become in the future.

But this does not happen automatically. Storytellers are not communicative puppets in these circumstances. Personal accounts are built up from experience and actively cast in preferred terms of reference and narrative frameworks (Garfinkel 1967; Sacks 1974, 1992). Michel Foucault (see Dreyfus and Rabinow 1982) has shown that discourses of experience in diverse institutional settings set conceptual limits to the shaping of subjectivity; nonetheless, the local and the particular continually insinuate themselves to construct differences. At the same time, the analysis of narrative practice does not devolve into the molecular documentation of storied utterances at the expense of story lines, nor should it reduce them to romanticized individual accounts (see Atkinson 1997). As a communicative genre, stories have both received and developed plots, characters, themes, and flow that harbor a significant narrative momentum of their own.

CONSTRUCTING THE INNER WORLD OF THE DEMENTIA SUFFERER

The inner world of the dementia sufferer was a matter of continuing concern in the support groups as participants told stories about the mind or mental status of a cognitively impaired family member or loved one. Familiar slogans drawn from the public culture of the AD movement regularly signaled the urgency of coming to terms with "what's going on in that head of his," as one caregiving spouse put it. Slogans such as "AD dims bright minds," "brain failure," and "the shell of a former self" conveyed the seemingly evident fact that an afflicted husband, wife, or parent just wasn't the same any more — that something "in that head" had gone seriously wrong. If support group participants hadn't already learned this from other sources, they were soon informed that the demented mind allegedly changes dramatically and, in time, is lost.

But what does it mean to lose a mind (as opposed to the brain)? How can one tell when the mind is gone? How is one to conceptualize its subjectivity? These are urgent questions because their answers organize thoughts, sentiments, and courses of action in relation to the individual in question. As a blunt group facilitator once put it to an overly zealous caregiver, "A person without a mind is just a piece of meat; only your memories keep you thinking of him as all there." As a warning to the caregiver, the facilitator added, "And you can't live forever on memories." The comments conveyed the ongoing need to have a sense of the other, as a precursor to forming attachments and organizing social interaction. Can the thoughts of a "piece of meat" actually be conceptualized? Does it make sense to have feelings for a mindless object, other than what might relate to memories? How does one behave toward someone who is no longer "there?"

Support group participants varied in how they dealt with such questions. There were caregivers who anxiously sought answers and seemingly grasped at any understanding that became available. Other caregivers came to the support groups with ready-made answers of their own, contributing to the local culture of knowledge about the inner world of the demented. Some support groups touted rather definite views of the demented mind, and participants were continuously held accountable to these views. Newcomers quickly learned that the personal stories that made the most sense and that were believed to be realistic were those that conformed to local understandings. Other support groups were relatively fluid in this regard—their shared understandings of the demented mind varied with the flow of storytelling and the comparison of relevant experiences. Discussions of the demented mind wended their way through these differences. The stories were composed as much in response to personal needs and biographical particulars as to locally shared understandings.

Let us compare related storytelling in two contrasting venues: a group that shared quite definite views of how the inner world of the demented operates versus a group that was relatively fluid in this regard, having little or no set understanding of the structure and workings of such a mind. A similar comparison later illustrates how the inner world of the caregiver is also locally produced. In both instances, the point is that the subjectivities of the caregiving experience are constructed within, not separate from, narrative practice, thereby forming considerably different inner worlds.

George's Inner World

Consider the way Marian, a relative newcomer, reflected on her husband George's "dimming" mind in a support group with a distinct view of how the inner world of the demented operates. At one point in a humorous discussion of the "stunts" the care receiver sometimes "pulls" in public, Marian tells about a recent restaurant outing with her husband and complains about his behavior. She is soon interrupted and told to "give the guy a break." Others communicate how they've "been there" too, and begin to elaborate on their views of how the minds of the demented work. As the exchange unfolds, note how Marian's story incorporates aspects of the group's understanding but still includes her own biographical twist. In the process, participants narratively co-construct George's mind, building the story of George's inner world out of the interplay of what is locally given and what is individually contributed. In a brief extract from a later meeting, we find Marian talking about George's mind in even more elaborate, yet locally understandable, terms. Helen, Rita, and Wilma are regular participants in the group; Evelyn is the facilitator.

Marian: It's difficult taking him [George] out. He pulls all kinds of stunts. Like he forgets where he's at and, uh, if he has to go to the john, well what d'ya do? [*Chuckling*] You can't go in there with him!

Helen: Cynthia [another participant] would! [*Laughter*]

Marian: [*Sarcastically*] Sure. You know what I mean. So you direct him to the door and hang around till he comes out. [*Pause*] If he comes out! [*Laughter*] Kind of embarrassing hanging around the men's room, too, if you know what I mean. [*Chuckles*] Anyway, Friday, we went to Big Boy's. He likes going there and it's cheap. [*Elaborates*] A glass of Coke and, bang, wouldn't you know it? He has to go to the bathroom. It sounds funny, but when you're in that situation, it can make you mad as hell. He can be *so* embarrassing. One time, he came out of the john and walked right into the kitchen with his pants halfway down. They started yelling at him and he got confused and yelled right back. You could hear him from way over on the other side of the restaurant. What could I say? The guy just lost it. [*Pause*] To me, he's just gone, or getting there fast. It makes me really mad, even if it's funny when ya look back at it. It may be a good story, but it's hell living through it, I'll tell ya. He can hardly remember my name, and who knows who he thinks I am, if he's thinking at all. Those tangles [neurological markers of AD] up there have tangled the guy up bad. [*Elaborates*]

Wilma: Now, Marian, give the guy a break. We've all had experiences like that. He's still got it up there, believe me, it's just that, well, he's getting things more and more confused. I know how it is with these guys. Ron [her demented husband] is still there, alright, and from what I can tell, believe me, he's worse off than George. [*Elaborates*] They begin to respond more and more to touch. Maybe the old noodle can't process like it used to but, believe me, they still have feelings.

Marian: Well, he [George] does respond to touch. Sometimes too much, if you know what I mean. [*Chuckles*]

Wilma: They all do, dear. Believe me. [*Laughter*]

Rita: I haven't been out with Mother in years. She just stays in her room or wanders around the house pretending that's she busy. She gets real agitated, but [*pause*] you know how when you give 'em a little peck on the cheek, their eyes light up? In her own way, it's working upstairs. You can sometimes actually read her thoughts in her eyes.

Evelyn: Marian. Try it. Try looking him right in the eyes and speak to him. Hold his hands. He'll come around. They all respond to touch. It's like the mind is connected to that somehow. Really! The mind works like that. If . . .

Wilma: If you can't communicate the usual way, I say try another way. Words aren't everything, you know. That old noodle doesn't just disappear. We all have the gift of touch and that doesn't leave us till we're dead and buried. [*Elaborates on the "phases" of dementia through which the sufferer ostensibly passes, which she claims to have read about somewhere (cf. Cohen, Kennedy, and Eisdorfer 1985, and Keady and Nolan 1994)*] Empty shell? Don't believe it. What do the doctors know? They're [the demented] right in there somewhere. Maybe they're lost because the brain ain't sparkin' or something, but they're there. You can't give up on them that easily, believe me.

Rita: That's what I was saying. I don't know what it is, but it works. [*Pause*] Well, most of the time. Remember a few weeks ago when Mother got lost and we finally found her a coupla blocks away? When I caught up with her, oh was she obstinate. I just couldn't persuade her to come along with me. The cobwebs had really set in there. But I gave her a big hug all the same, because I was so glad to see her. And bingo, she relaxes, and like she's lucid. Like wakes up.

Marian: Could be. The mind's a funny thing. I'm that way, too. I could be mad as hell, just a little affection and I'll melt. I guess George and I are a lot alike that way. When you think about it, maybe we're all like that. I think George is more of a back man; he loves his back rubbed. [*Elaborates*]

Wilma: You know, girls, we oughta teach them shrinks a thing or two about the mind. If you ask me, Henry's [mind] was always pretty closely connected with [*pause*], uh, down there. [*Winks and refers to Marian's comment about George*] He's a different kind of back man. [*Laughter*] And Rita, her Mother's secretly got hugs in her noodle. The old noodle's like that.

Evelyn: I think you really have to pay close attention to that. Words. Touch. Different ways of reaching into people.

Marian: Funny. Mother used to say something like that too. Something about the gift of touch. Didn't think much of it at the time.

These women, many of whom have met regularly for months to discuss their common situations, have formulated a working theory of the inner world of dementia, constituting its subjectivity in decidedly romantic terms (see Downs 1997 for other, professional, constructions). Although it is not a formal rendering of structure and operation supported by clinical or scientific evidence, their construction provides understanding and direction. Their version of the inner world of dementia is, like any conceptual formulation, a basis for talk and action, a point of departure for telling stories about experience and for rendering those stories intelligible. The stories, in turn, articulate the formulation that informs themes and plot lines, reflexively constituting the minds in question in narrative terms.

Let's pick this apart a bit. As Marian recounts a difficult episode, she notes with exasperation that George "just lost it," implicating both neurological and psychological understandings that she has come across. Wilma cajoles her to consider another way of thinking about what happened. Wilma reminds Marian that the group has had a great deal of experience in such matters and goes on to assure Marian that George is indeed "still there," but that he doesn't respond in the same way as before. She casually makes an important distinction — that the mind can be thought of as an entity expressed either in words or in feelings, or possibly both. Noting that "the old noodle doesn't process like it used to," Wilma informs Marian that, like other "guys," George now experiences more with feelings than with words. George's inner world is confused, but it isn't meaningless. As the disease progresses, the confusion may worsen, but "they respond more and more to touch." The disease, according to Wilma, doesn't destroy everything; the inner calculus of feelings, which ostensibly has an operating logic of its own, remains intact.

The construction of the inner world of the dementia sufferer in terms of "the gift of touch," which short-circuits the need to think of mind and communication as only renderable in words and sentences, has broader cultural significance. It borrows from a romanticized version of experience, which has traditionally been a cultural code juxtaposed to language and reason, to words and "mere" thoughts. While the mind that Wilma and others construct for George establishes a local rendition of this aspect of the disease experience, it reproduces a sense of mind that we can all recognize. As Wilma urges Marian to "give the guy a break," she in effect previews what George's inner world could be, as opposed to what it allegedly no longer is.

The women's discussion is not idle speculation. This particular extract is part of an ongoing conversation, sometimes humorous, often heartbreaking, that has led to a shared view of who their demented relatives are becoming. It would be unfair to their folk understandings to cast aspersions on their reasoning, for it is precisely those understandings that, like all understandings, serve to facilitate talk and interaction. It would be unjust to doubt that an inner world could be designed in terms other than the discourse of words and reason; after all, inner worlds are hardly subject to the immediate witness of independent observation. Instead, the inner world these women have constructed for the dementia sufferer has an ordinary validity. It renders their relatives' actions and their own responses meaningful and sensible.

As the discussion unfolds, the women playfully elaborate on the experiential linkages of the inner world they have constructed. Far from being limited to the head and the spoken word, the inner world of the dementia sufferer is articulated in stories of touch and affection. Excess touch can, of course, signal sexuality, and this humorous ramification explains the mind under consideration. As anecdotal as it is, evidence is marshaled in support of the unfolding story lines. The fact that Rita's mother's mind works is evidenced from hugs and "pecks on the cheek," which cause the eyes to "light up" and allow Rita to "read her [mother's] thoughts." Evelyn then conveys the conceptual implications of Rita's story, placing it in the broad context of an inchoate folk theory of mental linkages. The mind is connected to touch, just as it later links up with even bigger hugs and backrubs. Wilma elaborates further by dissociating the familiar slogan of "the empty shell" from the language of touch. "The old noodle doesn't just disappear" just because words do, Wilma explains. This launches Rita into a personal story warranting how the inner world can't possibly be mere "cobwebs" because a big hug seemed to communicate what persuasion couldn't.

This prompts Marian to begin telling her own story in the same terms. She communicates her personal experience in the discourse of sentiments. By noting that like George, she responds to affection, she implies that the inner logic of dementia, if viewed in terms of the language of touch and feelings, is less a language for the diseased than a common frame of reference available for detailing any of our lives. Perhaps the "mind is a funny thing" because it is a way of thinking and talking about the inner regions of experience, which, in the course of its rethinking and rearticulation, forms new and different stories about the regions in question (cf. Ryle 1949). Marian, Wilma, and the others are using words and stories to draw on what we know and share, assembling who we and others are in the best way they can.

Ivy's Inner World

Ivy Lewin's inner world generated a different kind of story in her daughter Karen's support group. Karen cared for her 81-year-old mother at home. It was a large home, and Karen had set aside a spacious bedroom for her mother, who had lived there for about five years at the time I began to participate in her support group. As in Marian's support group, Karen was one of a core of regulars who attended the group. She had become a regular participant ever since her mother was diagnosed with AD about three years after Ivy moved in with her.

During nearly a year of fieldwork in Karen's group, I found little or no evidence of any distinctly shared view of how the inner world of the demented operates. Susan, the facilitator, whose husband Raymond had been placed in a nursing home, simply encouraged participants to "share" their thoughts and feelings, drawing on her own home-care experience to make her points, offer advice, and invite comparisons. Occasionally, another participant, a veteran caregiver whose demented husband lived at home, would substitute for Susan in the role of facilitator, following the same script of encouragement and advice. There were many views expressed about "what it's like" for dementia sufferers as they grow forgetful and gradually lose control of their actions.

At times, participants entertained views much like those shared in Marian's group. The inner world of the demented, bereft of proper thought, was perceived to be filled with feelings, and the body was referenced as a surface of affective mental signs (see Gubrium and Holstein forthcoming). Karen once portrayed her mother's incessant "fidgeting" in these terms:

> Mother, bless her heart, has never been your typical rocking-chair type. She's always been that little old Jewish lady on the go. To me, she's just more of the same now. Damned plaques and tangles [neurological markers of AD] are robbing her of her mind, and she simply can't control all that energy. Always fidgeting, fidgeting. It kinda wells up in her and she's on the go again, like she's going to the market. [*Laughter*] Unfortunately, she doesn't have any sense of direction, or, anyway, she forgets where she's heading. [*Elaborates*] But she's never that far from me; the old vibes are still

there. They respond very well to touch and your tone of voice. The rare
one doesn't. I guess that's what they say anyway.

The portrayal was accepted for what it was, and in response, other
participants shared similar experiences. None insisted that there was a
particular way of thinking about the sufferer's inner experience, how
the mind of the demented is structured, or how it operates over time.
Karen's portrayal was taken to be as much a commentary about how
"they" respond, meaning the AD sufferer in general, as on how her
mother Ivy reacts to others, given her state of mind. For the purposes of
discussion at this point in the proceedings, the inner world of the dementia sufferer was a momentarily useful construct, forming a loose
narrative linkage with Karen's description of Ivy's fidgeting.

At other times, participants told contrasting stories, articulating a
different inner world. The "empty shell" metaphor could be so fore-
grounded that related stories conveyed a complete lack of subjectivity.
Stories detailed a person who was no longer there, only "someone [they]
once knew," a phrase that resonates with the title of a popular Alzheimer's Association videotape that portrays five disease sufferers and their
caregiving circumstances. In the following extract from such a discussion, note the painful admissions surrounding what is spoken of as "the
inevitable," meaning both the inevitable cognitive decline of the disease
sufferer and the inevitable "empty shell" that will result. Richard and
Ethel are elderly caregiving spouses.

> *Richard:* [*Quietly weeping*] I don't know what I'm gonna do. I'm losing more
> of her [his demented wife] every day. She's just drifting away from me. I can
> see it and can't do anything about it. We've never been what you'd call real
> affectionate. But she's all I have right now, except for her children [from
> another marriage] and I'm not real close to them. Never have been. [*Pause*]
> I try to reach out to her, but nothing seems to work. I mean nothing. I can't
> seem to do anything right to pull her out of it.
>
> *Ethel:* [*Reaches over and squeezes Richard's hand*] Come on, Richard, don't be
> so hard on yourself. They're not all alike. No one is. I know lots of people
> like that. They're not the huggy and kissy type, so ya gotta take her for what
> she is, that's all. It's inevitable.
>
> *Karen:* I agree one hundred percent. Some of 'em just drift away from us.
> No matter how hard you try to reach them, it just isn't gonna work. Mind's
> just gone. I'm afraid Mother's getting there and it isn't a pretty sight.
> Nothing is going tell me that she's the lady I used to know. It's all very sad,

and you have to ask yourself if you can go on like you have been, caring for [*pause*] what amounts to fading memories, right?

While Karen's group constructs and entertains varied subjectivities for the dementia sufferer, none of them is as locally privileged as those in Marian's support group. In Karen's group, the inner world of the dementia sufferer is occasionally conceived of as including both cognitive and affective areas, the latter's borders being undefined. On these occasions, storytelling conveys plots and themes centered as much on what the sufferer "is trying to say" as on what he or she "conveys with the eyes" or "the face." For such a subject, there are alternate communicative routes to the inner world. When "whatever you say" doesn't seem to work, a back rub, a kiss, or a hug might do the trick. Lucid moments might prompt a more cognitive than affective strategy, while a vegetative status may make it necessary to stay an affective course. On other occasions, neither the thinking nor feeling subject behind the mask of the disease is taken to experientially anchor what is "no longer you." On these occasions, participants communicatively tread the margins of the actual and the remembered, as the preceding extract illustrated. Indeed, as Karen suggests at the end of the extract, perhaps the inner world of the demented is ultimately a world composed entirely from others' memories, sustained as much by their inserting recollections into everyday caregiving as by the ostensible mind of the demented in its own right (see Gubrium 1986b).

In Karen's group, Ivy's mind has a more variable narrative organization than it would have in Marian's. In Karen's group, Ivy's mind is sometimes basically what it is taken to be for all dementia sufferers — that is, a mind whose "vibes" respond to tactile stimulation, facilitating communication through feelings. These are occasions for narratively framing stories about how and why touch works, how the mind is communicatively linked with what the eyes say and with what the body in general conveys to others. The occasions thematize the affective lessons of "what they don't say," including the very exceptional disease sufferer who ostensibly responds neither to touch nor to the tone of one's voice. There are other occasions, as the previous extract illustrates, when stories convey mere memories, in which the onus of the sufferer's inner world ultimately rests on storytelling about what the sufferer once was. Sadly, the moral of such stories can be that when the "mind" goes, so does the person. In its greater narrative constancy, Marian's group is perhaps also narratively more hopeful. Through stories centered on the gifts of touch, participants are continuously urged to look beyond what a spouse or parent can no longer convey in words to the tales the heart can speak in different terms if given the chance and properly cultivated.

Constructing the Inner World of the Caregiver

Caregivers are commonly referred to as the disease's "second victims," affirming that, in relation to the everyday subjectivities of the caregiving experience, there are always two inner worlds in question. Both the sufferer and the caregiver are disease victims. Storytelling in the support groups revealed varied structures for the inner world of the caregiver, which also was mediated by the local defining apparatus for the thoughts, feelings, and actions involved.

Of course, there was an important difference as well. Unlike the dementia sufferer, the caregiver's basic cognitive abilities were not in question. He or she continued to be able to speak about what was happening to the care receiver, even while the care receiver's inner world was communicated indirectly and was itself constructively linked to local senses of the disease sufferer's subjectivity. Unlike the disease sufferer, caregivers were also considered capable of intelligibly monitoring their own thoughts and feelings and communicating them both to themselves and to others. While caregivers were viewed as subject to errors in judgment in this regard, they were rarely seen as being unable to put things in the right perspective with proper counseling.

If there was no doubt that the caregiver had access to his or her inner world, there still remained the issue of whether that world was being correctly or authentically represented by those in question. When talk and interaction in the support groups turned to what the caregiver "is going through," which was never completely distinct from talk about what the disease sufferer was ostensibly experiencing, the inner world of the caregiver was deployed in relation to concerns about "how honest [the caregiver] is being with herself," whether the caregiver was "facing up to [his or her] feelings," or whether the caregiver was "denying" what everyone was believed to know. The absorbing immediacies of the AD experience were believed to be continuing interpretive challenges to the most perceptive and reflective persons. Because caregivers were daily in the "thick of things," it was said that they could misconstrue matters of distinct importance to them, such as their very own inner thoughts and feelings.

Especially poignant stories centered on how caregivers responded when the disease sufferer initially failed to recognize who they were.

For some caregivers, it was the first time they were seriously confronted by the very real possibility that both their own and the care receivers' interpersonal identities were in question and could be forever altered. Such stories could represent a narrative watershed: telling them readily led to the question of who the participants in the disease experience were, and whether former responsibilities continued to apply. If a disease sufferer neither recognized the caregiver — as, for example, a spouse of half a century — nor appeared to know who they themselves were, the moral underpinnings of the relationship were dramatically put into question. Could they continue to apply on the basis of the mere memory of historical rights and obligations? Were the mere shells of former selves owed the same attention and consideration as a cognizant wife, husband, or parent? In turn, could mere shells of former selves be viewed as holding significant others morally accountable for longstanding commitments? Such questions turned support group participants to the inner realm of their personal relations with the care receiver.

Dee's Inner World

In this regard, consider extracts from the proceedings of two contrasting support groups, which I will refer to, respectively, as Dee's and Sally's groups. Dee's group was facilitated by Ann and Ruth, veteran caregivers who could be rather forthright in describing what the caregiver goes through in the continuing home care of the demented. While participants in Dee's group rarely minced words in conveying their thoughts and feelings, they were also warmly solicitous and helpful in responding to the various questions raised and dilemmas presented in group discussion. In many ways, these were meetings of critically sincere friends, and newcomers quickly came to realize they had everyone's best interests at heart.

Participant observation indicated that Dee's group had a well-developed sense of the normal course of the disease experience for the caregiver. It was conveyed in terms of the burdens of the so-called 36-hour day that caregiving proverbially entailed and a multiphase chronology reminiscent of Elisabeth Kübler-Ross's (1969) stage model of dying. In the AD experience, the caregiver initially orients to the victim's cure and recovery, ignoring his or her own needs, with the result that caregivers devote what can seem like 36-hour days to the disease sufferer. While caregivers eventually acknowledge the inevitability of the sufferer's decline, they initially refuse to believe this applies to their afflicted family member and thus enter a stage of denial. Caregivers may feel that they are not doing enough for the afflicted and become guilt-ridden when they inadvertently place their own welfare ahead of that of the afflicted person. As domestic life goes from bad to worse, with no hope for recovery for the afflicted and no relief in sight from the burdens of care for the disease's second victim, caregivers are said to enter into a stage of depression. Soon, it is hoped, they move beyond that and enter into yet another stage, when it is realized that there is more at stake in the disease experience than the sufferer. At this stage, the inevitability of full-blown dementia is accepted; caregivers take stock of the impact of the disease on their own and other family members' lives. At this point, the possibility of institutionalization or nursing home placement is discussed for the "sake of all concerned."

Participants in Dee's support group regularly sorted and discerned their thoughts and feelings in relation to this model, deploying their subjectivity in relatedly structured narratives. This was not, however, the result of a wholesale enculturation in which what was related reflected the internalized by-product of a developmental code. Rather, talk and interaction showed that participants' practical reasoning could assemble the inner world of the caregiver in biographically different ways. Nonetheless, all the stories either played on, or responded to, what the typical caregiver was believed to go through in dealing with the individual and domestic effects of the "disease of the century."

A brief conversation between Ann and Ruth (the two facilitators), Dee, and two other participants suggested that the link between the local culture of the disease experience and the deployment of the caregiver's subjectivity was not automatic. Instead, it was formed from the interplay between what was locally shared and the invoked biographical particulars under consideration. In the next extract, we detail the group proceedings after an extended exchange between Ann, Ruth, and Belle about how similar their personal experiences in home care have been. Note how a shared recognition of what one goes through crops up throughout the discussion, referenced in terms of how one can "see what happens," how "we're all in this thing together," how one "knows [what is] coming," and how one goes through a stage of "feeling lonely and depressed." Even Dee, who starts off by presenting a mind of her own, shares in the group's developmental understanding of the *typical* caregiver's inner world.

> *Dee:* I don't know, Belle. Sure, I can see what happened . . . why you decided to start looking for a place [nursing home] for Harold [Belle's demented husband]. I guess if I was in your shoes, I wouldn't fight it

anymore either. You do have to start thinking about how you feel inside and what's happening to your family. God knows, the kids would have been ignored. [Dee has no children of her own.]

Dora: [*To Dee*] Well then, dear, what's your problem? We're all in this thing together. You're no different. You just think you are. I was like you once. [*Elaborates*] I did everything. I had no time to think. It was get this, do that, and take care of Ben [her husband] 24 hours a day. Well, I learned the hard way and nearly put myself in the hospital. Ben's on a waiting list [for nursing home placement] at Pine Crest. God help me, it won't come too soon.

Belle: I don't think I'm ready for that yet, but I know I'll have to pretty soon. I know it's coming. It's only a matter of time.

Dee: I don't think its that simple, Belle.

Anne: Oh, come on, Dee. That's what it is in a nutshell. You have to start thinking about yourself. [*Elaborates*] Look at you. You're all worn down, and I'll bet you're feeling lonely and depressed.

Dee: That's what I was trying to explain last time. I'm not really lonely, I'm . . .

Ruth: You're denying. We all try to deny it.

At this point, there was an extended discussion of denial, its workings, and how that had once applied to several other caregivers. The discussion made it clear that the story Dee was telling was not one that coincided with local understanding. In the context of denial, the story was in virtual need of retelling so that it coincided with what Anne later declared was what "we know all about." As Dee continued, she constructed a space for a distinct narrative. Notice, however, that she didn't question what everyone, Dee included, already knew was typical in the matter under consideration.

Dee: I don't think so. Seriously, if I was in the same situation as most people, maybe I'd be denying, but basically I'm here to learn how to cope with his [her husband] . . . you know, how to dress him and what's going to happen to him in the months ahead. [*Elaborates*]

Anne: Dee, you're forgetting that we know all about this.

Dee: I know. I know that's the way it works. I understand that. But you're forgetting one thing, too: he's all I have. He's a friend, a companion, even if he forgets who I am sometimes. It doesn't matter that much anyway, because I know he knows in his heart that it's me. [*Elaborates*] If we had had kids, maybe it'd be different. I'd probably be going through all the phases of this thing. [*Describes how she would have progressed through the phases*] But I don't have kids, and his family's not around, and I don't know who mine are.

We've been pretty much on our own and with each other all our lives. If I give him up, it'd be, well, giving up on life. It's not like I'm going to get back to my life after he's gone. What life are we talking about? Life with Gordon is all I've ever really had. Gordon's my family.

Acknowledging the stage model's general validity, Dee views herself as an exception to its developmental rule. For her, the issue is one of applicability, not denial. Adherents of the model assume that there is a course of progress in the caregiver's adjustment to the disease experience. In the normal scheme of things, the caregiver eventually breaks the clutches of denial. Indeed, at an unextracted point of the proceedings, the group's two facilitators explained that one of their goals was to help others do just that. Dee, however, thought of herself differently. She linked her subjectivity with her particular domestic circumstances and constructed a contrasting story.

Dee narratively disentangled her experience caring for Gordon from the prevailing model of caregiver adjustment. Instead, she combined caregiving with the story of a life that she and Gordon had built alone. This obviated the typical competing familial obligations that informed the model. The impact of caregiving on others in the family network, especially as it affects one's own well-being and related ability to be responsible to all concerned, was a primary consideration. As Dee stated at the start of the first extract from this discussion, she would have had to start thinking of "what's happening to [her] family" if she had had children—who, she added, "would have been ignored." In contrast, Dee's particular story purportedly fell outside the purview of "the way [Dee acknowledged] it works," which established narrative grounds for particularizing local culture. She, in effect, was an exception to the local constituting rules concerning responsibility, inner experience, and the taken-for-granted borders of the familial. Her exceptional status proved the rules, allowing Dee's difference to stand rationally juxtaposed with the typical organization of the caregiver's inner world.

Sally's Inner World

Contrast this with a support group that had little or no prevailing understanding of caregiver adjustment. By and large, proceedings were made up of shared thoughts and feelings from the previous weeks' happenings on the home front. Participants made use of a diverse history of shared examples against which they assessed and interpreted individual caregiving experiences. Still, as with the other groups, participants felt the need to understand what was happening to their lives. Answers to questions centered on what they were "going through" were drawn from continuing interpersonal comparisons with little or no overall standard (or model) for evaluation.

This presented a contrasting narrative organization for communicating personal experience, highlighted in caregiver Sally's extended remarks at an evening's meeting. Responding to participants' comments about how it felt when the care receiver failed to recognize the caregiver as a family member, Sally related the story of her own thoughts and feelings. Toward the end of the following extract, note how she even served as a kind of narrative model for herself, as she told herself ("Sal") the inner meaning of the relationship under consideration.

I can't say that it's been the same for me as Violet [another participant]. Of course, you do think about what all this means sometimes. Like this last week, Al [her husband] turned around . . . just like that . . . and asked me, "Who are you? What are you doing in here?" It was like I was a stranger in the house or something. God, did that set me back. They say it wakes you up and makes you realize what it's all about. I got scared. I remember how Cora [a participant] reacted when her mother yelled at her about not wanting a stranger running around in the bedroom. I felt like that. How could Al think I was someone else? It was real hard to take. I remembered what Cora said, and it snapped me back a bit. They [AD sufferers] get confused sometimes. They don't know how to express things and so it comes out all twisted around, like they don't know who they are, even. It's not their fault. I remembered that, and that calmed me down a bit, and I thanked Cora for having shared that. [*Pause*] I think what a person has to do is keep in mind what we've heard from everyone here tonight. Down the road, well, I know if I stand back and think back to myself and what happened, I'll say to myself, "Hold on there, Sal. Remember what happened last week or last month and how it made you feel, and tell yourself how you should feel right now." You learn from experience, all the experiences, and that helps to answer things that keep coming up in your mind, like what's happening to your marriage or if you even have one to speak of . . . you know, what you owe to each other after all those years.

CONCLUSION

Drawn from the larger body of narrative material collected in the study, these illustrations offer considerable food for thought concerning the subjectivities of the AD experience.

First, there is the issue of whether we can continue to think about inner worlds as constitutively separate from their diverse social contexts. It is a rather common practice to conceptualize and formulate approaches to inner worlds as if they were principally self-contained entities, even while much has been made of their social shaping and development. Thus, we model "the" caregiver's adjustment and we metaphorically structure or destructure "the" disease sufferer's mind (Gubrium 1987). Reasonably, given such understandings, we move ahead if we can to help, change, support, or otherwise ameliorate related personal suffering and address, or come to terms with, the mental status of the afflicted. At the same time, it is evident that what we understand and communicate about these inner worlds is narratively organized; what we believe and say are part of the stories we tell about who we and others are, were, and will become. Indeed, stories are the very empirical grist of this knowledge and communication, which, in turn, are constitutively embedded in the varied circumstances of storytelling. The narrative material presented here suggests that inner worlds are as much a part of these circumstances as they are individual experiential entities in their own right.

A second issue relates to the cultural mediation of experience. AD only became a widely shared framework for assigning personal meaning to the cognitive experiences of later life in the 1970s. Narratively, what became a disease experience — as opposed to one of the natural facts of old age — provided a new framework for formulating stories about the inner worlds in question. Such stories were laced with the language of brain failure, progress in treatment, psychosocial adjustment, and other medicalized themes and terms of reference.

This cultural space helped to make AD newly meaningful to those concerned, filling related experience with new kinds of understanding. The affliction, of course, is one thing; its diverse meanings are, in many ways, something else — formulated, organized, and managed through their own distinct dynamic. The social organization of related storytelling that emerged in the late 1970s not only gave experiential birth to a diagnosable experience but also provided variably urgent diagnostic identities for those concerned. In addition to constructing new subjectivities for late life, AD gave the concerned much more to worry about. As the opportunities for telling related stories flourished in a variety of venues, such as support groups, the inner worlds and personal distresses of the disease experience took shape. It is this diverse cultural space that has given narrative presence to the everyday subjectivity of what is ordinarily thought and felt about becoming demented or caring for afflicted persons.

Third, there is the issue of intervention. Producing an inner world with a developmental logic, which Dee's group shared and perpetuated, suggests a considerably different form of intervention strategy than would be implicated by an inner world constructed through continuing interpersonal comparisons, such as in Sally's group. If a general folk model is a recipe for wholesale intervention, these differences move us in rather different directions, fueled by the practical needs of particulars. The narrative materials suggest that both general models and particularized understandings are constructive and narratively conveyed, neither privileging the general nor the particular in everyday understandings of the inner worlds in question. Narrative practice suggests that intervention is best understood in relation to local variations in the cultural space that has developed around the disease experience. These domains — some highly medicalized, others psychosocial, and still others antiprofessional — make distinct forms of intervention phenomenologically sensible and experientially necessary.

It is clear that the sensibilities of intervention will also be constructed in relation to this relatively new cultural space. As such, those concerned will act to transform their inner worlds, perhaps alleviating their related troubles by way of stories of "the gift of touch," "closing the books on the shell of a former self," "taking care of the second victim," and "going through all the phases of this thing." In other words, doing something about these inner worlds is itself a set of stories, part and parcel of the narrative opportunities made available in the new cultural space provided by AD in the late 1970s.

References

Allport, Gordon W. 1942. *The Use of Personal Documents in Psychological Science.* New York: Little, Brown.

Atkinson, Paul. 1997. Narrative Turn or Blind Alley? *Qualitative Health Research* 7:323–44.

Cohen, Donna, G. Kennedy, and Carl Eisdorfer. 1985. Phases of Change in the Patient with Alzheimer's Disease. *Journal of the American Geriatrics Society* 32:11–15.

Cortazzi, Martin. 1993. *Narrative Analysis.* London: Falmer Press.

Coulter, Jeff. 1989. *Mind in Action.* Atlantic Highlands, N.J.: Humanities Press.

Dégh, Linda. 1995. *Narratives in Society*. Helsinki: Academia Scientarum Fennica.

Denzin, Norman K. 1989. *Interpretive Biography*. Newbury Park, Calif.: Sage.

Dollard, John. 1935. *Criteria for the Life History*. New Haven: Yale University Press.

Downs, Murna. 1997. The Emergence of the Person in Dementia Research. *Ageing and Society* 17:597–607.

Dreyfus, Hubert L., and Paul Rabinow. 1982. *Michel Foucault: Beyond Structuralism and Hermeneutics*. Chicago: University of Chicago Press.

Garfinkel, Harold. 1967. *Studies in Ethnomethodology*. Englewood Cliffs, N.J.: Prentice-Hall.

Gubrium, Jaber F. 1986a. *Oldtimers and Alzheimer's: The Descriptive Organization of Senility*. Greenwich, Conn.: JAI Press.

———. 1986b. The Social Preservation of Mind: The Alzheimer's Disease Experience. *Symbolic Interaction* 6:37–51.

———. 1987. Structuring and Destructuring the Course of Illness: The Alzheimer's Disease Experience. *Sociology of Health and Illness* 3:1–24.

———. 1997[1975]. *Living and Dying at Murray Manor*. Charlottesville: University Press of Virginia.

Gubrium, Jaber F., and James A. Holstein. 1994. Grounding the Postmodern Self. *Sociological Quarterly* 34:685–703.

———. 1997. *The New Language of Qualitative Method*. New York: Oxford University Press.

———. 1998. Narrative Practice and the Coherence of Personal Stories. *Sociological Quarterly* 39:163–87.

———. Forthcoming. The Nursing Home as a Discursive Anchor for the Body. In *Gray Areas: An Anthropology of the Nursing Home*, ed. Phillip Stafford. Santa Fe, N.M.: SAR Press.

Hinchman, Lewis P., and Sandra K. Hinchman. 1997. *Memory, Community, Identity: The Idea of Narrative in the Human Sciences*. Albany: SUNY Press.

Keady, J., and M. Nolan. 1994. Younger Onset Dementia: Developing a Longitudinal Model as the Basis for a Research Agenda and as a Guide to Intervention with Sufferers and Carers. *British Journal of Nursing* 4:309–14.

Kübler-Ross, Elisabeth. 1969. *On Death and Dying*. New York: Macmillan.

Linde, Charlotte. 1993. *Life Stories: The Creation of Coherence*. New York: Oxford University Press.

Lyotard, Jean-François. 1984. *The Postmodern Condition: A Report on Knowledge*. Minneapolis: University of Minnesota Press.

Murray, Henry. 1938. *Explorations in Personality*. New York: Oxford University Press.

Pollner, Melvin. 1987. *Mundane Reason: Reality in Everyday and Sociological Discourse.* New York: Cambridge University Press.

Richardson, Laurel. 1990. Narrative and Sociology. *Journal of Contemporary Ethnography* 19:116–35.

Riessman, Catherine Kohler. 1990. *Divorce Talk: Women and Men Make Sense of Personal Relationships.* New Brunswick: Rutgers University Press.

———. 1993. *Narrative Analysis.* Thousand Oaks, Calif.: Sage.

Rose, Nikolas. 1990. *Governing the Soul: The Shaping of the Private Self.* London: Routledge.

Ryle, Gilbert. 1949. *The Concept of Mind.* Chicago: University of Chicago Press.

Sacks, Harvey. 1974. On the Analyzability of Stories by Children. In *Ethnomethodology*, ed. Roy Turner, 216–32. New York: Penguin.

———. 1992. *Lectures on Conversation.* Cambridge: Blackwell.

Shaw, Clifford. 1930. *The Jack Roller: A Delinquent Boy's Own Story.* Chicago: University of Chicago Press.

———. 1931. *The Natural History of a Delinquent Career.* Chicago: University of Chicago Press.

Stafford, Philip B. 1992. The Nature and Culture of Alzheimer's Disease. *Semiotica* 92:167–76.

Thomas, W. I., and Florian Znaniecki. 1927 [1918–20]. *The Polish Peasant in Europe and America.* New York: Knopf.

Wells, Charles E., ed. 1977. *Dementia.* Philadelphia: F. A. Davis.

Wittgenstein, Ludwig. 1953. *Philosophical Investigations.* New York: Macmillan.

PART IV

Politics, Policy, and the Perspectives of the Caregiver and Patient

Since the recovery (described in Chapter 1) of the original file of Auguste D., Alzheimer's first patient, her haunting photograph has begun to attain iconic status in professional lectures on the disease around the world — indicating the significance attached to the perspective of the patient. It is, after all, the sufferings of the patient and caregiver that biomedicine aims to alleviate. Yet in practice, the perspectives of patients and their caregivers are often difficult to discern. In part, this is because the disease makes it difficult for patients to articulate, and for professionals to hear, a coherent perspective. But another difficulty lies in the political climate of the public policy arena in which the professional perspectives of biomedical scientists, lobbyists, and policy makers tend to overshadow the everyday concerns of patients and caregivers. The chapters in this section seek to elucidate both the difficulty and the crucial importance of the perspectives of caregivers and patients if we are to formulate effective and ethically sound policies.

Understanding the perspective of the caregiver and patient must begin with recognition that the concept of Alzheimer disease (AD) has multiple meanings, determined by one's experience of the disease and the particular problems it presents in a given context. For biomedical researchers struggling to win National Institutes of Health support for their work, the disease presents itself as both a daunting scientific challenge and an opportunity to build a career. Public policy makers and analysts experience the disease as one of many claims on an increasingly scant pool of resources. Caregivers, as Gubrium's chapter in the previous section showed, experience the disease in terms of their concrete, everyday struggles to meet the immense physical and emotional burdens of caring for the demented patient. In a similar way, Stephen Post's chapter demonstrates that the meaning of AD for the patient (in the context of our culture) lies in its profound threat to the integrity of the self.

The history of the Alzheimer's Association, the subject of the chapters by Patrick Fox and Katherine Bick, is central to understanding both the difficulty and importance of the caregiver perspective because the association has aspired to translate that perspective into public policy. In so doing, the association played a pivotal role in making AD a major public health issue in the early 1980s. Founded in 1979 by the merging of seven organizations around the country, the Alzheimer's Association combined the grassroots support and energy of families and caregivers with the professional authority and political savvy of scientists and federal officials to lobby the federal government to assist with the material burdens of caregiving and to mount an extensive research program to discover treatments and ultimately a cure for AD. Thus, from the outset, the association has had to balance the interests of caregivers, biomedical researchers, and federal officials. Where the interests of caregivers have been identical with those of researchers and interested federal officials (e.g., winning federal support for a massive biomedical research effort), the association has been able to translate caregiver interests into policy. Where the interests of caregivers have been unrelated to, or in conflict with, those of biomedical researchers and federal officials (e.g., establishing federally funded long-term care insurance), it has been far less successful.

Fox's chapter explores in detail the creation of the association around a disease-specific strategy to win funds for basic biomedical research on AD, and argues that this tremendously successful strategy has contributed to the failure to attain the association's policy objectives regarding support for caregivers in the form of policies such as universal health coverage and long-term care insurance. Caregiver input in the form of lobbying Congress was a major part of the strategy to win funds for research. At numerous congressional hearings and media events, caregivers told personal stories of the crushing emotional, physical, and financial burdens AD imposed, lending the lobbying efforts a tremendous moral appeal — an appeal that Robert Butler, former NIA director and one of the principal architects of this strategy, termed the "politics of anguish." But when it came to policy aimed to assist with the burdens of caregiving, the disease-specific approach was counterproductive. The disease-specific strategy rested on an argument that finding effective treatments and ultimately a prevention or cure for AD was the most effective way to address the social and personal burdens the disease imposed. More importantly, the strategy, which was pursued by advocates for other diseases as well, splintered the constituency that would be necessary to support policies such as universal long-term care insurance that would benefit caregivers of persons suffering from all sorts of chronic conditions.

Katherine Bick discusses prospects and challenges for continued success in winning funding for research in an era of constricting budgets. Bick argues that the "golden era," when demonstrating that a disease caused a significant amount of suffering and that scientists had reasonable prospects for progress in understanding and treating it were sufficient to attract generous levels of federal funding, is over for health voluntary organizations. In the current fiscal environment, the issue is "setting priorities" for the NIH — which translates into choosing which items *not* to fund among a pool of worthy research programs. In this new era, the approach of traditional health voluntaries patterned after the American Cancer Society have been challenged by the more aggressive, populist approach of organizations like the AIDS advocacy group ACT UP. The traditional approach of the health voluntaries, which the Alzheimer's Association emulated, was to raise the awareness of the public and of Congress about the ravages of a given disease, then endorse the proposals of science and policy elites for formulating a research program. The newer organizations have found success by marshaling their constituents' hunger for the delivery of effective treatments now, sometimes against the will of scientific and policy elites. Bick suggests that, in order to succeed in the new environment, health voluntary organizations will have to be more responsive to the needs of the people whose interests they represent than to the professional authority of "the experts."

Stephen Post takes the need to pay attention to the perspectives of patients in a different direction, pointing to the possibilities for well-being and human fulfillment that remain even in dementia. Post criticizes what he calls our "hypercognitive society," characterized by an intensive emphasis on rationality, productivity, self-control, and intellectual growth as the exclusive means to human fulfillment. A hypercognitive society devalues or ignores the relational, aesthetic, and spiritual aspects of life — sources of human well-being that remain open even to persons who are deeply demented. Ethical debates about AD, particularly regarding end-of-life issues, have been dominated by "personhood" theories rooted in hypercognitive values that deny the demented full moral status as persons. In this ethical discourse, physician-assisted suicide is becoming increasingly attractive as an apparently reasonable solution to the problem of dementia. Post argues that debates about ethics and policy must recognize the continued selfhood of the demented and should look for ways in which their well-being can be enhanced through an environment that fosters the emotional, aesthetic, and spiritual opportunities that remain open to them. Such care will not involve technological medical interventions to prolong the lives of persons beyond the moderate stage of dementia, but will provide aesthetic therapies and spiritual support aimed at enhancing the qualities that the patient retains. Post argues that "being with," rather than "doing to," is the most appropriate approach in caring for the demented in a manner that respects their status as persons.

11

The Role of the Concept of Alzheimer Disease in the Development of the Alzheimer's Association in the United States

Patrick J. Fox

Biological, clinical, and epidemiological characterizations feature prominently in social scientific analyses of human disease and infirmity. In some instances, these conceptualizations are viewed critically as sociohistorically derived representations of biomedical phenomena (cf., Lock and Gordon 1988; Nicolson and McLaughlin 1988; Wright and Treacher 1982). Analytic attention is focused on social processes within which the ontological status of disease comes to be characterized, altered, and accepted by medical and nonmedical groups within specific social and historical conditions. In other instances, biomedical constructs are viewed as part of the "background" or context for explaining the conditions and factors that lead to the development of organized social and policy responses to disease entities (e.g., Rettig 1977; Strickland 1972). Such studies approach biomedical conceptualizations as having social utility because they are depictions of reality.

In this chapter, I depart from these analytic approaches to biomedical constructs of disease. Instead, I examine ways in which the biomedical characterizations of Alzheimer disease (AD) are strategically related to the emergence of a social movement dedicated to the eradication of the disease. This line of inquiry explores the link among cultural apparatus (e.g., systems of ideas, rhetoric, symbols), the structure and goals of the movement, and the mobilization of efforts to achieve policy change (cf., Laruna, Johnston, and Gusfield 1994). In particular, it stresses the ways in which cultural forms are used as ideological resources for transforming personal troubles into shared grievances, and the processes that result in organized social and political responses to alter these grievances (McAdam 1994).

By examining the emergence of this disease-based social movement, I highlight the importance of what have been termed "cognitive frames," "ideological packages," "cultural discourses" (Tarrow 1994), or "strategic frames" (Zald 1996) in generating collective representations that are a basis for participation in social movements and identification of political opportunities. A second level of inquiry emphasizes the centrality of social structural conditions and the mobilization of various political, economic, and organizational resources toward the advancement of social and institutional change (McCarthy and Zald 1987). This approach links social institutions with "resource mobilization" strategies to explain the factors that facilitate the emergence, growth, and accomplishments of collective action. Bringing the two lines of inquiry into focus is one way to account for processes that give rise to the emergence of disease-based social movements, as well as to illuminate the public and institutional policy outcomes of movement formation (McAdam 1994; McCarthy and Zald 1987).

I draw on these insights to illustrate how biomedical conceptualizations of AD provided a strategic framework for social movement structures and goals, and for the development of public policies to deal with the consequences of this disease. Although the line that separates social movement activity from interest group activity is rarely clearly demarcated empirically, organized collective activity focusing on AD began as a social movement that was organized in response to the perception that inadequate societal resources were available to assist people affected by the disease. As Walker (1991) argued, the entrenched interest-group system generally does not allow for the expression of concern about emerging new problems. But shifts in biomedical conceptualizations of AD allowed it to be characterized as an emerging new problem in American society that justified organized social and political action.

I narrow my analysis to conceptualizations advanced in the late 1970s and early to mid-1980s because it was in these years that the modern medical meanings of AD in the United States took shape and came to be publicly understood. It was also during this time that groups of people began to publicly identify the disease's effects on their personal lives and to collectively organize a social movement and then interest groups as a response to these experiences. Biomedical conceptualizations of AD served as resources for defining clinical and epidemiological dimensions of the disease, as well as for cognitive frames to identify common interests around which to organize group action among participants. At the end of the 1980s, federal policy responses to AD favored biomedical research and disfavored the health and social service needs of affected groups.

The AD movement generally can be characterized as having followed a "grassroots" model (Rucht 1996) in its formative stage. This model is characterized by a relatively loose, informal, and decentralized structure; an emphasis on unruly, radical protest politics; and reliance on committed adherents. The AD movement diverged from a pure grassroots model in that unruly, radical protest politics were not characteristic of the tactics used by adherents to achieve their goals. While the AD movement possessed both a relatively loose, decentralized structure and groups of committed adherents, its focus on influencing policies through the use of existing political and bureaucratic structures more closely resembled an interest-group model (Rucht 1996).

THE NATIONAL INSTITUTE ON AGING AND ALZHEIMER DISEASE: FINDING AND FUNDING A CAUSE

The U.S. Congress established the National Institute on Aging (NIA) within the National Institutes of Health (NIH) by the Research on Aging Act of 1974 (Public Law 92–296). The NIA was to develop "a plan for a research program on aging designed to coordinate and promote research into the biological, medical, psychological, social, educational, and economic aspects of aging." In the 1960s and 1970s, opponents of a separate institute for aging research claimed that there were inadequate numbers of competent investigators interested in aging research, that too many institutes were proliferating, and that the NIH was already supporting an adequate aging research effort (Lockett 1983).

A compromise was reached between those supporting a narrowly defined focus on biomedical research for the institute and those supporting a broader mission including psychosocial and behavioral research. The final bill that was passed by Congress (H.R. 14424) retained the language of the Senate version calling for biomedical, social, and behavioral research. However, President Nixon vetoed the bill in his interest to reduce the size and complexity of the federal government. In

1973 the bill was reintroduced essentially unchanged and was again passed by Congress in 1974. The bill was sent to President Richard Nixon's desk slightly less than two months before he would leave office as a result of Watergate. Not wanting to further alienate a Congress that was involved in considering his impeachment, Nixon signed P.L. 93–296 on May 31, 1974 (Lockett 1983).

As the first director of the NIA, Robert Butler was interested in the importance of countering misconceptions about "senility." He had been a practicing psychiatrist and brought with him an interest in correcting public perceptions that every elderly person is functionally and cognitively disabled. He wanted to emphasize that many conditions that lead to dementing disorders or memory loss are not necessarily natural aspects of aging and to correct the misconception that all such problems were irreversible.

The NIA initially struggled to identify an area into which it could direct research efforts. As had historically been the case for other institutes within the NIH, it was important for NIA to develop areas of research specialization. From the beginning, the NIH resisted a separate institute for aging research. First, the NIH argued against duplication of administrative services and costs and was against the proliferation of research. Second, the NIH was skeptical of the possibilities of major breakthroughs in understanding the complex process of aging. "The agency already had a 'life process' institute, the (NICHD) National Institute of Child Health and Human Development. The logical argument was that many diseases of the elderly are rooted in the social, physical, and nutritional environment of childhood and adulthood. To break away from the process of human development was not rational" (Lockett 1983, 184). Third, opposition to the development of a separate institute for the study of aging was evident from the wider scientific community. The fear that funds for aging research would divert funds from other established research areas intensified the opposition from members of the scientific community (Lockett 1983).

In the same year that the NIA was legislatively created (two years before Butler was appointed director), Dr. Robert Katzman, a neurologist at Albert Einstein Medical Center in New York, prepared a paper for presentation at the Houston Neurological Symposium sponsored by the University of Texas Health Science Center. In the paper that he prepared with Toksoz Karasu (1975), he made two suggestions that attempted to eliminate the conceptual separation between AD and senile dementia (SD). The first suggestion, which was derived from existing epidemiological data, was that "senile dementia" was the fourth or fifth leading cause of death in the United States. The second suggestion, based on prior scientific work, was that SD and AD were the same entity (Katzman and Karasu 1975). By suggesting an identity between SD and AD, the estimate of the number of potential cases of the disease in the general population substantially increased. This suggestion challenged the assumption of inevitable cognitive decline associated with growing old by explicitly linking "senility" to AD.

In an editorial in the April 1976 *Archives of Neurology*, Katzman reiterated his projection that AD ranked as the fourth or fifth most common cause of death in the United States. Concerns voiced by researchers in the 1950s regarding increases in the population of institutionalized elderly persons with AD in the United States were echoed by Katzman in relation to the community resident elderly. And with the deinstitutionalization movement of the early 1960s in the United States, cognitively impaired elderly persons living in the community provided more visible reminders of the effects of disabling conditions such as AD that increasingly had to be managed outside of institutional settings, usually by family members.

Demographic changes in the age composition of the population also provided fertile ground for the growth of a social movement dedicated to fighting AD. The proportion of persons 65 and older in the U.S. population had steadily increased since the beginning of the twentieth century. In 1910 only 4.3 percent of the population was 65 and older, and by 1970 that proportion had grown to almost 10 percent. By 1980 the proportion of those 65 and older in the population was over two and a half times greater than in 1910 (U.S. Bureau of the Census 1990). Unlike any previous period in American history, the conditions were ripe for the emergence of a social movement dedicated to the eradication of a disease that primarily affects elderly people. Katzman's relatively simple projections would be echoed in subsequent political activities and, tied to estimates of long-term care costs for elderly persons, would emerge as a primary justification for increasing federal support for AD research. They also formed the catalyst for subsequent efforts to define the disease as a major social and health problem and for mobilizing resources to address the defined problem. Katzman was a major "issue entrepreneur" (McCarthy and Zald 1987) for the AD cause.

The emerging movement was also important for increasing the legitimacy of the NIA within the NIH. The NIA needed a social collectivity that could organize to advocate for increased funding for a disease the new institute could call its own. The disease-specific approach had worked for other institutes within the NIH, and it was likely that it could work again. Although the NIA would provide the necessary organizational structure for biomedical research development, it was not able to sustain a constituency to advocate for increased AD research funding. The creation of an organization that could mobilize and sustain an independent social movement was crucial if AD research efforts were to multiply.

Butler focused his efforts on representing the NIA to Congress and on developing a public constituency to advocate for AD research. He was aware of a number of grassroots organizations that addressed issues associated with taking care of brain-impaired persons. But the organizations were geographically dispersed and primarily focused on activity in their local areas. A catalyst was needed to bring their dispersed group efforts into collective action.

Katzman had attempted to organize an AD lay organization in 1974; it finally materialized in December of 1978 as the Alzheimer's Disease Society. The organization, and others around the country, provided the structure needed to facilitate resource aggregation (McCarthy and Zald 1987) (i.e., labor and money) for the nascent AD movement.

Other community-based organizations in the United States focusing on problems associated with the care and treatment of brain-impaired persons included the Family Survival Project in California, the Massachusetts Society Against Dementia in Massachusetts, the Association for Alzheimer's and Related Diseases (AARD) in Minnesota, the Alzheimer's Disease Association in Ohio, the Chronic Organic Brain Syndrome Society (COBSS) in Pennsylvania, and the Alzheimer's Support Information Service Team (ASIST) in Washington. Three of the seven groups were started by researchers. The others were started by family members whose relatives had AD or a related disorder and who had repeatedly experienced difficulty in obtaining medical, emotional, social, and financial support.

Dr. Miriam Aronson, a colleague of Katzman's at Albert Einstein College of Medicine, had visited the California, Minnesota, and Washington groups to explore the idea of forming a national organization and to assess the progress of other groups in developing programs for demented persons and their families. The groups were supportive of the idea of a national group, contingent on working out the specific details of the organizational structure. For Katzman's group, it was clear that targeting AD as the focus of the organization was of primary importance. In commenting on a meeting she attended of the Association for

Alzheimer's and Related Dementias in Minneapolis, Aronson noted that "everyone seems to be in agreement regarding the name including Alzheimer's disease and regarding the need for a national effort" (memo from M. Aronson to R. Katzman, 24 September 1979). A meeting had already been scheduled by the NIA and the National Institute of Neurological and Communicative Disorders and Stroke (NINCDS) to bring these groups together to discuss the possibility of forming a national organization. Aronson felt that "it is imperative that our Alzheimer's Disease Society prepare a proposal to be presented at the October 29th NIA meeting." The proposal would cover the structure, by-laws, financial complications, potential benefits, proposed location, and leadership (memo from M. Aronson to R. Katzman, 24 September 1979).

Robert Butler was instrumental in bringing these groups together, because in his view they had to form a national organization to be effective. He was also interested in claiming AD as one of the major research areas for the NIA so that funding for research could be channeled through the new institute. The active involvement of the NIA in promoting AD research was critical in mobilizing the resources that would be necessary to organize and sustain a social movement dedicated to eradicating the disease. But sustaining a social movement is not easy, and disagreements regarding the goals and mission of the organization would seriously threaten the emerging movement.

From Conflict to Consolidation: Organizing the Alzheimer Disease Social Movement

On October 29, 1979, Robert Butler, in conjunction with Donald Tower at NINCDS, persuaded representatives from the dementia support groups to come to Washington, D.C., for a meeting. After a lengthy discussion, the name Alzheimer's Disease and Related Disorders Association (ADRDA) was agreed upon.

Different opinions as to the purpose of the organization emerged. Disagreements regarding the organization's structure and purposes arose during attempts to develop and ratify a set of by-laws. Some felt that the organization was overly focused on AD and that the "related disorders" were being ignored. They pointed to Katzman's recommendation that the major efforts of the ADRDA in the areas of public information and research be targeted toward AD. While Katzman felt that the services of the ADRDA-sponsored family support groups should be made available to anyone, regardless of disease, he thought that public education and scientific research activities should focus only on AD and a limited number of researchable related disorders that might illuminate aspects of the disease.

But other participants in the movement, especially those who had experience in caring for relatives with cognitive disabilities, wanted a broader focus that would provide assistance for people with all types of brain impairments and their caregivers. The issue of expanding the organization's efforts beyond AD remained the most troublesome problem for caregiver groups from Pittsburgh, Seattle, and San Francisco.

The decision to adopt a disease-specific focus for the ADRDA resulted from the acceptance of a "new" biomedical definition of the disease. The transformation of cases of "senility," "organic brain syndrome," "senile psychosis," and other nondescript diagnostic labels into cases of AD, which had been advocated by Katzman and other researchers during over seventy years of scientific work, was finally beginning to take hold. The transformation of "senility" to AD and the ADRDA emphasis on the disease signaled the acceptance of their norms and provided a clear direction for the association to proceed.

Concerns regarding a disease-specific focus of advocacy efforts also arose from members of the ADRDA Medical and Scientific Advisory Board. In conjunction with the NIA, the fledgling organization wasted no time in initiating efforts to increase congressional awareness of the disease. In July 1980, Senator Thomas Eagleton, a long-time supporter of aging-related research who had been instrumental in establishing the NIA (Lockett 1983), chaired a joint congressional hearing on the impact of AD on the nation's elderly.

During the hearing, Jerome Stone outlined the broad goals of the ADRDA: stimulating research into the causes of, and treatments for, AD; medical professional education; public education; advocacy for long-term care services for victims and families; formation of family support groups nationwide; and the development of epidemiological data on the disease. Although recommendations regarding professional education and revising the financing of long-term care were raised, it was evident that the primary goal of the hearing was to stimulate support for research at the NIH into the causes and treatment of AD. A difference of opinion arose, however, as to whether the research should be disease-specific and what types of research should be emphasized.

In their formal testimony, Carl Eisdorfer and Robert Butler supported the general need for both basic and clinical research. In response to a question, however, Eisdorfer promoted the expansion of clinical research, not categorical funding:

My concern is not so much targeted research for a given disease — and I hope my friends in the society do not get angry with me for saying it — I am less concerned with targeted research for Alzheimer's, diabetes, and so on than I am for doing something about the profile of clinical research. I am fairly clear that I think we would make a disastrous thing if we shifted from a strong basic research profile. But at the same time, the way we are structured now, it is very difficult to do clinical research in the U.S., for a whole variety of reasons, with no criticism of the National Institutes; they were never created for that. (U.S. Senate 1980, 105)

Butler agreed with Eisdorfer on the importance of clinical research, but admitted that 90 to 92 percent of the NIA's AD research budget was for basic science research, a distribution similar to that of the other NIH institutes (U.S. Senate 1980). Mirroring the dominant attitude within the scientific community, the NIH had been strongly committed to basic research and relatively cautious about disease-specific clinical research.

The choice of a categorical approach to advocacy was disruptive to the ADRDA. The differentiation of diseases was difficult for certain members to accept as the primary focus of the new organization. In a letter to the ADRDA board following the joint hearing, Bobbie Glaze, the ADRDA program development chairperson and a witness at the hearing, commented on the written testimony that had been submitted by Martha Fenchak, vice-president of ADRDA:

In reviewing this statement, we became aware that nowhere was there mention of our national association (ADRDA), but there was reference to "their affiliates," San Francisco Family Survival and Seattle ASIST. There was one slight mention of Alzheimer's disease — "one of the early forms of early senility." These, and several other factors, became a curious consideration when coming from the Vice President of our national association. (Memo from B. Glaze to ADRDA board members, 18 August 1980)

In a memo to Jerome Stone and Lonnie Wollin (who helped Katzman organize the New York-based Alzheimer Disease Society) following the hearing, John Mitchell, an ADRDA board member, reflected a similar sentiment:

It is apparent that Ms. Fenchak's statement pertained to senility in general with a very slight mention made of Alzheimer's disease on page 4. Furthermore, she refers to the Family Survival Project of San Francisco and ASIST of Seattle as being "affiliates of [Pittsburgh] COBSS" and "assures you (the committee) that there is national support of this movement." In my opinion since this was a joint hearing with the Appropriations Subcommittee this statement seriously impairs the goal, policies and objectives of ADRDA. The name of the game is Alzheimer's, not Senility. (Memo from J. Mitchell to J. Stone and L. Wollin, 7 August 1980)

The conflicts reflected the fact that "Alzheimer's disease" was beginning to replace "senility" in the consciousness of these Americans as the label for cognitive impairments associated with age. The disease was becoming part of the routine definition of the cause of cognitive impairments in the elderly that laypersons on the board of the newly formed organization were using as a guide for the group's activities. But the philosophical differences among the seven groups were not resolved, and the San Francisco-based FSP and the Seattle-based ASIST groups formally withdrew from the ADRDA in 1980 (minutes of the ADRDA board of directors, 15 August 1980 and 8 November 1980).

Interest in the ADRDA soared after a letter from a family member of an AD victim outlining the problems in caring for someone with the disease was published in October 1980 in "Dear Abby," the nationally syndicated newspaper advice column. The "Dear Abby" column aroused a tremendous response. ADRDA received between thirty and forty thousand letters from people in all regions of the United States. The letter stimulated the formation of local support groups. In San Diego, for example, Joy Glenner and her husband George, who was an AD researcher at the University of California, recall that the letter prompted a woman whose husband had been diagnosed with AD to put a notice in the local newspaper inviting anyone who had a relative with AD to meet at a certain church to form a self-help family support group. "And we arrived on the scene just at the time that she had taken the initiative. My husband got in touch with her and said, 'I would like to help you.' We went to the church and 26 families came to that first meeting and we collected $12.58 in a paper cup. I just kept going to the newspapers and we got more notices put in the paper and the next month 58 families showed up. The following month over 70 families came" (J. Glenner, personal communication, 13 May 1986).

During this period the number of AD-related projects within the NIA was growing. The reputation of the scientists and the quality of the proposals resulted in increasing numbers of NIA proposals being funded. NIA funding had increased an average of 39 percent per year between 1976 and 1980 (U.S. Department of Health and Human Services 1984), and the new institute's credibility and legitimacy grew within both the NIH and Congress. The development of scientific credibility was essential because in the political struggle that led to the creation of the NIA, the paucity of researchers in the field of aging research was repeatedly used as a rationale to deny the need for a separate aging institute (Lockett 1983).

Beginning in the 1980s, primarily as a result of ADRDA-initiated activities to increase public awareness, a series of congressional hearings documenting the devastating effects of AD, as well as the need for increased research funds, were conducted (U.S. Senate 1980; U.S. House of Representatives 1983a, 1983b, 1985a, 1985b, 1985c, 1986a, 1986b, 1986c, 1986d). In addition to the press releases the NIA issued regarding advances in AD research, the ADRDA began to disseminate more actively human-interest stories illustrating the devastating effects of the disease on family members (ADRDA 1985). These activities kept AD in the public consciousness and helped to recruit new allies to the cause.

While the ADRDA and the NIA were working closely to advance the cause of AD research, the efforts of the ADRDA's Washington lobbyist resulted in increased access to representatives and senators (R. Katzman, personal communication, 12 November 1985; J. Stone, personal communication, 30 October 1986). The ADRDA developed a two-pronged public awareness campaign aimed at local communities and government leaders (Ruscio and Cavarocchi 1984). Chapter and affiliate members contacted their senators and representatives advocating support of AD-related legislation. ADRDA covered 15 states in 1979. By 1986 there were 125 chapters and affiliates in 44 states that utilized between 25,000 and 35,000 volunteers (U.S. Senate Subcommittee on Aging 1980).

Princess Yasmin Aga Kahn, the daughter of film star Rita Hayworth, who had been diagnosed as having AD, was a highly visible advocate. Yasmin Kahn had been recruited to serve on the board of the ADRDA, and her notoriety was instrumental in gaining entree to the offices of congressmen (R. Katzman, personal communication, 12 November 1985). The association of celebrities such as Yasmin Kahn with the ADRDA signaled the emergence of a public culture of AD. This high level of public awareness (Gubrium 1986) was reinforced by the revelation in 1995 that former President Ronald Reagan had developed AD.

As an active supporter of the AD social movement, Butler was concerned that resources that could potentially be directed to the AD research enterprise might instead be directed to competing disease interests. The NIA needed to court congressional allies who could facilitate the mobilization of economic resources for the expansion of the fight against AD. By one measure, the NIA was extremely successful: in 1979, it had spent approximately $4 million on research into AD; by 1991, it was spending $155 million—a 37-fold increase. The larger research budget and the passage of legislation related to the disease were largely due to concerted efforts by members and allies of the AD movement to call congressional and public attention to the "disease of the century" (Thomas 1983). NIA staff were able to develop a resource base in conjunction with the scientific community and, through the formation of the ADRDA, to raise issues associated with AD to a level of national prominence.

Largely due to the efforts of the NIA and the ADRDA, the interests of scientists in increasing funds for biomedical research emerged as the primary focus of federal AD policy. But political and economic forces in the 1980s also facilitated this type of policy development. Unprecedented federal budget deficits and an administration that was ambivalent, if not hostile, toward federal spending for social welfare promoted a public policy that was in concert with the interests of an elite group of biomedical researchers but that failed to develop programs to meet the needs of caregivers. Although people with the disease and their care providers were supportive of research that might lead to treatments, they needed services and financial support to help them cope with the immediate problems of daily life. But policy development to address those needs would have to wait.

THE FRUITS OF POLITICAL ACTION: THE EMERGENCE OF ALZHEIMER DISEASE POLICY

As a result of the activities of the NIA and the ADRDA in the early 1980s, policymakers and the public were becoming increasingly aware of the problem of the "fourth or fifth leading cause of death in the United States." With demographers discussing the "graying of America," pressure to develop public policy to address AD was mounting. But increasing federal budget deficits provided the Reagan Administration with an economic argument for proceeding with its ideological preference for limiting the growth in spending for social services. This political ideology was a crucial determinant of the emergence of an AD public policy that emphasized funding scientific research.

With the federal budget deficit having grown by 163 percent between 1981 and 1983, the Reagan Administration introduced a broad range of policy changes. The goals of the administration were to "reduce the size and influence of government, restore economic prosperity, and improve national security" (Palmer and Sawhill 1984). National security would be spurred by increasing defense spending, economic prosperity would be realized by lowering taxes, and reducing the size and influence of government would be realized by shrinking social welfare spending. To achieve the latter, public funding for a variety of categorical public health and social service programs was restructured and reduced. Multicategorical grants for health and social services were converted into smaller block grants to state governments, which could use the funds for broad programmatic areas with few restrictions or reporting requirements. Under the Omnibus Budget Reconciliation Act of 1980, the federal share of the Medicaid program was cut and Medicare payments were tightened, although the rising cost of hospital care and physicians' services more than compensated for these attempts to control spending (Newcomer and Harrington 1983; Harrington 1983). States were given broad authority to restrict Medicaid program eligibility, reduce the number and type of covered services, and limit payments to hospitals.

To stimulate economic growth, the Economic Recovery Tax Act of 1981 reduced taxes on the private sector. The loss of tax revenues proved to be so great, however, that the business tax cuts were substantially revoked by the Tax Equity and Fiscal Responsibility Act of the following year. When the economy picked up as inflation and unemployment rates declined, the deficit nonetheless continued to grow, and "the prospect of balancing the budget in the foreseeable future disappeared once the administration realized the full impact of its tax and spending decisions" (Sawhill and Stone 1984). These political and economic conditions limited policy options regarding AD. They also contributed to the success of scientists, the NIA, and the ADRDA in directing federal AD policy toward funding biomedical research.

FEDERAL ALZHEIMER DISEASE POLICY: CRISIS FOR THE FUTURE, PROBLEM FOR THE PRESENT

Beginning in 1980, a series of congressional hearings were held to obtain information regarding AD and efforts to deal with it (U.S. Senate 1980; U.S. House of Representatives 1982, 1983a, 1983b, 1985a, 1985b, 1985c, 1986a, 1986b, 1986c, 1986d). The personal crises engendered by the disease were repeatedly reaffirmed during these hearings. Family members provided testimony documenting the horrors associated with watching a relative deteriorate with little hope of financial or service support. Caregivers recounted in painful detail the emotional and financial burdens they experienced.

Help with caring for people with AD was also emerging as a women's issue, because women typically were the ones to care for ill or infirm family members (U.S. House of Representatives 1983a). Although caregiving as a women's issue was not a major focus of the hearings, suggestions were made regarding the range of services needed to adequately address the problem of community care for demented patients. Detailed proposals for the expansion of services appropriate for the care of afflicted patients were presented (U.S. House of Representatives 1983a). Inadequacies in coverage provided by government and private insurance as well as in the provision and financing of home health care, adult day care, adult day health care, skilled nursing care, homemaker/chore assistance, respite care, and other long-term care services were documented (U.S. House of Representatives 1983a, 1985a, 1986a, 1986b, 1986c, 1986d).

A recurrent focus of discussions between witnesses and committee members at the hearings was the practical funding and personnel requirements for biomedical research and training. In all but one of the twelve hearings conducted from 1980 to 1986, the focus of discussion was policy development to address biomedical research needs. Researchers provided information regarding the characteristics of the disease, its projected burden on the economy, and the research and training needs for medical and health professionals.

The primary rationale used by advocates to support increased biomedical research funding was that the costs of caring for persons with AD would increase dramatically in the future with the aging of the "baby boomers." Spending more now for biomedical research in the hope of stemming the tide of the disease, they argued, could save untold billions of dollars for long-term care in the future (U.S. House of Representatives 1983a). As Lonnie Wollin commented during a House hearing on AD: "If you don't fund substantial research, you will have this problem for a long time. The only analogy would be polio. Had the money gone into treatment, we would have a magnificent portable iron lung, but no cure for the disease" (U.S. House of Representatives 1986c).

Researchers and representatives of government bureaucracies repeatedly cited the enormous costs that American society would have to bear in the future if a treatment or cure for AD was not found. In testimony given between 1983 and 1986, the annual costs of care for victims of the disease was estimated to be between $25 and $30 billion. It was also suggested that the future costs of the disease could potentially bankrupt the government as the baby boom generation reached senescence (U.S. House of Representatives 1983a, 1983b, 1986c). The cost of caring for people with the disease was estimated at $100 billion for 1990 (Rice et al. 1992); by the year 2030 the national cost of caring for victims of the disease was predicted to balloon to $750 billion (ADRDA 1987). The cost-saving argument implied that given adequate resources, medical science would be able to develop treatments or a cure for the disease that would forestall the need for significant long-term care expenditures by the time the baby boom generation began to reach senescence early in the twenty-first century.

Advocates for the AD cause implicitly established a twenty-year time table for the fruits of their faith in medical science to be realized. In spite of new discoveries about the disease, there was still no way to conclusively diagnose it while the patient was alive, no consensus as to its cause, and no effective methods to treat, much less cure it. But there were also no paradigms to compete with the biomedical model. Funding biomedical research seemed a far more attractive option than establishing entitlement programs to provide long-term care for patients and support services for their families. Biomedical research costs would be much easier to control than expansions in long-term care entitlements, and reform of long-term care was a struggle that few congressional policymakers cared to embark upon. Besides, increasing the funding for disease research was in line with the goals of the ADRDA, the major advocacy group representing the interests of persons with AD.

The long-term-care cost estimates and the cost-savings argument became a commodity in the public crisis marketplace. Increased funding for biomedical research emerged as a politically and economically expedient policy, tangible evidence of federal action to address the "disease of the century."

ALZHEIMER DISEASE AND THE POLITICAL ECONOMY OF HEALTH AND AGING

Conceptions of the relationship between health and old age permeate political and economic decisions that are reflected in health policies affecting elderly people. In American society, these conceptions usually include three interrelated assumptions. First, aging tends to be characterized as a process of biological and physiological decline and decay. Second, some elderly persons are viewed as deserving, while others are seen as undeserving. Third, old people and old age are a problem to society that is of crisis proportions and is a major contributor to the healthcare crisis that is said to be occurring (Estes et al. 1984). These perceptions "flow largely from those who have the greatest power to influence the dominant definition of societal problems and to specify policy interventions and resource allocations to address those problems" (Estes 1983).

The decision by the founders of the ADRDA to focus the organization's efforts on AD was made because of a desire to find treatments and a cure, and because of the realities of biomedical research funding in the United States. The emergence of AD as the metaphor for dementia associated with aging resulted in a challenge to the notion of the inevitability of decline in old age that traditionally has been equated with "senility." The stereotype of elderly people as forgetful, unable to manage their everyday affairs, and totally dependent on others for survival because of cognitive impairment is one of the most feared connotations associated with growing old. The suggestion by medical men and women that AD was the primary cause of senile dementia emphasized that cognitive changes associated with aging were not inevitable. Rather, they are manifestations of specific disease processes that can be identified, studied, and perhaps controlled. From this biomedical viewpoint, aging is characterized as a period in which certain diseases are more likely to emerge than others, rather than as a process of inevitable biological and physiological decline. The reconstitution of senility cum AD signaled the transformation in the public mind of the meaning of brain impairment associated with age from an inevitability to a possibility. Instead of an inevitable by-product of growing old, cognitive impairments associated with aging became attributable to a pernicious disease entity afflicting a certain percentage of elderly persons irrespective of social, psychological, or physical characteristics. The acceptance of the definitional transformation was politically crucial because it conferred power on biomedical researchers and medical professionals and spread their norms to others (Edleman 1977).

Although the medical conception of AD challenged the notion of inevitable cognitive decline associated with aging, in conjunction with the categorical approach to increasing research funds, it reinforced two other assumptions that undergird the political economy of health and aging in American society. The categorical emphasis on AD that was necessary for resource aggregation to support biomedical research tacitly reaffirmed the assumption of the "deserving" and "undeserving" elderly. The policy of the ADRDA was to provide family support services to anyone who needed them. The emphasis on AD for advocacy and public education efforts resulted in the implicit differentiation of the "deserving" and the "undeserving" elderly on the basis of disease type. The deserving elderly are those with AD and those with related dementing disorders. Both groups have the direct benefit of support services, but those with AD are more "deserving" because research resources are directed toward curing the specific disease with which they are afflicted. The "undeserving" elderly are those who do not have a dementing disorder and who are not targeted for research or services, even though services that benefit persons with AD and related disorders (e.g., personal care, homemaker/chore assistance, etc.) can benefit persons with a wide variety of chronic illnesses. The split between the deserving and undeserving engendered by the categorical approach to funding research on specific diseases was an outgrowth of interest-group politics that dominates American political culture.

The third assumption that undergirds the political economy of health and aging in American society — that old people and old age are a major contributor to the healthcare crisis that is said to be occurring — leads to a crisis mentality. It emphasizes spiraling healthcare costs and the inability of government to control those costs that is a by-product of health care offered as a commodity in the marketplace (Rodberg and Stevenson 1977). The assumption that old people and old age are a problem of crisis proportions to society was tacitly reflected in the primary rationale used for increasing biomedical research funding — to save future long-term-care costs. The crisis is going to get worse, the argument goes, and aged persons with AD are going to be a greater burden on society, so we need to find a cure to solve the problem.

The strategy worked, but disagreements that were evident in the formative stages of the ADRDA, which placed the interests of those promoting biomedical research in competition with those promoting public policy addressing the immediate problems of people who care for victims of the disease, continued (Boffey 1985). In spite of the inclusion of "related disorders" in the name, the primary goal of the ADRDA was the promotion of AD research. Reflecting this, in 1988 the name of the organization was changed to the Alzheimer's Association.

The continuation of the ADRDA's primary mission of supporting biomedical research is reflected in the policy recommendations of their yearly "National Program to Conquer Alzheimer's Disease" (ADRDA 1987; Alzheimer's Association 1988, 1989, 1990, 1991, 1992). From the late 1980s to the early 1990s, the program recommendations reflect consistent themes that have been the cornerstone of the organization since its inception. These themes are oriented toward research, education, association chapter development, public policy advocacy to meet the needs of patients and families, and improving services to patients and caregivers.

Reflecting the concerns expressed by those involved in the founding of ADRDA, the recommendations for increasing research funding contained in the policy statements consistently refer to finding treatments and a cure for AD and related disorders. Reflecting the unintended differentiation between the deserving and undeserving elderly inherent in the categorical approach, AD remains the rallying point around which the association advocates for increased research funds. Policy recommendations concerned with other goals of the organization, although focused on AD, are more explicit in terms of specifying the need for help for both persons with AD and those with a related disorder.

Recognizing and reacting to the competition of the disease crisis marketplace, the association began in 1989 to include explicit comparisons between the social costs of AD and research funding levels. These comparisons provided a benchmark that highlighted the association's success in achieving its goal of increasing federal, state, and private support for research. In the organization's 1989 program report, $30 per AD patient was reported as being spent on research; in 1990, it increased to $32 per patient; in 1991, to $60; and in 1992, to $70 per patient (Alzheimer's Association 1989, 1990, 1991, 1992).

Reflecting the earlier concerns of scientists who feared that funds for aging research would divert funds from other established research areas, the association's program statements also began in 1989 to compare AD to other diseases in terms of the social cost/research funding formula. The commodification of the disease was in full swing. The established killers, cancer and cardiovascular disease, as well as a newcomer, AIDS, began to be compared with AD as the association continued to press its research funding agenda. People with AD were just as deserving as people with cancer, heart disease, and AIDS of a portion of the federal biomedical research and health and social service dollar. And the association was dedicated to insuring that their constituencies — patients, caregivers, and researchers — got their fair share.

The association also continued to press for modifications of the long-term-care service delivery and financing system. In this arena, the policy statements of the association reflected a concern with the long-term-care needs of all persons with chronic diseases, especially those caused by AD and related disorders. Advocating for the interests of persons with AD and related disorders; their caregivers; and providers of education, health, and social services, the association consistently outlined recommendations in their program statements for the federal government to develop a comprehensive long-term-care social insurance system for persons of all ages. The association's specific recommendations focused on long- and short-term goals and varied from year to year in response to pending legislation related to the interests of the association's constituents. In the association's 1992 recommendations, the focus shifted from long-term-care reform to advocating for the enactment of comprehensive healthcare reform covering both the acute and long-term-care needs of Americans of all ages. This philosophical shift in the association's advocacy approach mitigated the differentiation of categories of the deserving and undeserving elderly that was implicit in policy statements of prior years.

While emphasizing the crisis mode of the healthcare system in the context of AD continued to be an association hallmark, it became linked for the first time in the association's history to the larger issue of healthcare coverage for all Americans. The nesting of the interests of persons with AD and their caregivers within the larger issue of universal health care in the United States signaled a change from the categorical approach for research funding that had served the association well for many years. Although federal policies and funding continue to reflect the interests of the association in finding treatments and a cure, the linking of the care needs of persons with AD to those of other persons with similar needs provides the potential for the emergence of common interests that transcend the disease-specific approach that has been used so effectively in the United States to increase research funds for AD and a variety of other diseases.

DIVERSE INTERESTS AND THE ALZHEIMER'S ENTERPRISE

The basic goal of medical science in relation to AD is one of the noblest forms of human endeavor — to treat and cure disease. But it is also a business, and thus it involves powerful economic interests involved in the marketplace of disease diagnosis and treatment. As the interests of research scientists and businesses that will profit from the development of treatments for the disease must be understood, so too must the interests of those afflicted with the disease and those who care for them. If the recent emergence of AD as a social and health problem is any indication, scientists will be organized to protect their interests. Businesses that can profit from developing treatments for the disease can also be relied upon to protect their interests. But the interests of the mass of people who have the disease are less clearly protected, especially in light of governmental inaction in developing a plan for universal medical care in general, and long-term care in particular.

The time line implied by advocates of research into AD was that significant treatments or even a cure would occur by the first decade of the twenty-first century. Even using modest estimates of the prevalence of dementia in people over age 65 (e.g., 9 to 12 percent), as the baby boom cohort reaches senescence, the proportion of Americans with dementing illnesses will be larger than ever before in U.S. history. If treatments that significantly reduce the morbidity associated with AD are not available, the issue of how to provide care for this group of people increases in importance.

Family members shoulder the primary burden of caring for demented relatives (Rice et al. 1993). In the early stages of the AD movement, their frustration, anger, and sadness motivated them to form into voluntary groups in California, Massachusetts, Minnesota, New York, Ohio, Pennsylvania, and Washington, and, subsequently, into the national Alzheimer's Disease and Related Disorders Association. The explicit link between the organization of disaffected people and the direction of the movement provided by government bureaucrats and medical researchers is a large part of how medical research priorities are established within the American political arena. The movement was influenced by medical men and women who provided a concrete direction that not only supported their career interests but also was legitimized by scientific expertise and ideology. The danger of this system is that the interests of researchers, couched in terms of the interests of patients and families in finding treatments and a cure for AD, may overshadow the interests of caregivers in obtaining services and other types of support to immediately assist them in the care of demented relatives.

The role of caregiver in American society has been traditionally filled by women. As the participation of women in the labor force increases, women may not be as willing or able to assume caregiving roles as the baby boomers begin to age. The Alzheimer's Association clearly recognizes the needs of caregivers and victims of the disease because they form the constituency whom the association ultimately represents.

The focus of advocacy adopted by the organization is directed through the lens of those interested in promoting a disease-specific focus for resource aggregation to establish careers, build organizations, compete for resources, and ultimately to discover treatments and a cure for the disease. The hope for treatment advances is the foundation of the faith in medical science as the route to the solution of the problem of

AD. But as research on other diseases such as cancer demonstrates, progress in developing treatments and cures, especially for chronic diseases affecting the brain, is excruciatingly slow. Cancer has proved especially difficult to treat and cure, AIDS is a dreaded newcomer that promises to be multifarious, and diseases of the brain are likely to be among the most complex of all. The human capacity for solving problems of disease is more often than not overshadowed by the complexity of diseases and their biological mechanisms. But the search for treatments and a cure provides hope to millions that one day AD will only be an unpleasant memory. A potential by-product of this pace is the entrenchment of the treatment and research enterprise as overly self-serving. This is especially a concern when funds earmarked for researching a disease are greater than those earmarked to help care for victims of it.

The categorical approach to research funding for diseases results in two things. First, constituencies must be mobilized to create political pressure to advocate for the direction of resources to a specific disease. A by-product of this approach is that people come to: (1) see their interests defined in terms of a specific disease; and (2) define their self-interest in terms of the interests of medical researchers who can find treatments and a cure. The stakes are then played out among competing diseases for research support.

Second, the categorical approach tends to mitigate the possibility of a broad coalition of people representing many diseases organizing to advocate for insurance coverage to meet a larger portion of the healthcare needs of all Americans. As was the case in the formative stages of the AD movement, those interested in ADRDA advocacy efforts extending beyond research support for AD attempted to surmount the limitations imposed by the categorical approach. The splintering of interest groups along disease lines tends to inhibit the organized political action that is necessary to advance the cause of universal healthcare coverage for all Americans.

People with chronic illnesses have similar needs with respect to managing their everyday lives. Homemaker/chore, personal care, and similar types of assistance are valuable for persons with arthritis, AIDS, chronic heart failure, chronic obstructive pulmonary disease, ischemic vascular dementia, and so on as well as AD. But the development of interest groups for political advocacy is a cornerstone of American political life. That feature of the political system promotes the separation of interests as people readily support disease-specific approaches because of their personal experience of having a disease or from knowing someone who has it. The emotional power of these experiences is compelling and provides the energy for people to become involved and support an organization dedicated to a disease.

Faith in medical science as the route to finding the cure for a disease that significantly changes the stability and certainty of an individual's lifetime behavior patterns is the basis for much of the effort of the AD movement. The reductionism of medical science, as investigators attempt to search for treatments and a cure for the disease in the physical substratum of the brain, continues a long tradition concerned with searching for the keys to the human mind in the biological structure and function of the human brain. The practical question that remains is whether the approach can result in significant progress in the two areas that are the yardstick against which medical progress is ultimately measured — successful treatments and cures.

References

Alzheimer's Association. 1988. *National Program to Conquer Alzheimer's Disease 1988.* Chicago: Alzheimer's Disease and Related Disorders Association.

——. 1989. *National Program to Conquer Alzheimer's Disease 1989.* Chicago: Alzheimer's Disease and Related Disorders Association.

——. 1990. *National Program to Conquer Alzheimer's Disease 1990.* Chicago: Alzheimer's Association.

——. 1991. *National Program to Conquer Alzheimer's Disease 1991.* Chicago: Alzheimer's Association.

——. 1992. *National Program to Conquer Alzheimer's Disease 1992.* Chicago: Alzheimer's Association.

Alzheimer's Disease and Related Disorders Association (ADRDA). 1985. Alzheimer's no longer a silent epidemic. *ADRDA Newsletter* 5.

——. 1987. *National Program to Conquer Alzheimer's Disease 1987.* Chicago: Alzheimer's Disease and Related Disorders Association.

Boffey, P. M. 1985. Alzheimer's disease: Families are bitter. *New York Times,* 7 May.

Edleman, M. 1977. *Political Language: Words that Succeed and Policies that Fail.* New York: Academic Press.

Estes, C. L. 1983. Fiscal austerity and aging. In *Fiscal Austerity and Aging: Shifting Government Responsibility for the Elderly,* ed. C. L. Estes, R. J. Newcomer, and Associates. Beverly Hills, Calif.: Sage.

Estes, C. L., L. E. Gerard, J. Sprague Zones, and J. H. Swan, 1984. *Political Economy, Health, and Aging.* Boston: Little, Brown and Co.

Gubrium, J. 1986. *Oldtimers and Alzheimer's: The Descriptive Organization of Senility.* Greenwich, Conn.: JAI Press.

Harrington, C. 1983. Social Security and Medicare: Policy shifts in the 1980s. In *Fiscal Austerity and Aging: Shifting Government Responsibility for the Elderly*, ed. C. Estes, R. Newcomer and Associates. Beverly Hills, Calif.: Sage.

Katzman, R., and T. Karasu. 1975. Differential diagnosis of dementia. In *Neurological and Sensory Disorders in the Elderly*, ed. W. Fields. New York: Stratton Intercontinental Medical Book Corp.

Larana, E., H. Johnston, and J. R. Gusfield. 1994. *New Social Movements: From Ideology to Identity*. Philadelphia: Temple University Press.

Lock, M., and D. Gordon, eds. 1988. *Biomedicine Examined*. Dordrecht: Kluwer.

Lockett, B. 1983. *Aging, Politics, and Research: Setting the Federal Agenda for Research on Aging*. New York: Springer.

McAdam, D. 1994. Culture and social movements. In *New Social Movements: From Ideology to Identity*, ed. E. Larana, H. Johnston, and J. R. Gusfield. Philadelphia: Temple University Press.

McCarthy, J., and M. Zald. 1987. Resource mobilization theory. In *Social Movements in Organizational Society*, ed. M. Zald and J. McCarthy. New Brunswick, N.J.: Transaction Books.

Newcomer, R., and C. Harrington. 1983. State Medicaid expenditures: Trends and program policy changes. In *Fiscal Austerity and Aging: Shifting Government Responsibility for the Elderly*, ed. C. Estes, R. Newcomer, and Associates. Beverly Hills, Calif.: Sage.

Nicolson, M., and C. McLaughlin. 1988. Social constructionism and medical sociology: A study of the vascular theory of multiple sclerosis. *Sociology of Health and Illness* 10(3): 234–61.

Palmer, J. L., and I. V. Sawhill, eds. 1984. *The Reagan Record*. Cambridge, Mass.: Ballinger Publishing.

Rettig, R. 1977. *Cancer Crusade: The Story of the National Cancer Act of 1971*. Princeton: Princeton University Press.

Rice, D. P., P. J. Fox, W. Max, P. A. Webber, D. A. Lindeman, W. W. Hauck, and E. Segura. 1992. The Economic Burden of Alzheimer's Disease. Unpublished manuscript, Institute for Health & Aging, School of Nursing, University of California, San Francisco.

———. 1993. The economic burden of caring for people with Alzheimer's disease. *Health Affairs* 12(2): 164–76.

Rodberg, L., and G. Stevenson. 1977. The health care industry in advanced capitalism. *Review of Radical Political Economics* 9:104.

Rucht, D. 1996. The impact of national contexts on social movement structures: A cross-movement and cross-national comparison. In *Comparative Perspectives on Social Movements*, ed. D. McAdam, J. McCarthy, and M. Zald. New York: Cambridge University Press.

Ruscio, D., and N. Cavarocchi. 1984. Getting on the political Agenda. *Generations* (Winter): 12–14.

Sawhill, I. V., and C. F. Stone. 1984. The economy: The key to success. In *The Reagan Record*, ed. J. L. Palmer and I. V. Sawhill. Cambridge, Mass.: Ballinger Publishing.

Strickland, S. P. 1972. *Politics, Science and Dread Disease.* Cambridge: Harvard University Press.

Tarrow, S. 1994. *Power in Movement.* New York: Cambridge University Press.

Thomas, L. 1983. Quote appearing in ADRDA advertisement, *New York Times*, 21 June.

U.S. Bureau of the Census. 1970. *Statistical Abstract of the United States: 1970, 91st ed.* Washington D.C.: U.S. Government Printing Office.

———. 1990. *Statistical Abstract of the United States: 1990, 110th ed.* Washington D.C.: U.S. Government Printing Office.

U.S. Department of Health and Human Services. 1984. *NIH Data Book*, pub. no. 84–1261, Public Health Service, National Institutes of Health. Washington D.C: U.S. Government Printing Office.

U.S. House of Representatives, Select Committee on Aging. 1982. *Oversight Conference on Aging: A Preconference Assessment.* Pub. no. 97–320. Washington, D.C.: Government Printing Office.

U.S. House of Representatives, Select Committee on Aging, 98th Congress. 1983a. *Senility: The Last Stereotype.* Pub. no. 98–390. Washington, D.C.: U.S. Government Printing Office.

———. 1983b. *Alzheimer's Disease: Is There an Acid Rain Connection?* Pub. no. 98–400. Washington, D.C.: U.S. Government Printing Office.

———. 1985a. *Alzheimer's Disease: A Florida Perspective.* Pub. no. 98–476. Washington, D.C.: U.S. Government Printing Office.

———. 1985b. *Caring for Our Nation's Alzheimer's Victims.* Washington, D.C.: U.S. Government Printing Office.

U.S. House of Representatives, Committee on Science and Technology, 99th Congress. 1985c. *Alzheimer's Disease Research.* Pub. no. 135. Washington, D.C.: U.S. Government Printing Office.

U.S. House of Representatives, Select Committee on Aging, 99th Congress. 1986a. *Setting a Federal Agenda for Alzheimer's Disease.* Pub. no. 99–569. Washington, D.C.: U.S. Government Printing Office.

———. 1986b. *Alzheimer's Disease and Related Disorders: The Government's Response.* Pub. no. 99–588. Washington, D.C.: U.S. Government Printing Office.

———. 1986c. *Alzheimer's Disease: Burdens and Problems for Victims and their Families.* Pub. no. 99–542. Washington, D.C.: U.S. Government Printing Office.

————. 1986d. *Alzheimer's Disease: Pennsylvania Perspective.* Pub. no. 99–548. Washington, D.C.: U.S. Government Printing Office.

U.S. Senate, Subcommittee on Aging of the Committee on Labor and Human Resources, and U.S. House of Representatives, Subcommittee on Labor, Health, Education and Welfare of the Committee on Appropriations, 96th Congress. 1980. *Impact of Alzheimer's Disease on the Nation's Elderly.* Washington, D.C.: U.S. Government Printing Office.

Walker, J. 1991. *Mobilizing Interest Groups in America.* Ann Arbor: University of Michigan Press.

Wright, P. G., and A. Treacher, eds. 1982. *The Problem of Medical Knowledge: Examining the Social Construction of Medicine.* Edinburgh: Edinburgh University Press.

Zald, M. 1996. Culture, ideology, and strategic framing. In *Comparative Perspectives on Social Movements,* ed. D. McAdam, J. McCarthy, and M. Zald. New York: Cambridge University Press.

12

The History of the Alzheimer's Association

FUTURE PUBLIC POLICY IMPLICATIONS

Katherine L. Bick

The Alzheimer's Association was originally named the Alzheimer's Disease and Related Disorders Association (ADRDA), a cumbersome name cobbled together to address the concerns of the founding organizations for the preservation of their respective identities. At the organizational meeting held at the National Institutes of Health (NIH) in 1979 at the invitation of the National Institute of Neurological and Communicative Disorders and Stroke (NINCDS) and the National Institute on Aging (NIA), the original seven groups were clearly diverse in their origins and in the goals they considered key to their mission. While the political advantages of consolidation were obvious to most of the participants, there were some who thought that the price might be too high in terms of the loss, or at the least subordination, of their specific missions. In Chapter 11 of this volume, Patrick Fox discusses this early history more extensively. The organization changed its name to the Alzheimer's Association in 1988 to reflect its unequivocal focus on Alzheimer disease (AD) and to enhance public recognition of its mission.

In the historical sense, the Alzheimer's Association is a relative newcomer in the world of health voluntary organizations. Such health voluntaries are formed by persons personally affected by a particular disease; they mobilize to get their plight across to the broader public, who, as a rule, are not concerned with the suffering of others in general. Initially, such founders are usually driven more by altruism — the urge to alleviate for others the difficulties they have encountered in their own misfortune — than by an urge for power. In fact, as Alexis de Tocqueville noted over one hundred and fifty years ago (1835–39), Americans have a particular propensity for forming themselves into voluntary associations to improve the public good, at least as they perceive that good. The original founders of the ADRDA were typical in that they included members with family afflicted with cognitive problems due to brain injuries, others with late-life dementias, and scientists and physicians with both personal and scientific interests in the study of dementias.

In the United States, the path for those affected by AD and other dementias was well marked by such prominent groups as the March of Dimes, the American Cancer Society, and the American Heart Association earlier in the century. In the beginning these organizations were influenced largely by scientists and physicians with expertise in the appropriate research strategies, who cooperated with politically astute and socially prominent public citizens. They rapidly became major political forces, successful in reaching policy makers in Congress and in the Executive Branch. In particular, the American Cancer Society and the American Heart Association worked intensively with both Senator Lister Hill of Alabama and Representative John Fogarty of Rhode Island in the 1950s. This mutually supportive relationship ensured the fiscal health of the NIH for the next twenty years or so and was responsible for the formation of a number of new Institutes at NIH during that time. Many Washington insiders were quite aware of the white-gloved successes of the great ladies of health research such as Mary Lasker and Florence Mahoney. They were effective advocates for research into conditions that were common and feared by both members of Congress and voters. This pattern was copied successfully by the ADRDA early in its history, as Patrick Fox has informed us, and was certainly key in raising public and political awareness of AD as a disease and support for research and care of the victims and their families.

In more recent times, the high-minded approach taken by the early health voluntaries and copied by the Alzheimer's Association has given way to a more radical, populist strategy. One of the best-known examples of this change is the very successful campaign conducted by ACT UP, an activist organization founded by gay men to force more attention and more funding for research on AIDS. The successes of the radical groups have prompted other, usually more traditional patient advocacy groups, to follow a similar path. For example, breast cancer advocates have adopted some of the techniques pioneered by the AIDS activists, although without some of the more in-your-face tactics of the early days of ACT UP. The recent U.S. Balanced Budget accord contains a proposal to allow the U.S. Postal Service to issue a postage stamp that will retail for a few cents more than its face value, with the overage earmarked for federally funded breast cancer research. Certainly this is an innovation that must have all the various "special interests" gnashing their teeth because they didn't think of it first. A "special interest" could be defined by Washington pundits as "the other guys trying to muscle in on the attention and dollars that might go to your cause."

It is apparent that the rise of public interest in health-related research is linked temporally, if not causally, with the increasing role played by federal, tax-derived funds that began after World War II. Before World War II, the major players and sources of money for research into diseases and health concerns were the great private philanthropic foundations. The monies that originally funded these foundations were often made in the late-nineteenth- and early-twentieth-century expansionist age in the United States by what some historians have called the "Robber Barons." A prominent example has been the Rockefeller Foundation, whose interests in medical matters inspired a number of scientifically based attacks on diseases. The Carnegie Institution in Washington, D.C., sprang from the wealth amassed by Andrew Carnegie, one of the more colorful examples of a "Robber Baron." While some have deplored the ease with which what they considered unethical business practices were laundered by these philanthropies, others suggested that their influence in stimulating research and research training was key to the post–World War II blossoming of biomedical research in the United States. From the late nineteenth century through the pre–World War II period, private foundations were major supporters of biomedical research in the United States (Fitzpatrick and Bruer 1997). Currently, opinion makers and fundraisers speculate about how they can best pique the interest of the current crop of multimillionaires, as well as those with lesser fortunes, in founding like venues to endow contemporary health research. Fitzpatrick and Bruer (1997) recommend that a coordinated national partnership among foundations, government, and corporations form the framework for support of biomedical research in the twenty-first century.

A similar history occurred in Europe. It is generally believed that the close collaboration between Germany's vigorous chemical industry and their renowned academic centers was responsible for the prominence of German science in the early part of the twentieth century. Indeed, Nissl and his friend Alois Alzheimer could not have studied the nervous system as they did without the aniline dyes synthesized by the German industrial dye chemists. A key event in the late-twentieth-century renascence of research interest in AD was the CIBA Foundation symposium held in London in 1969 and published in 1970 (Wolstenholme and O'Connor 1970). Furthermore, it would be hard to imagine British medical research today without the funds and, inevitably, the direction setting of the Wellcome Trust. Similarly, the role of Eli Lilly and Company and its support of the Alzheimer Haus in Marktbreit, Germany, is a contemporary example of the continued presence and importance of nongovernmental corporate support.

For many years the research departments of the most prominent and successful chemical and pharmaceutical giants were home to many of our leading scientists. For example, when David Bowen came back to England after his graduate and postdoctoral studies in the United States in 1968, he returned to a position with Unilever Research with the Nobel Laureate A. J. P. Martin. Later Bowen joined Alan Davison's newly established neurochemistry research group at the Institute of Neurology, Queen Square, London.

One of the apparent consequences of the post–World War II rise of federal funding for biomedical research in the United States was a concomitant decline in the proportion of more basic studies supported by the pharmaceutical industry. As federal funds have become constricted over the last fifteen years, industry has reassumed its leadership role, and now supports more biomedical research in the United States than does the public sector. This phenomenon has occurred as a consequence of major investments in the opportunities opened up by the burgeoning knowledge of molecular biological approaches.

The success of the wartime Manhattan Project and the later achievements in weapons technology engendered by the Cold War gave politicians and scientists alike confidence that science could solve all problems. For a time this belief was strengthened by the successes of the U.S. and Soviet space programs, despite the caveats voiced by many scientists that these were engineering or technological achievements and not science. In Washington jargon, science and technology became almost one word, as if they were synonymous. Indeed, the White House office devoted to such issues is still called the Office of Science and Technology Policy, and it has most frequently been headed by those whose interests are closer to technology than to science.

Of course, the great triumphs of medical research trumpeted by its advocates have also been largely technological, even when based on increasingly accurate biological knowledge of cell function. Coronary artery bypasses, carotid endarterectomies, and other examples that could be cited are fundamentally technological. To balance the picture, however, one should mention the remarkable advances in cancer chemotherapy, hypertension control, and atherosclerosis prevention that derive almost entirely from new understanding of the basic cellular biochemistry involved in control of differentiation and metabolism.

It is also incumbent upon us not to overstate the advances in human welfare that will come from a more complete knowledge of the human genome. New insights are fascinating, and for a time, the excitement of knowing where a gene that causes a particular disease is located may lead us into making extravagant predictions of what this means to the ordinary person. My experience with the search for the Huntington gene and its gene product has been somewhat chastening; no person at risk for Huntington disease is much better off today as a result of those advances than he or she was in 1983. Dare I say that the same might be said thus far about the genes that are involved in AD? This is not to denigrate the extraordinary advances in our understanding of the biology of diseases, but only to caution that there is likely to be a long road between the announcement of a disease-specific gene's location and the discovery of a therapy that will make a difference to those afflicted with the disease. Cancer research has still to live down the Nixon era War on Cancer hyperbole, although much of that criticism is unjustified today.

These issues are important in considering public policy implications of science research, its funding, its direction setting, and who sets the directions. I remember very vividly hearing the late Honorable William Natcher, then chairman of the U.S. House of Representatives Subcommittee on Appropriations for the NIH, give Vincent DeVita, a distinguished cancer researcher and then director of the National Cancer Institute (NCI), a very hard time over his recital of the great scientific advances that had been made in the past years with the money appropriated by Mr. Natcher's committee. Mr. Natcher, a staunch supporter of the NIH, lectured DeVita for some minutes about the need to spend public monies on what the public needs (i.e., a cure for cancer, not more insight into oncogenes, etc). That was an early sign that the activism of the smaller groups, whose focus was on *cures now*, but who were not in the inner circles of power, was making an impact on the political picture in the United States.

Many of these smaller groups were initially considered fringe groups with little understanding of "how things were done" and were tolerated and even patronized by the policy makers in both the political and scientific worlds. The remarkable growth in stature and influence shown by the National Organization for Rare Diseases is but one example of many that could be cited. More recently, the rise to prominence of the Parkinson disease advocacy groups has been equally influential in the Washington corridors of power.

It has become even clearer that the leadership in policy making exerted by the "experts" in the various fields was being challenged successfully. The institution of a "parallel track" for testing AIDS drugs was instigated by AIDS activists, most of them involved in ACT UP, and implemented by a particular coterie of scientists, government regulators, and an enlightened pharmaceutical company (Levi 1991). Many of the AIDS researchers active in clinical trials of drugs for AIDS were initially horrified and confidently predicted that dire consequences would inevitably follow the departure from controlled clinical trial methodology. They were wrong! A similar argument was used successfully to allow other drugs for desperate conditions, including AD, to use the parallel track methodology to speed up the delivery of treatments to patients with life-destroying diseases. Although the Food and Drug Administration has maintained that it was planning to institute such a plan on its own, many who were active in the debate remain convinced that it would not have happened as quickly without ACT UP.

Shortly before his assassination in 1963, in a speech at the celebration of the centennial of the National Academy of Sciences, John F. Kennedy said, "Scientists alone can establish the objectives of their research, but society, in extending support to science, must take account of its own needs" (Greenberg 1971, 288). What concerns us now, in the waning days of the twentieth century, is the definition of society and its needs. As I have said above, it is no longer seen to be adequate to consider the views of the experts and the elites of U.S. society as representative of the needs of the people. In 1965 Kenneth M. Watson, a physicist, said in "A Comment on the Motivation for Studying Particle Physics" in *Nature of Matter* that "there is a current saying among government supporters of research that scientific research is the only pork barrel for which the pigs get to determine who gets the pork" (Greenberg 1971, 151). That has changed forever, and the change is causing a good deal of angst amongst the "pigs."

In the science press, the current debate about priority setting is portrayed as an argument about "politics" versus "science" in federal funding of research. The researchers fear that their treasured system of using peer review to decide what research is important and feasible is threatened by increasing calls for allocating taxpayer-derived funds according to societal needs, such as how many people are affected by a given disease. While the record attests that peer review is invaluable in decisions about what should be supported within any particular field, it is of no help in deciding among different areas of research. An effort to begin the dialogue about the national setting of science priorities by scientists in various disciplines was begun by the National Academy of Sciences under the impetus of Frank Press (1995). Most observers have commented that it seems to have had very limited impact on the ongoing debates in the U.S. Congress. The scientific community appears to have paid his effort little more than lip service.

In invited testimony before the Subcommittee on Health and Safety of the U.S. Senate Committee on Labor and Human Resources on May 1, 1997, Dr. Harold Varmus, Director of NIH, responded to very pointed questions about the process of priority setting at the NIH. In the "good old days," such a hearing would have been unheard of and deemed unnecessary. In today's world, the old ways are no longer viable. Dr. Varmus spoke of "this important, contentious, and complex issue" and explicitly addressed the creative tension between "the need to respond to public health needs as judged by the incidence, severity, and cost of specific disorders" and the "commitment to support work of the highest scientific calibre" (Varmus 1997).

At bottom, the real issue is the fact that work of high scientific merit is supported in one area and not in another because there is not enough money to support all the excellent science that has been proposed. Whose area is neglected has become the sticking point. Rep. Ernest Istook of Oklahoma said, "Federal funding for medical research is skewed, failing to focus on those diseases that cause the most suffering and death in America. . . . It's time to reexamine how Congress sets its priorities. . . . Members of Congress have a constitutional duty to ensure that tax dollars are spent properly and to set policy" (Istook 1997).

Indeed, Congress is not finished with its examination of biomedical research priority setting. *Science* reported on October 31, 1997, that Speaker of the House Newt Gingrich had created a panel, chaired by Rep. George Nethercutt of Washington, to examine priorities in the NIH's $13 billion budget. The Senate appropriated funds for a similar review by the Institute of Medicine of the National Academy of Sciences.

This is clearly a change from the oft-lamented "golden age" of biomedical research funding when Hill and Fogarty asked Director James A. Shannon how much was needed by the NIH and then doubled it. Whether this actually happened is unlikely, but it is part of the received folklore. In today's atmosphere, researchers do not need to be reminded that priority setting, at least in Congress, is rarely a process governed by logically derived and presented arguments. The setting of priorities, in the context of the Appropriations Bills, is more often conducted in the corridors of power by lobbyists than in the formal hearings in the great rooms of Congress. Although the term is often used pejoratively, a "lobbyist" is most often a successful educator in the legislative process; all advocates for research on diseases and disorders need their expertise.

The research community has weathered other challenges. The history of the recent past to which I have alluded gives me confidence that the quest for biomedical knowledge will go on without serious detriment. Scientists have a long tradition of adherence to behavioral norms in which the health of the enterprise is seen to be the primary good; adaptation to changing conditions, including more intense competitive pressures, is the response that garners rewards and promotes survival. It is inevitable that some areas will flourish and others, perhaps equally promising, will be temporarily neglected. While this is probably not a life-or-death issue for the whole of biomedical research, it can have disastrous consequences for particular fields and for individual researchers, especially those who are just beginning their careers.

A more challenging task faces the activist patient-advocacy groups. Somehow they must negotiate past the heady days of success in changing policy and increasing funding for their disease or condition — success that their supporters have come to expect as their due — in order to cope with a situation in which the fiscal realities of balanced budgets must constrain their winnings. Their traditions are being built on the fly, and this observer, at least, is not entirely confident that "the tragedy of the commons," Garrett Hardin's (1968) apt phrase, will not overtake and destroy some of the gains in public esteem that health voluntaries have made in the past fifty years.

But our concern is with the Alzheimer's Association. In all fairness, I do not expect these groups to become so strident that they risk a backlash from the contemporary federal patrons of research. A fine line must be walked to keep one's public, the patients, and their families content enough with progress to continue support, while at the same time convincing the political establishment that real breakthroughs are just around the corner and that more money should be appropriated from the public purse, despite the other needs that press upon our society. More and more, setting priorities will be a matter of what will be tossed out of, rather than added to, the basket. And that is not likely to be an appetizing prospect — either for those who must make the policies or for those who must live with them. Leadership of an activist health voluntary is going to be a ticklish task in which expertise and savvy, both scientific and political, will count for more than the urge to make a difference, however noble such motivations may be.

Several key issues are likely to have an impact on the future of the Alzheimer Association. Scientific progress will necessitate rethinking the goals of such organizations. Even a happy event, such as the polio vaccines were for the March of Dimes, is a trying time for an organization. Given the structural and emotional investments already in place, voluntary disbanding never seems to be an option.

The political success of the Alzheimer's Association message has been bolstered by the predictions of increasing numbers of persons at risk for development of the disease. When we entered the twentieth century, about 4 percent of the population was over 65; as we leave it, about 13 percent of our people are over 65. Percentages are not as impressive as actual numbers to most of us. Thirteen percent translates into almost 20 million people. As more people live longer, the fastest rate of increase has been in the oldest old, those at greatest risk for developing cognitive declines severe enough to require institutionalization. But recent data from the National Health Interview Survey indicate the good news that while more of us live longer, we are also staying healthier. Of those 65 to 74, 89 percent report no disability; even after 85, 40 percent are still fully functional (Rowe 1997). Rowe comments that there are at least 1.4 million fewer older people with disabilities than there would have been if the health of the elderly had not improved since 1982. While this compression of morbidity in the later years is good news for all of us, it may require some change of emphasis in the messages of the health voluntary organizations. Will it be as persuasive to the policy makers in Congress to refocus attention on the need to carry on research to enhance the numbers of people who age "successfully" — without the currently expected frailties of old age — as it has been to concentrate on cures to relieve the human suffering of the AD patients and their families?

The worldwide constrictions in the ability and will of governments to address all the problems that their citizenry demands will mean that competition for an increasing share of the pie may become lethal if not constrained by enlightened leadership that promotes collaboration. Biomedical research is an international endeavor — a fact easily understood by its practitioners, but not always so evident to the political powers-that-be. The United States is the leader in health research as it is in many other areas of science and technology. That leadership is directly attributable to the far-sighted advice given by scientist-statesmen like Vannevar Bush at the end of World War II and followed up by the U.S. government in its generous support of research and research training in those postwar years. Those activities laid the groundwork for the successes we have enjoyed over the past twenty years. It is at this moment uncertain whether this impetus will be sustained for the future. The announcement in the president's 1998 State of the Union speech of the administration's proposal for a new biomedical research initiative to move the country into the next millennium is certainly an encouraging sign. Whether Congress will share the president's enthusiasm and appropriate the needed funds is an open question. Recent press reports do not inspire confidence that they will.

Like all organisms, health voluntary organizations have a life cycle, complete with the growing pains of adolescence. How they come out of this phase and become mature and productive depends largely on the leaders and their ability to carry the rank and file with them. Can they achieve the transition to societal responsibility without losing their enthusiasm and dedication? And how is societal responsibility to be defined and by whom? A short-term perspective is always easier to convey to the body politic. In the case of biomedical research, however, it is clear that a longer view must be maintained. While it is true that we have learned more in the past five years about the brain than had been learned heretofore, that is more an indictment of our previous ignorance than of our perspicacity now. I remain concerned about reports that effective therapies for AD should be available in five years, ten years, and so forth. While all of us hope and expect that this is true, the caveats and uncertainties that the researchers express are often lost or deemphasized in the public reports. As I mentioned earlier, the road from understanding the biological causes of disease to developing an effective cure or even treatment is unpredictable. It may be gratifyingly short and straight, or it may be long, tortuous, and tortured.

All of these issues must be faced in an environment in which public discourse has become more public, more discordant, and often even vituperative. The late Senator Sam Rayburn said all politics are local, and the bloodiest fights are among those who are within the clan. Fragmentation of advocacy groups is an ever-present danger in competitive times. We are certainly in competitive times and are likely to remain so, at least for the next few years. For young investigators, five to ten years is a lifetime. Despite all the problems, challenges, and opportunities, I remain confident that the Alzheimer's Association will weather this period and evolve with the changing times to remain a vital partner with the investigators in the search for solutions to the devastation caused by the dementias.

References

De Tocqueville, Alexis. 1835–39. *Democracy in America*. 1945 Reprint. New York: Vintage Books.

Fitzpatrick, S. M., and J. T. Bruer. 1997. Science funding and private philanthropy. *Science* 277:621.

Greenberg, D. S. 1971. *The Politics of Pure Science*. New York: New American Library.

Hardin, Garrett. 1968. The tragedy of the commons. *Science* 162:1243.

Istook, E. 1997. Quoted in *Dana Alliance Member News* (September/October): 5. New York: Dana Alliance for Brain Initiatives.

Levi, Jeffrey. 1991. Unproven AIDS therapies: The Food and Drug Administration and ddI. In *Biomedical Politics*, ed. K. Hanna. Washington, D.C.: National Academy Press.

Press, Frank. 1995. *Allocating Federal Funds for Science and Technology*. Washington, D.C.: National Academy Press.

Rowe, John W. 1997. The new gerontology. *Science* 278:367.

Setting Research Priorities at the NIH. 1997. Pamphlet available from the Office of the Director, NIH, 9000 Rockville Pike, Bethesda, MD 20892.

Varmus, Harold. 1997. Testimony before the Subcommittee on Public Health and Safety, Committee on Labor and Human Resources, United States Senate, May 1.

Wolstenholme, G. E. W., and M. O'Connor, eds. 1970. *CIBA Foundation Symposium on Alzheimer's Disease and Related Conditions*. London: Churchill.

13

The Concept of Alzheimer Disease in a Hypercognitive Society

Stephen G. Post

Is the difference between Alzheimer disease (AD) and the cognitive decline associated with normal aging qualitative or quantitative? Does AD dementia differ from the normal loss of capacities associated with aging only in its order of magnitude? The senile plaques and neurofibrillary tangles present in great quantities in the brains of people with AD are also present to a lesser degree in the normal brains of older persons. Would anyone who lives long enough, then, reach that threshold of incapacitation that we define as AD?

My comments emerge from a background in moral philosophy and comparative religious ethics. I contextualize the concept of AD within what I have previously called a "hypercognitive" culture and society, in which nothing is as fearful as AD because it violates the spirit (*geist*) of self-control, independence, economic productivity, and cognitive enhancement that defines our dominant image of human fulfillment. Deep forgetfulness represents such a violation of this spirit that all those with dementia are imperiled. Yet AD is also much more than *deep forgetfulness*, a term I use to encourage compassion and solidarity; it is human development in reverse, an "outliving of the brain," and an assault on human dignity.

In order to clarify any ambiguity, my interest in the well-being of persons with AD includes a strong recommendation against the use of any life-extending medical treatments (including antibiotics and artificial nutrition and hydration) beyond the moderate stage of the disease. Traditional hospice, which developed around the oncology model, is best suited for the patient who is lucid and for whom death is predictably imminent. Unfortunately, only a small number of terminal-stage AD patients are cared for in hospices. We must offer AD patients hospice-level medical care (including palliation), coupled with special techniques to enhance quality of life, long before the terminal stage of the disease.

For patients beyond the moderate stage of AD, optimal care is "being with" rather than "doing to." Emotional, relational, and aesthetic well-being can be enhanced in a way that involves family members, giving them a sense of meaning and of purpose, and that provides an alternative to preemptive assisted suicide or euthanasia. In the PASSAGES program at Heather Hill, a nursing home in Chardon, Ohio, my colleagues and I advocate a paradigm shift away from the technological protraction of morbidity toward acts of caring solicitude that draw on and support patients' remaining capacities: healing arts therapies in the categories of the fine arts (music, art, dance/movement, poetry, drama); caring touch (therapeutic touch, massage); and spirituality (ritual based on deeply learned religious backgrounds). Clergypersons from the relevant spiritual traditions are needed to support bereaved family members. They need to understand that their support and caring is often best expressed by entering into the culture of dementia care to facilitate the well-being of loved ones.

I recommend this approach to care based on considerations of quality of life (including the burden of technology to the deeply forgetful, who lack insight into its purposes), the prior indications of many persons with AD while competent, and the "best interests" of patients, as discerned by caregivers.

In this chapter, I draw out the implications of interpreting AD against the ubiquitous background of a hypercognitive culture. Hypercognitive values blind us to possible approaches to well-being in persons with AD. Ultimately, these values lead us toward the justification of preemptive assisted suicide as the only reasonable solution to dementia — a practice I do not personally condone.

THE ELITE EXCLUSIVISM OF THE BIOETHICAL MODEL OF PERSONHOOD

Among philosophical bioethicists, hypercognitive values drive the strong modernist trend to deny that people with advanced dementia are "persons." Instead, they are defined as "nonpersons" because they lack various empowering cognitive capacities. Many but not all bioethicists focus not on what these human beings are, but on what they are not. Such bioethicists will allow that those with severe dementia are still living human beings — but they are not persons, and they therefore lack the moral standing of the cognitively intact.

I wish to assert that people with severe dementia *are* persons, however disabled, weak, and disempowered. In the words of theologian Gilbert Meilaender, "Those who never had or who have now lost certain distinctive human capacities should not be described as nonpersons; rather, they are simply the weakest and least advantaged *members* of the human community" (1996, 33).

In *The Moral Challenge of Alzheimer Disease*, I warn against the tendencies of a "hypercognitive culture" to exclude the deeply forgetful by reducing their moral status or by neglecting the emotional, relational, aesthetic, and spiritual aspects of well-being that are open to them even in the severe stage of the disease (Post 1995). I associate hypercognitive values with the Enlightenment notion of salvation by reason alone and suggest that this imperils people with dementia. Very simplistically, "I think, therefore, I am," implies that if I do not think, I am not. In essence, the values of rationality and productivity blind us to other ways of thinking about the meaning of our humanity and the nature of humane care. As one medical anthropologist notes, our response to people with AD is interpreted and responded to in the context of socially constructed images of the human self and of its fulfillment (Herskovitz 1995).

In reflecting on people with severe dementia (in contrast, for example, to those in the persistent vegetative state, a condition that some people in end-stage AD enter), I have grown wary of personhood theories of morality, for these assert a higher moral status to human beings who are self-legislating moral agents. In fairness, those philosophers who emphasize the superior status of the cognitively intact have not all excluded the person with severe dementia from moral considerabilty. A leading proponent of personhood theory has argued that while people with severe AD are not "persons" in the strict sense of moral agency, they are still "persons" in various social senses within particular communities and thus are generally afforded moral dignity (Engelhardt 1996, 150). But theologian David H. Smith writes that even such a "conferred" or "social" sense of persons means that "at some point someone entering into a dementia begins to count less than, or have a different status than, the rest of us" (1992, 47). He describes caring for his AD-affected mother-in-law and contends that personhood theories can diminish our sensitivity to the well-being of those with AD: "Used as an engine of *exclusion*, the personhood theory easily leads to insensitivity, if not to great wickedness" (47). A decade ago, for example, four Austrian nursing aids allegedly killed forty-nine elderly demented residents in a long-term care setting (Protzman 1989).

In some respects, then, by labeling the most deeply forgetful as AD-affected, we admit the possibility of their being placed in a social wastebasket. This is especially possible in a hypercognitive cultural context in which the weaknesses of those with AD are contrasted with our images of fulfillment.

Fortunately, bioethicists of "personhood" are practically irrelevant, although ideas can have consequences. Nobody would approach a family in the throes of medical decision making about their loved one with advanced dementia and proclaim that he or she is a "nonperson" (the rough equivalent of "shell" or "husk").

It remains morally, socially, and politically salutary to define those groups that are the most oppressed, the most ghettoized, and the most vulnerable, as persons in need. The Judeo-Christian tradition of prophetic ethics chiefly asserts the moral principle of protecting the most vulnerable and "least" among us (Harrelson 1986). Identifying an AD-affected group allows us to marshal the moral passions of those who wish, both vocationally and professionally, to serve the destitute with a "preferential option."

The most basic moral problem in AD care is that many people want to separate themselves from the presence of those with dementia. Love (synonymous with "care," the Jewish *chesed*, or the Christian *agape*), a basic solicitude or anxiety about the well-being of the other, can overcome the tendency to exclude the forgetful. Love, which family caregivers so often profoundly manifest, is often best expressed by "being with" the forgetful in "attentive presence," rather than by "doing to" medically. This solicitude is the very heart of moral life.

NAMING ALZHEIMER DISEASE IN A HYPERCOGNITIVE CULTURE

Whatever biological realities distinguish AD from normal aging, the fact is that this threshold of discontinuity, which is ultimately somewhat arbitrary, separates "them" from "us" and shields us from facing the fact that we are all a little demented by age 70. "They," however, eventually become so demented that we designate them, not as people who are the most deeply forgetful, but as people with AD. We lean on the notion of AD scientifically and socially in order to emphasize our discontinuities with the most forgetful and the weakest among us. Dementia can be labeled as AD only if it is understood as a significant departure from normal aging. Because we have managed to convince ourselves that normal aging is relatively dementia-free and even youthful, significant dementia can be conceptualized as disease.

Were ours *not* a hypercognitive culture, would we fear dementia enough to label it AD at a certain threshold? If we in the West did not place so much value on autonomy, the Enlightenment ideal of independent rational choice, would we be worried enough about the interdependence of dementia to label it AD? Anthropologist Charlotte Ikels contends that in Chinese culture, where there is a relatively greater emphasis on the affective domain coupled with a highly interdependent view of human experience, there is a greater acceptance of dementia and less readiness to label it as disease (Ikels forthcoming). If we were not a culture that imposes the image of a youthful and fully intact mind on the old-old, would we so stigmatize dementia as to label AD as, in the words of Lewis Thomas, "the disease of the century?"

There is no definition of either health or disease that does not include some quiet background of cultural values. To some extent, the naming of a disease tells us something about what a culture most despises. The designation of AD as a disease and its rise to prominence in the culture tells us a great deal about what our culture most likes and most dislikes. In fact, we so dislike the very idea of becoming deeply forgetful that preemptive assisted suicide becomes suddenly a rational strike on behalf of normalcy.

All the metaphors and resources of a war against a disease can be applied to AD — the embodiment of all we despise — with the support of a social movement and political pressures. To prevent, delay onset, or cure AD becomes a public health goal of much greater focus than merely enhancing the cognitive capacities of elderly people, some of whom would be viewed as more senile than others. The disease AD constitutes an assault on the compression of morbidity and a youthful old age that runs smoothly right up to the endpoint of death. We can get angry at this disease that robs the elderly of the temporal glue between their past, present, and future; yet many would argue that we would more or less all lose that temporal glue were we to live long enough.

None of the above should suggest that I doubt the objective element of neurological deterioration that defines AD. I do, however, remain confused as to whether this deterioration is ultimately a normal and ubiquitous reality of growing very old. Perhaps the only way to demonstrate the discontinuities between normal aging and AD is epidemiolog-ical. For example, is there in fact an epidemiological plateau after the eighth decade of life, so that those who enter their 90s will more than likely retain their cognitive capacities? Then the claim can credibly be made that the normal human brain should continue to function remark-ably well (e.g., the renowned French woman who died in good cognitive condition at age 123; George Burns, who died at age 100 while cog-nitively intact). If there is no epidemiological plateau, and it can be said that everyone who lives long enough will manifest AD, it becomes more difficult to define AD as a disease rather than as a normal aspect of growing old that is sometimes regrettably seen in middle-aged people.

Accepting the notion that severe forgetfulness is a disease (rather than senility writ large) may well be directly proportional to the domi-nance of hypercognitive values within a culture. Moreover, the fear of forgetfulness, which stirs the pot of AD genetic testing, would also be proportional to such dominance.

The Moral Challenge of Entering the Culture of Dementia

Whatever the final word on the definition of AD, morality and eth-ics require that we enter the world of the severely demented, respect the mystery of the person, and humbly facilitate whatever "resurrection" is possible (Weaver 1986). Although emotional, relational, aesthetic, and spiritual well-being are all possible to some degree, hypercognitive val-ues blind us to these possibilities. Our theories of personhood highlight what is not, rather than what is.

The aesthetic well-being open to people with AD is obvious to anyone who has watched art or music therapy sessions. In some cases a person with AD may still draw the same valued symbol very deep into the illness, as though a sense of self is retained through art (Firlik 1991; Clair 1996). The abstract expressionist de Kooning painted his way through much of his struggle with AD, and various art critics com-mented that his work, while not what it had been, was nevertheless impressive. As Kay Larson, former art critic for *New Yorker* magazine wrote, "It would be cruel to suggest that de Kooning needed his disease to free himself. Nonetheless, the erosions of Alzheimer's could not eliminate the effects of a lifetime of discipline and love of craft. When infirmity struck, the artist was prepared. If he didn't know what he was doing, maybe it didn't matter — to him. He knew what he loved best, and it sustained him" (Larson 1997). A review of de Kooning's late art indicates a loss of the sweeping power and command of brush that was typical of his work in the 1950s; however, there is also a quality to the late work that should not be diminished.

Chaplains can engage people with AD and their caregivers in a clinically relevant ministry. Chaplain Debbie Everett of Edmunton said at a national meeting of the U.S. Alzheimer's Association, "If a deeper experience of life could be realized by myself through a greater awareness of touch, music, human presence, love, smell, color, play, laughter, nature and so on, what could this mean in the lives of those with Alzheimer's disease? In discovering how better to meet the spiritual needs of these people, in essence I found what spirituality means in a wider context beyond intellect, in the realm of our bodies and emotions." She added that if part of spirituality in eastern and western religions includes an awareness of the present moment, then there may even be something to learn from people with AD: "The paradigm shift that I advocate in the care of those affected by AD is to discover and appreciate a wider range of communication possibilities" (Everett 1997, A4).

Consider Oliver Sacks' compelling description of a patient with severe Korsakoff's dementia: "Seeing Jim in the chapel opened my eyes to other realms where the soul is called on, and held, and stilled, in attention and communion. The same depth of absorption and attention was to be seen in relation to music and art: he had no difficulty" (1970, 38). Sacks goes further regarding Jim: "But if he was held in emotional and spiritual attention — in the contemplation of nature or art, in listening to music, in taking part in the Mass in chapel — the attention, its 'mood,' its quietude, would persist for a while, and there would be in him a pensiveness and peace we rarely, if ever saw during the rest of his life at the Home" (39).

Without asserting the existence of a soul that lies beneath the confusion of dementia, Sacks does assert "the undiminished possibility of reintegration by art, by communion, by touching the human spirit: and this can be preserved in what seems at first a hopeless state of neurological devastation" (39).

PHYSICIAN-ASSISTED SUICIDE IN ALZHEIMER DISEASE: A HYPERCOGNITIVE IMPERATIVE

The ultimate hypercognitive assault on AD-related forgetfulness is physician-assisted suicide (PAS). The United States has only recently entered the debate over PAS. Holland has for several years refrained from prosecuting for PAS and euthanasia.

Advocates of PAS support legalization to reduce, in principle, patient suffering and enhance the rights of patients to retain control over their destinies. The person with a progressive, irreversible dementia such as AD falls within these concerns.

The social and historical significance of AD-PAS is very considerable. Local focus groups of AD caregivers in Greater Cleveland indicate moral differences of opinion. As one caregiver stated, "It is really a matter of positive, not negative pride in who and what I am. The state has no business telling me that I can't avoid a future that peels away my soul. Don't get moralistic about this." Another said, "Why restrict this to PAS when it is precisely when I am too far gone to make decisions and do things for myself that I would want to die." Some indicated that AD-PAS is unacceptable because (a) no one can know ahead of time what the subjective experience of dementia is like, (b) it is inevitably biased by hypercognitive cultural values, (c) it is likely to lead to requests for voluntary AD-euthanasia (defined as mercy killing) and eventually to nonvoluntary euthanasia, and (d) it is likely to demoralize the movement to enhance long-term AD care.

One argument states that emerging laws should allow people with AD preemptive PAS in order to avoid discrimination (i.e., assisted suicide while the patient is still competent to make such a serious choice and to then implement it with assistance). This argument need not be based on a conviction that PAS is morally compelling in most cases. Rather, it is a somewhat grudging appeal to nondiscrimination in the light of legalization of PAS.

The availability of PAS would allow the person with AD to preemptively avoid decline into severe dementia. The case of Janet Adkins illustrates this. One of her physicians described her as a 54-year-old married woman who developed memory impairment about two years before her death. Cognitive deficits included problems in reading comprehension and word-finding, making it "impossible for her to continue her career as a teacher and her avocation as a pianist" (Rhode, Peskind, and Raskind 1995, 187). No longer able to play her classical favorites, but still able to play tennis well, she sought the assistance of Dr. Kevorkian while she was still competent.

In the Netherlands, where PAS is legal, the health system provides ample hospice and long-term care (de Wachter 1992); even so, about 10 percent of requests come from patients with chronic degenerative neurological disorders. Battin writes of progressive dementia: "This is the condition the Dutch call *entluistering*, the 'effacement' or complete eclipse of human personality, and for the Dutch, *entluistering* rather than pain is a primary reason for choices of [active] euthanasia" (Battin 1992). She points out that in the Netherlands, PAS is based on intolerable suffering as determined by the patient. Suffering includes fear of the loss of personal identity. The Dutch system, in theory, allows PAS or voluntary euthanasia only while the patient remains competent, although some reports indicate that euthanasia is occurring after the patient becomes incompetent.

In contrast to MS patients, who often remain aware of their circumstances until death, patients with AD reach a point in the progression of disease when they "forget that they forget" and no longer have insight into their situation. Some may argue that the inevitable cessation of requests for PAS due to loss of cognitive capacity makes PAS unnecessary for AD patients. They eventually drift into the "pure present" and do not experience physical pain. Such a benign image of AD underestimates the anxiety and behavioral difficulties associated with this decline and disturbingly suggests that the intact self has no moral authority over the inevitable decline of the deeply forgetful self. Patients with a diagnosis of AD fear pain less than the loss of self, a condition of such indignity in the minds of some that life would not be worth living.

Should legislation or judicial precedent permit PAS, it is arguable that people with AD must have the same legal right of access as those who are, by a narrower definition, in the "terminal condition." AD is perceived by many people in our society as a death before death—a partial to full death of the mind while the body lives on. While this view is simplistic, advanced dementia often approximates the condition of having no self-identity (no temporal connections between past, present, and future).

Even if some percentage of patients do adjust emotionally to their condition, not all do. Further, those who take pride in being fully capacitated and having intact selves will not be content with state interference in a highly personal decision.

Yet, such an opening for preemptive AD-PAS could affect societal and familial resolve to provide optimal long-term and end-of-life care. AD-PAS is cheaper than long-term AD caregiving. PAS may alleviate pressure on managed care to develop long-term care and hospice for end-stage AD patients. The American Geriatrics Society's Ethics Committee raises this same sort of concern: "Legalization of physician-assisted suicide might thwart society's resolve to expand services and resources aimed at caring for the terminally ill, dying patient" (1995). This hospice concern is directly relevant to patients with end-stage AD and bears on long-term AD care generally, which is underfunded in the United States (Volicer and Hurley forthcoming).

The exclusion of people with AD from access to PAS could be based on a concern that both long-term care and hospice for end-stage AD patients are deeply inadequate. Rejecting PAS for AD patients forces society to focus on developing these alternatives more fully. This is by no means a new line of argument among critics of PAS. Why persist with expensive long-term care and AD-specific hospice when life can be cheaply ended in a manner consistent with autonomy?

The complex and acrimonious debates around AD-PAS will continue. My point is that AD-PAS is especially attractive in a hypercognitive culture; in alternative cultures, the idea of PAS as the answer to dementia would never arise.

ENVOI

Writing in 1727, Jonathan Swift described Gulliver's travels to the Luggnaggians, a polite and generous people. Gulliver inquires about their Immortals (or "Struldbrugs"), rare children born with a red dot on their foreheads. He is at first elated to hear of these cases of human immortality, for such persons would have no "depression of spirits caused by the continual apprehension of death" (Swift 1945 [1727], 210). Sadly, it turns out that these Immortals "have no remembrance of anything but what they learned and observed in their youth and middle age, and even that is imperfect" (214). The least miserable among them are the ones who "entirely lose their memories" (215). Further, "In talking they forget the common appellation of things, and the names of persons, even of those who are their nearest friends and relations. For the same reason they can never amuse themselves with reading, because their memory will not serve to carry them from the beginning of a sentence to the end; and by this defect they are deprived of the only entertainment whereof they might otherwise be capable" (215).

Strikingly, Gulliver observes that Immortals are "despised and hated by all sorts of people" (216). The king tells Gulliver to bring a couple of Immortals to his own country "to arm our people against the fear of death" (216).

Swift was partly responding to utopian scientific images of the much-extended life span. He was also, however, commenting on our propensity to despise the forgetful. He bequeathed his small fortune to found a hospice for the mentally incapacitated. I think we should follow Swift by creating a specialized hospice-like care system for people with AD, free of any stipulations about the imminence of death and available to all those beyond the moderate stage of disease.

References

American Geriatrics Society Ethics Committee. 1995. Physician-assisted suicide and voluntary active euthanasia. *Journal of the American Geriatrics Society* 43:579–80.

Clair, A. A. 1996. *Therapeutic Uses of Music with Older Adults.* Baltimore: Health Professions Press.

Battin, M. P. 1992. Euthanasia in Alzheimer's disease? In *Dementia and Aging: Ethics, Values, and Policy Choices,* ed. R. H. Binstock, S. G. Post, and P. J. Whitehouse, 118–37. Baltimore: Johns Hopkins University Press.

De Wachter, M. A. M. 1992. Euthanasia in the Netherlands. *Hastings Center Report* 22(2): 23–30.

Engelhardt, H. T. 1996. *The Foundations of Bioethics.* New York: Oxford University Press.

Everett, D. 1997. Forget me not: The spiritual care of people with Alzheimer's. Proceedings of the Sixth National Alzheimer's Disease Education Conference. Chicago: Alzheimer's Disease and Related Disorders Association.

Firlik, A. D. 1991. Margo's logo. *Journal of the American Medical Association* 265:201.

Harrelson, W. 1986. Prophetic ethics. In *The Westminster Dictionary of Christian Ethics,* ed. J. F. Childress and John Macquarrie, 508–12. Philadelphia: Westminster Press.

Herskovits, E. 1995. Struggling over subjectivity: Debates about the "self" and Alzheimer's disease. *Medical Anthropology Quarterly* 9(2): 146–64.

Ikels, C. Forthcoming. The experience of dementia in China. *Culture, Medicine and Psychiatry.*

Larson, K. 1997. Willem de Kooning and Alzheimer's. *The World and I* 12(2): 297–99.

Meilaender, G. 1996. *Bioethics: A Primer for Christians.* Grand Rapids, Mich.: Wm. B. Eerdmans.

Post, S. G. 1995. *The Moral Challenge of Alzheimer Disease.* Baltimore: Johns Hopkins University Press.

Protzman, F. 1989. Killing of 49 elderly patients by nurse aids stuns Austria. *New York Times,* 18 April, 1A.

Rhode, K., E. R. Peskind, and M. A. Raskind. 1995. Suicide in two patients with Alzheimer's disease. *Journal of the American Geriatrics Society* 43:187–89.

Sacks, O. 1970. The lost mariner. In *The Man Who Mistook His Wife for a Hat and Other Clinical Tales*, 23–42. New York: HarperCollins.

Smith, D. H. 1992. Seeing and knowing dementia. In *Dementia and Aging: Ethics, Values, and Policy Choices*, ed. R. H. Binstock, S. G. Post, and P. J. Whitehouse, 44–54. Baltimore: Johns Hopkins University Press.

Swift, J. 1945 (1727). *Gulliver's Travels*. Garden City, New York: Doubleday.

Volicer, C., and A. C. Hurley, eds. Forthcoming. *Hospice Care for Patients with Advanced Progressive Dementia*. New York: Springer.

Weaver, G. D. 1986. Senile dementia and resurrection theology. *Theology Today* 43(4): 444–56.

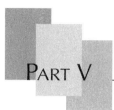

PART V

Progress and Its Problems

The Future of Alzheimer Disease

Inside every large problem are a dozen small ones struggling to get out. This corollary to Murphy's law might well seem applicable to progress in Alzheimer disease (AD), except that in this case it is difficult to discern if the problems solved are bigger than the ones set loose. The chapters in this section consider the tremendous prospects for progress in the biomedical science of AD, particularly in the area of molecular genetics. But they also consider the sorts of challenges this progress may create in the realms of politics and ethics.

Larry Altstiel and Steven Paul provide a cogent description of recent progress. Their chapter describes how molecular biology has revolutionized AD research, surveying the current state of the field and the prospects for developing therapeutic agents that not only relieve some of the symptoms of cognitive decline but also slow disease progression and reduce its incidence. The identification of specific gene mutations and proteins involved in AD, the development of a transgenic mouse to test new drugs that models both AD pathology and cognitive decline, and explorations of the role of estrogen in the maintenance of the neurons affected by AD — all these provide ample reason to hope that new and effective therapeutic strategies will be developed in the foreseeable future. Although these strategies are a result of the "new biology," Altstiel and Paul point to their connection to the foundational clinical studies carried out by Alzheimer and his contemporaries. They conclude that the tradition of painstaking clinical observation is as important in the age of molecular biology as it was in Alzheimer's time.

For all its obvious promise, what sort of problems might such progress create? In the first place, there are problems that may be characterized as the inadequacy of politics and policy to keep up with the exponential growth of knowledge and technical capacity. Scientific progress in understanding the biological mechanisms of AD, creating diagnostic technologies, and developing treatment strategies occurs at a dizzying rate. But consensus — or even informed discussion — about what to do with new knowledge and technology comes slowly at best. Robert Cooke-Deegan's chapter describes the tremendous progress in the field of molecular genetics in the last few years, and he agrees with others that it is poised to make even greater strides in the near future. But he also discusses how such progress raises daunting challenges to existing policy arrangements, such as the potential for tests to determine genetic susceptibility to AD to segregate private-sector long-term care insurance markets in the United States, undermining the system just as it is about to undergo the strain of the aging of the baby boom generation. He discusses how entirely new issues, which policy makers have scarcely begun to consider, are created as well — issues such as the potential claim of volunteer subjects of genetic studies to a share of the profits that are increasingly being reaped in the development of new biotechnologies that have been developed only through the use of their tissues and family histories.

Beyond these issues of how best to manage the fruits of scientific progress, it is possible to ask more fundamental questions: Is there a fundamental antipathy between biomedicine's rational, reductive, and instrumental approach to the complex problem of dementia and the sort of relational, spiritual, and aesthetic approach that Stephen Post argues (see Chapter 13) is necessary to respect the human integrity of the demented? Does the intense focus of resources and the fixing of all hope on the development of effective treatment at the molecular level impoverish the cultural and spiritual resources needed to care for the demented? Peter Whitehouse explores these issue by raising the specter of the postmodern — arguing that there are both limits and dangers to our knowledge and our ability to control the world in order to solve the problem of dementia. Noting that dominant approaches to dementia have historically alternated between the social and the biological, Whitehouse considers whether, despite the heady prospect for progress of molecular biology, social approaches to the problem of dementia may again become prominent. He concludes by suggesting that "quality of life" may be a concept that can frame dementia in a way that allows us to bring the resources of biological, social, and spiritual approaches to bear on the problem.

It may seem like perverse antitriumphalism to raise such issues at a time when molecular science seems poised to deliver such important insights and interventions. Indeed, such questions are clearly not in the mainstream; they are asked only in academic discourse, and not all that often even there. But they are essential questions; for whatever progress is made, dementia, and more generally the problem of suffering and death, will remain with us as a fundamental challenge to the meaningfulness of human life. In the coming decades, if biomedical science does not deliver on the high hopes it has raised, it is quite possible that in mainstream discourse, such questions will be raised with a vengeance.

None of this should be taken to suggest that investigations into the biological mechanisms of dementia are unimportant or that scientific progress is undesirable. But unless it is accompanied by wise and responsible policy making and a renewed emphasis on spirituality, aesthetics, and community as the wellsprings of human meaning, scientific progress will be hollow. It is not that biomedical science needs to be pushed to the margins but that space must be made to explore these other aspects of dementia. The typical strategy for creating such space is to encourage academic study in the appropriate disciplines — the social sciences, history and the humanities, ethics, and philosophy. Indeed, we hope and expect that knowledge will be developed along these lines. But we also believe that a discourse that is able to address fully the challenge of AD requires transcending traditional disciplinary boundaries to create a common ground where scholars from the natural and social sciences, the humanities, and the arts can bring their various perspectives to bear on one another in a creative tension that serves as both challenge and exhortation to the task that lies before us. It is our hope that this book, and the conference on which it was based, serves as a small step toward creating such a space.

14

Alzheimer Disease and the New Biology

Larry Altstiel and Steven Paul

Clinical research begins with the definition of a "case." This generally starts as an empirical collection of clinical signs and symptoms that evolves over time into an accepted description of a distinct disease entity or syndrome. Clinical nosology is an iterative, almost evolutionary discipline that often leads to improved methods of diagnosis for a given disease entity. Equally important, it is a necessary prerequisite for unraveling the exact etiology and associated pathophysiology of the patient's illness, thus facilitating the ultimate goal of finding processes or mechanisms that are amenable to intervention.

Alois Alzheimer's description of the illness that now bears his name remains in use some ninety years after his pioneering descriptive studies (Alzheimer 1907). Alzheimer disease (AD) is a progressive, dementing illness that usually occurs in late life but with variable age of onset. Approximately 4 percent of persons over the age of 65 have AD, and by age 85 the prevalence may range from 25 to 45 percent (Breitner et al. 1988; Evans et al. 1989). The incidence of the disease doubles approximately every five years after age 65 (Beard et al. 1995). Current AD therapy is directed toward symptomatic treatment of cognitive deficits and appears to have little effect on either disease incidence or progression. Given the emergence of AD as a critical public health problem in an ever-aging population, development of agents that may slow the disease's progression or reduce its incidence is of paramount importance.

As initially noted by Alzheimer, the brains of AD patients are remarkable for generalized atrophy, numerous plaques (senile plaques) that have an amyloid core surrounded by dystrophic neurites, cerebrovascular amyloid, and neurofibrillary tangles (Alzheimer 1907; Glenner 1989). The amyloid deposits are formed from a 40–42 amino acid peptide (Aβ), which is in turn derived from a larger precursor protein, the β-amyloid precursor protein (APP) (Kang et al. 1987). Compelling evidence has implicated Aβ deposition as a principal factor in AD pathology. Rare families have been found in which mutations in the APP gene results in an autosomal-dominant form of early onset AD. These mutations in APP flank the amino acids, which must be cleaved in order to produce Aβ, the primary constituent of the plaque (Selkoe 1996). Mutations in the presenilin genes (PS-1, PS-2) have been identified and appear to be responsible for additional forms of early-onset autosomal-dominant AD (Van Broeckhoven 1995). The mutated forms of PS-1 and PS-2 appear to alter processing of APP in a manner that leads to accumulation of the more amyloidogenic forms of Aβ (Borchelt et al. 1997). While the role of Aβ as a direct cause of AD has not been unequivocally established, there is compelling evidence that Aβ accumulation may both be directly neurotoxic and promote chronic neurodegeneration (Selkoe 1996). Moreover, patients with Down syndrome, who have an extra copy of chromosome 21 (the location of the APP gene), almost invariably develop AD pathology (Mann et al. 1986). Taken together, these findings from both patients with early-onset AD and patients with Down syndrome suggest that aberrant Aβ deposition is an important early event in the pathogenesis of AD.

While the exact mechanisms of Aβ synthesis and APP processing are not completely understood, it is generally assumed that the proteolytic processing of APP occurs via a series of proteases that cleave the precursor protein in discrete regions. The γ secretase, for example, cleaves APP at the C-terminal end of the Aβ sequence, whereas the β-secretase cleaves proximal to the N-terminus. Importantly, an α-secretase cuts within the Aβ sequence itself and leads to production of a soluble form of APP (APP$_s$) and a nonamyloidogenic fragment of APP (Selkoe 1996; Lendon, Ashall, and Goate 1997). Thus, drugs that inhibit the γ or β secretases, or stimulate α-secretase, could reduce Aβ production and thereby alter (perhaps slow) the progression of AD.

The identification of specific gene mutations that cause AD has prompted the recent development of animal models that have relevant AD pathology. These models have greatly accelerated the pace of research in APP processing and deposition. One such model, developed by

Eli Lilly and Company and Athena Neurosciences, is a transgenic mouse that overexpresses a human APP gene mutation (APP 717 $_{val \rightarrow phe}$), which is responsible for an autosomal-dominant form of AD. Expression of this gene, under the control of the platelet derived growth factor promoter, results in high brain levels of Aβ, and over time these mice develop senile plaques in a gene-dose dependent manner (Games et al. 1995). Moreover, these mice also develop deteriorating performance on a number of tests of cognitive performance. A recent series of compounds discovered by Lilly and Athena scientists that appear to decrease Aβ production *in vitro* dramatically reduce the formation of Aβ as well as the number of cortical senile plaques. Thus, the transgenic mouse models have facilitated the discovery of compounds that may be used to test the hypothesis that reduction of Aβ burden may beneficially affect AD.

The principal risk factors for AD are age and having a first-degree relative with AD (Breitner et al. 1988). Thus, AD risk has a significant genetic component. In addition to the previously mentioned mutations in the APP genes, additional genes have been found to cause familial AD. Hyslop and colleagues found that mutations in genes coding for proteins called presenilins can cause an autosomal-dominant form of AD (Sherington et al. 1995; Rogaev et al. 1995). These genes, PS-1 (located on chromosome 14) and PS-2 (located on chromosome 1), appear to alter some aspects of APP processing, which may result in increased Aβ burden (Selkoe 1996; Van Broeckhoven 1995; Borchelt et al. 1997). Transgenic animals expressing mutant presenilin have been developed and should provide an important tool for development of AD therapy. It is important to note that the rare forms of autosomal-dominant AD caused by genetic mutations have relatively early onset, which may begin in some affected patients in the late 30s to mid-40s. Thus an understanding of the function of both the normal and mutated forms of these genes will provide important insight into the factors that initiate AD.

In addition to those genes that are involved in rare autosomal-dominant forms of AD, there are genes that affect the likelihood of developing AD. These genes are not sufficient to cause AD, but rather they affect the risk of developing the disease by a given age. The best characterized of these genes is apolipoprotein E (ApoE). ApoE is a plasma protein that is involved in cholesterol transport (Weisgraber 1994). In humans there are three common isoforms of ApoE, denoted E2, E3, and E4. Apo-E3 is the most common form with an allele frequency of approximately 0.8. The next most common isoform is E4 with a frequency of 0.15. E2 is relatively rare with a frequency of about 0.05

(Gerdes et al. 1992). It has been known for some time that individuals who have one or two copies of the E4 allele have an elevated risk of cardiovascular disease, which is dependent on gene dose (Davingnon, Gregg, and Sing 1988; Van Bockxmeer and Mamotte 1992). In addition, more than one hundred separate studies have shown that the E4 allele is a major risk factor for AD (Roses 1996). Persons who are homozygous for the E4 allele (E4/E4) have approximately ten to fifteen times greater risk of developing AD than do persons who do not have an E4 allele. In contrast, the presence of an E2 allele appears to reduce the relative risk of developing AD. The risk conferred by the E4 allele is gene-dose dependent and appears to involve lowering the age of disease onset (Roses 1996). Thus, the effect of E4 allele dosage is most prominent among relatively young patients and less pronounced in older patients. There is also significant age stratification in population allele frequencies because of censoring due to increased cardiovascular risk conferred by E4.

The function of ApoE in the brain is a topic of intense investigation and debate. The mechanisms by which ApoE affects processes central to AD remain unknown. In addition to the increased relative risk of developing AD conferred by ApoE genotype, recent studies have shown that certain polymorphisms in the ApoE gene promoter-enhancer regions are also associated with an increased risk for developing AD (Budillo et al. 1998). These results suggest that in addition to genotype, levels of ApoE expression may play a role in the expression of AD pathology. Recently we have provided evidence that ApoE may directly affect Aβ deposition. Mice overexpressing a APP transgene (PDAPP) were crossed with mice that had either normal ApoE, or both copies of the ApoE gene rendered nonfunctional. The progeny of crosses between PDAPP-containing mice and mice with normal ApoE developed Aβ plaques at about 6 months of age. However, mice lacking a functional ApoE gene had only little or no plaque development (Bales et al. 1997). While these results do not explain the ApoE isoform-dependent risk for developing AD, they do suggest that ApoE does influence Aβ deposition. Although ApoE genotype affects the relative risk of developing AD, it is not a diagnostic test. ApoE genotyping alone does not have sufficient predictive value for the accurate diagnosis of AD (NIA/ADWG 1996).

The powerful techniques of molecular biology and genetics have provided a rapidly growing database on the complexity of AD etiology and have initiated new approaches to pharmacological intervention. Clinical epidemiological studies have also provided important insights into AD etiology. A growing body of evidence indicates that postmenopausal women who are taking estrogen replacement therapy (ERT) have a significantly decreased risk of developing AD (Henderson 1997). In addition, a number of small studies also suggest that ERT may partially ameliorate the symptoms of AD (Henderson 1997). Estrogen appears to be involved in the maintenance of cholinergic neurons (which are primarily affected in AD) (Luine 1985; Gibbs and Pfaff 1992) and may alter APP processing in a manner that lowers Aβ production (Jaffe et al. 1994). These results suggest that estrogen may beneficially affect processes thought to be involved with AD. Nevertheless, the use of estrogen carries a small but significant risk for the development of breast and uterine malignancies.

Selective estrogen receptor modulators (SERMS) are compounds that have tissue-selective agonist/antagonist properties. Several SERMS act as estrogen receptor antagonists in breast and gonadal tissue; while acting as estrogen receptor agonists in the cardiovascular system, bone, and possibly brain (Grese et al. 1997; Mitlak and Cohen 1997; Bryant and Dere 1998). An agent that acts as an estrogen receptor agonist in the brain while acting as an estrogen receptor antagonist in breast and gonadal tissue could have a desirable profile as an experimental therapeutic agent. These compounds are currently being studied for AD prevention.

Recent research has begun to unravel the complex etiology of AD. The combined influence of a number of fields, ranging from molecular genetics to epidemiology, have identified a number of causes and risk factors for AD and have provided several new approaches for rational pharmacological intervention. However, the remarkable work of Alois Alzheimer remains one of the principle examples of how clinical research, a combination of thoughtful clinical observation and painstaking descriptive efforts, can result in mechanistic explanations for the observed clinical signs and symptoms of a disease, in this case AD. The tools of clinical diagnosis have become more powerful, and the revolutionary developments in molecular biology and genetics have allowed detailed examination of AD etiology and pathogenesis that could not have been imagined by scientists of Alzheimer's generation. Nevertheless, the fundamental value of clinical investigation, such as the search for meaningful clinicopathologic correlations as exemplified by the work of Alzheimer, remains unchanged.

References

Alzheimer, A. 1907. Über eine eigenartige Erkrankung der Hirinde. *Allgemeine Zeitschrift für Psychiatrie und Psychich-Gerichtich Medizin* 64:146–48.

Bales, K. R., T. Verina, R. C. Dodel, Y. Du, L. Altstiel, M. Bender, P. Hyslop, E. M. Johnstone, S. P. Little, D. J. Cummins, P. Piccardo, B. Ghetti, and S. M. Paul. 1997. Lack of apolipoprotein E dramatically reduces amyloid beta-peptide deposition. *Nature Genetics* 17:263–64.

Beard, C. M., E. Kokmen, P. C. O'Brian, and L. T. Kurland. 1995. The prevalence of dementia is changing over time in Rochester, Minnesota. *Neurology* 45:75–79.

Borchelt, D. R., T. Ratovitski, J. van Lare, M. K. Lee, V. Gonzales, N. A. Jenkins, N. G. Copeland, D. L. Price, and S. S. Sisodia. 1997. Accelerated amyloid deposition in the brains of transgenic mice coexpressing mutant presenilin 1 and amyloid precursor proteins. *Neuron* 19:939–45.

Breitner, J. C. S., E. A. Murphy, J. M. Silverman, R. C. Mohs, and K. L. Davis. 1988. Age-dependent expression of familial risk in Alzheimer's disease. *Am J Epidemiol* 128:536–48.

Bryant, H. U., and W. H. Dere. 1998. Selective estrogen receptor modulators: An alternative to hormone replacement therapy. *Proc Soc Exp Biol Med* 217:45–52.

Budillo, M. J., M. J. Artiga, M. Recuero, I. Sastre, M. A. Garcia, J. Aldudo, C. Lendon, S. W. Han, J. C. Morris, A. Frank, J. Vazquez, A. Goate, F. Valdivieso. 1998. A polymorphism in the regulatory region of APOE associated with risk for Alzheimer's dementia. *Nature Genetics* 18:69–71.

Davignon, J., R. E. Gregg, and C. F. Sing. 1988. Apolipoprotein E polymorphism and atherosclerosis. *Arteriosclerosis* 8:1–21.

Evans, D. A., H. H. Funkenstein, M. S. Albert, P. A. Scherr, N. R. Cook, M. J. Chown, L. E. Herbert, C. H. Hennekens, J. O. Taylor. 1989. Prevalence of Alzheimer's disease in a community population: Higher than previously reported. *JAMA* 262:2551–56.

Games, D., D. Adams, R. Allessandrini, R. Barbour, P. Berthelette, C. Blackwell, T. Carr, J. Clemens, T. Donaldson, F. Gillespie, T. Guido, S. Hagopian, K. Johnson-Wood, K. Kahn, P. Liebowitz, I. Lieberburg, S. Little, E. Masliah, L. McConlogue, M. Montoya-Zavala, L. Muke, L. Paganini, E. Penniman, M. Power, D. Schenk, P. Seubert, B. Snyder, F. Soriano, H. Tan, J. Vitale, S. Wadsworth, B. Wolozin, and J. Zhao. 1995. Alzheimer-type neuropathology in transgenic mice over-expressing V717 β-amyloid precursor protein. *Nature* 373:523–27.

Gerdes, L. U., I. C. Klausen, I. Sihm, and O. Faergeman. 1992. Apolipoprotein E polymorphism in a Danish population compared to findings in 45 other populations around the world. *Genetic Epidemiology* 9:155–67.

Gibbs, R. B., and D. W. Pfaff. 1992. Effects of estrogen and fimbria/fornix transection on p75NGFR and ChAT expression in the medial septum and diagonal band of Broca. *Exp Neurol* 116:23–39.

Glenner, G. G. 1989. The pathology of Alzheimer's disease. *Ann Rev Med* 40:45–51.

Grese, T. A., J. P. Sluka, H. U. Bryant, G. J. Cullinan, A. L. Glasebrook, C. D. Jones, K. Matsomoto, A. D. Palkowitz, M. Sato, J. D. Termine, M. A. Winter, N. N. Yang, and J. A. Dodge. 1997. Molecular determinants of tissue selectivity in estrogen receptor modulators. *Proc Natl Acad Sci USA* 94: 14105–110.

Henderson. V. W. 1997. Estrogen replacement therapy for the prevention and treatment of Alzheimer's disease. *CNS Drugs* 5:343–51.

Jaffe, A. B., C. D. Toran-Allerand, P. Greengard, and S. E. Gandy. 1994. Estrogen regulates metabolism of Alzheimer's β precursor protein. *J Biol Chem* 269:13065–68.

Kang, J., H. G. Lemaire, A. Unterbeck, J. M. Salbaum, C. L. Masters, K. H. Grezeschik, G. Multhaup, K. Beyreuther, and B. Muller-Hill. 1987. The precursor of Alzheimer's disease amyloid A4 protein resembles a cell-surface receptor. *Nature* 325:733–36.

Lendon, C. L., F. Ashall, and A. M. Goate. 1997. Exploring the etiology of Alzheimer's disease using molecular genetics. *JAMA* 277:825–31.

Luine, V. 1985. Estradiol increases choline acetyl transferase activity in specific basal forebrain nuclei and projection areas of female rats. *Exp Neurol* 89:484–90.

Mann, D. M., P. O. Yates, B. Marcyniuk, and C. R. Ravindra. 1986. The topography of plaques and tangles in Down's syndrome patients of different ages. *Neuropathol Appl Neurobiol* 12:447–57.

Mitlak, B. H., and F. J. Cohen. 1997. In search of optimal long-term female hormone replacement: The potential of selective estrogen receptor modulators. *Horm Res* 48:155–63.

National Institute on Aging/Alzheimer's Disease Working Group (NIH/ADWG). 1996. Apolipoprotein E genotyping in Alzheimer's disease. *Lancet* 347:1091–95.

Rogaev, E. I., R. Sherrington, E. A. Rogaeva, G. Levesque, M. Ikeda, Y. Liang, H. Chi, C. Lin, K. Holman, T. Tsuda, L. Mar, S. Sorbi, B. Nacmias, S. Placentini, L. Amaducci, I. Chumakov, D. Cohen, L. Lannfelt, P. E. Fraser, J. M. Rommens, P. H. St. George-Hyslop. 1995. Familial Alzheimer's disease in kindreds with missense mutations in a gene on chromosome 1 related to the Alzheimer's disease type 3 gene. *Nature* 376:775–78.

Roses, A. D. 1996. Apolipoprotein E alleles as risk factors in Alzheimer's disease. *Ann Rev Med* 47:387–400.

Selkoe, D. J. 1996. Amyloid β-protein and the genetics of Alzheimer's disease. *J Biol Chem* 271:18295–98.

Sherington, R., E. I. Rogaev, Y. Liang, E. A. Rogaeva, G. Levesque, M. Ikeda,

H. Chi, C. Lin, G. Lin, K. Holman, T. Tsuda, L. Mar, J-F Foncin, A. C. Bruni, M. P. Montesi, S. Sorbi, I. Rainero, L. Pinessi, L. Nee, I. Chumakov, D. Pollen, A. Brookes, P. Sanseau, R. J. Polinsky, W. Wasco, H. A. R. Da Silva, J. L. Haines, M. A. Rericak-Vance, R. E. Tanzi, A. D. Roses, P. E. Fraser, J. M. Rommens, P. H. St. George-Hyslop. 1995. Cloning of a gene bearing missense mutations in early-onset familial Alzheimer's disease. *Nature* 375:754–60.

Van Bockxmeer, F. M., and C. D. S. Mamotte. 1992. Apolipoprotein e4 homozygosity in young men with coronary artery disease. *Lancet* 340:879–80.

Van Broeckhoven, C. 1995. Presenilins and Alzheimer's disease. *Nature Genetics* 11:230–32.

Weisgraber, K. H. 1994. Apolipoprotein E: Structure function relationships. *Advances in Protein Chemistry* 45:249–302.

15

The Genetics of Alzheimer Disease

Some Future Implications

Robert Mullan Cook-Deegan

The genetics of Alzheimer disease (AD), as well as genetics in general, will eventually lose its novelty and become a science that is taken for granted. Genetic techniques will be thought of, not as ways to look one by one for a gene that transmits diseases that are clearly passed within a family as Mendelian traits, but rather as tools for studying the inherited components of all diseases, including common ones. Part of this genetic dissection will identify genes that interact with other genes and genes that influence the action of (or are influenced by) hormones and growth factors, behavior, social factors, and environmental risks. AD genetics is a case study of genetics in this transition. It began by identifying genes inherited in families as autosomal dominant traits and has moved on to identify genetic risk factors that may interact with environmental factors to produce the same disease phenotype.

Dr. Pollen recounted the search for genes associated with AD in *Hannah's Heirs* (1996). I nonetheless want to review some of the history that seems particularly pertinent to trends portending the future of AD genetics, starting with scientific background and moving into policy issues. Some of the social implications associated with genetic testing have been anticipated and written about in the bioethics literature; others have received less attention.

The definition of genetics has been broadened by molecular biology. Whereas genetics used to be the study of inheritance (the transmission of measurable characters from one generation to the next), it is now the study of DNA structure. Genetics is expanding further to include the regulation of gene expression, and it will continue to grow. In the past, inheritance patterns were studied to infer the transmission of Mendel's genetic elements; now, we often start with DNA and look for correlations with clinical phenotype, environmental risk, or behavior. What began as the study of genes inherited from our mothers and fathers now includes mutations passed as lineages within an organism (i.e., changes in cancer cells, lymphocytes, and others). And in recent years, the vacuous debate about nature versus nurture has finally begun to give way to the use of molecular genetics to understand function. We no longer assume we are measuring fixed genes in static Mother Nature; rather, we can now also use genes to help understand how a mother nurtures.

Until the mid-1970s, most neurologists believed that genetics had little to do with AD. *Brain's Diseases of the Nervous System*, the compendious neurology textbook, pointed to an instance of twin discordance to justify the straightforward conclusion that AD "is not inherited" (Walton 1977). A disorder was either genetic or not—and genetic meant simple Mendelian. Since so many common diseases have been shown to have Mendelian forms (i.e., families in which a condition is inherited as dominant, recessive, or X-linked traits), a contemporary medical text would not likely make the same mistake.

Recognition that the same disease can be inherited in some cases and not in others tells us that there are multiple pathways to the clinical phenotype (disease) and genetic mutation is one of them. The Alzheimer story demonstrates clearly that genetic methods can move well beyond positional cloning of Mendelian mutations causing disease. AD was an early success of positional cloning—in fact, it was several success stories. The chromosome 21 story involved genetic linkage followed by the hunt for mutations in a candidate gene. The chromosome 14 story included genetic linkage followed by positional cloning. The chromosome 1 story was genetic linkage with almost simultaneous positional cloning, assisted by sequence similarity to the chromosome 14 gene.

The Apolipoprotein E (ApoE) story is different. It started with linkage to chromosome 19 but moved quickly to genetic susceptibility and is now using genetics to guide epidemiology (for example, the recent clues that, among those with the E4 allele, head trauma is associated with AD). The interaction of the ApoE risk factor with the chromosome 12 timing factor may prove to be one of the first discoveries of two genes interacting to influence disease risk.

McKusick's catalog of human genes began as *Mendelian Inheritance in Man* (1966) because it focused on the inheritance of those diseases clearly transmitted through families. It is now more and more filled with genes identified first by the direct analysis of DNA and subsequently by function (with or without disease association). The catalog is becoming a collection of loci, with more and more loci identified by studying DNA first and phenotype only later. The definition of *locus* shows this subtle shift; that is, it changes from alluding to a postulated gene invoked to explain Mendelian inheritance, to referring to a known variation in DNA that may or may not have a known phenotypic correlate. Many of the human genes discovered first by study of DNA do not behave as classic Mendelian characters at the level of phenotype, although of course they are inherited in Mendelian fashion when studied at the level of DNA sequence.

There are several reasons for the shift from the study of characters inherited as Mendelian traits to the direct study of DNA variation. Genes for most of the obvious and common Mendelian traits have been linked and cloned because they were logical early targets for genetic study. The hunt for Mendelian traits often started with large pedigrees (such as those in which the presenilin genes were discovered), but newer genetic techniques may focus on sibling pairs, lineage by descent, and other ways of inferring mutational change without resort to large pedigrees. New technologies and the data accumulating about genes in databases make it easier to start from DNA structure than from clinical phenotype, thereby enabling the rapid discovery of genes in ways that initially do not entail a description of phenotypes or tracing lineages through large families.

AD genetics illustrates this shift. In the early AD gene hunts, the crucial resources were newly available genetic markers and large Mendelian families. When my mentor, James Austin of the University of Colorado, proposed to hunt for an autosomal dominant Alzheimer gene in 1976, there were about 70 markers on human chromosomes. Most could be tested only one at a time because they were protein polymorphisms measured by enzyme assays or electrophoretic separation of peptides. Most markers were uninformative because they rarely varied often enough within a family to distinguish paternal from maternal chromosome inheritance; they provided little of the information needed to correlate phenotype with chromosomal location. In many respects, the odds of success were so low that it was folly to pursue genetic linkage under those conditions. The only hope was to find a family so large that the statistical power would overwhelm the technical limitations. The crucial element was pedigree construction: finding such families; gathering samples for analysis; and carefully recording genetic relationships, clinical diagnosis, and pathological confirmation.

The genetic approach had at least three virtues. First, it did not seem much worse than other approaches to AD, all of which were unpromising. Second, the existence of autosomal dominant families suggested that there was a broken gene lurking in the genome — so there was definitely something to be found. Even though the odds were against finding genes by wandering into the genetic wilderness, the history of science records many lucky trailblazers. And finally, pedigree construction at least laid the foundation for subsequent studies in an area where the technology was advancing rapidly. Even if the first genetic trails were primitive, molecular geneticists were constructing the infrastructure for an elaborate system that would enable the success of a genetic strategy. The autosomal dominant families identified in the 1970s were ripe for analysis when the new tools for genetic linkage came along (detailed by Botstein et al. 1980). By enabling multiple genotypes to be tested in parallel from the same sample, using vastly more informative markers and without needing to guess at candidate genes, that genetic linkage map made finding human genes much more likely to succeed.

The methods of genetic linkage and positional cloning were applicable to many diseases, but each family was uniquely touched by AD. As Tolstoy observed about Anna Karenina's unhappiness, every family's disease is a different story. It turned out that different families carried different genetic mutations producing the same Alzheimer phenotype.

AD was an early example of a condition found linked to multiple genes, demonstrating that the same clinical symptoms and pathology (at least, at first blush) was caused by different mutations. This forced the field to move away from a simple linear model of causality. Gene discoveries that showed that different families harbored different AD genes undermined the conception that the disease was unitary. The subsequent story of susceptibility factors retreats still farther from the simple Mendelian framework. Instead, genetic factors contribute to the disorder and make it more likely to occur, or they reduce the age of onset — but, by definition, the genes are not acting alone. The future of AD genetics seems likely to look more like the complex story of genetic susceptibility than the continual discovery of new Mendelian forms.

If we turn to other disorders, we can glimpse the use of genetics to illuminate how environmental factors interact with genes to change phenotype. One of the early successes in looking for Archibald Garrod's postulated inherited errors of metabolism was the correlation of defects in tyrosine hydroxylase with impaired brain development during childhood, or phenylketonuria. Here the genetic defect was triggered by the environmental factor dietary phenylalanine. Although the interaction of genes and environment has been known since the early history of modern medical genetics, environmental triggers are often forgotten because of a sense that genes are destiny. We need continual reminders that genes often predispose but are rarely dispositive.

The salient attribute of the human brain is its ability to learn and adapt to environmental changes. One central scientific question for the future is how — not whether — this occurs. We know from the start that genes influence learning and adaptation, but we also know that they can not act alone. While genes help set the context for behavior, environment is just as necessary for brain development. Environmental cues, nongenetic biological factors, and social structures that set a context for human development are critical, and genetics should help us understand them. Genetics will play several distinct roles. It will play its classic role of explicating inheritance by identifying phenotypes that affect behavior and correlate with genotypes. Molecular genetics will also be central to looking at how genes are turned on and off, and how DNA information is regulated in response to environmental cues. Finally, genetics will identify genotypes that confer specific risks that have been obscured by lumping together disparate pathogenetic pathways. Genetic subtyping, for example, is likely to guide testing of drugs that work better in one subgroup than in another.

The elaboration of human genetics will be a long and fruitful effort, and we know from the outset that the story will be complicated. We know, for example, that a few hundred thousand genes cannot specify trillions of neural connections in all their detail. We also know, however, that the 46 human chromosomes consistently (with a few tragic exceptions) specify a fully functioning human brain, whereas chimpanzee chromosomes specify a chimp's brain. Thus, a long-standing controversy bred of false dichotomy — pitting nature against nurture — must ultimately come a cropper to advancing knowledge. Future students of biology are likely to see this debate as a quaint relic driven by assumptions embedded in ideology (i.e., the desire for progressive social engineering on the left, and invisible hands optimizing social choice in the face of fixed human nature on the right). The strong forms of both genetic determinism and environmental determinism will die at the hands of science.

We know that environmental factors influence AD, and genetics may help ferret them out. One of my early scientific collaborations involved identical twin sisters with the disease. While this was not a big discovery, it was worth publication because it violated the conventional wisdom that AD was not inherited, and this case was of interest in part because the twins had originally been reported as discordant (Cook et al. 1981). The discrepancy was caused by more than a decade's difference in the age of onset. The case was about identical twins, but the underlying message is that something in the environment shifted the age of onset despite the shared genes. If these twins got AD from environmental causes, the concordance suggested a shared genetic susceptibility. If what they inherited was a genetic form of the disease, then that genetic form's expression could be influenced by something else. In the end, these two explanations amount to the same thing: genes interacting with the environment.

Were they alive today, those twins might give us a more precise clue. We might identify a mutation in one of the known AD genes or in the ApoE or chromosome 12 loci. Future AD studies that hearken back to classical genetics (i.e., twin studies, adoption studies, sibling pair studies, and lineage by descent) will be looking for correlation to environmental factors *in addition to* DNA inheritance. Although such studies are surprisingly rare now, we will see more of them in the future because they can bring the power of genetics to bear on environmental factors.

There is another future of AD genetics beyond the scientific findings. It concerns the way the science is done. The future of AD genetics is likely to differ as markedly from today as the field from which it sprung, molecular biology, differs from its past. It is hard to know just what "molecular biology" means these days because it is so pervasive and dominant in biomedical research. It usually means the study of proteins and DNA, but its original meaning was quite different. Warren Weaver of the Rockefeller Foundation coined the term *molecular biology* to describe a 1938 grants program that used physical and chemical techniques to study biological questions. It was a program to import physicists and chemists, along with their precise methods, into biology. The early molecular biologists knew they would study protein structure, but only a few suspected that DNA would prove an even bigger story.

In its first six decades, molecular biology has stopped being a grant program for enticing physical scientists to enter biology and has turned into a field of its own. It has become an expansive field with its own methods to be learned by apprenticeship. Molecular biologists run gels and centrifuges — novel and difficult physical techniques a few decades ago. Today physical separation and analytical techniques such as electrophoresis or spectroscopy are an inherent part of biology, learned within molecular biology laboratories rather than imported into them. Because the current era of gene-hunting, robotic genomics, and genetic informatics traces its lineage directly to Warren Weaver's vision, it is worth noting molecular biology's origins. AD genetics seems similarly destined to be absorbed into the mainstream, seeming unremarkable to those entering the field from here on.

Today's pharmaceutical industry grew from a combination of physiological screening techniques, organic synthetic chemistry, and rigorous clinical investigation. Organic chemistry was the core field that enabled the scientific transformation of drug discovery. As John Swann's book on the history of the pharmaceutical industry (1988) recounts, today's giant firms distinguished themselves from previous pharmaceutical ventures by using science to augment serendipity, clinical guesswork, and folk remedy. The industry is now turning its considerable resources to genomics. AD genetics is following this trend. It is no accident that Glaxo Wellcome hired as its research and development director an AD geneticist, Ausen Roses.

As Patrick Fox notes in Chapter 11 of this volume, for several medical, demographic, and social reasons, AD moved from the remote margin into the mainstream of biomedical research during the late 1970s and 1980s. By coincidence, or perhaps in part because of the success of the new methods, AD got hot just as molecular biology was carrying out its blitzkrieg on biomedical research. Funding for AD research was driven by both external factors and scientific factors: (1) rediscovery that most cases of senility were neuropathologically indistinguishable from AD, (2) Dr. Katzman's editorial (1976) pointing out the disease's prevalence and impact (see also Chapter 6 above), and (3) the coalescence of support groups into a social movement as Fox describes. The forces pushing AD into public attention (and congressional funding for biomedical research) were many and varied, but the research money was channeled mainly into molecular neuroscience and genetics. That seemed the fastest way to satisfy a desire for progress. In many respects, AD genetics closely parallels the modern era of understanding AD, because the expansion of research happened just as genetics was beginning to reach full flower.

In 1976 it was possible for a freshman medical student to read seven decades of world literature on AD in a summer (i.e., a total of a few hundred articles, comparable to a month's worth of publications today).

Most of the AD literature then was a battle between "lumpers" and "splitters" within neuropathology, psychiatry, and neurology (i.e., those who look for common categories that join disparate findings versus those constantly looking for new and more refined categories). Neuropathologists gave names to subtypes of plaques and tangles; neurologists and psychiatrists listed constellations of symptoms and clinical signs. The data to support the biological validity or prognostic significance of such differences were scant, but there was little else to write about. The splitters won, temporarily, by separating AD from late-onset dementia until Katzman and others reunited them. Most of the other taxonomic battles were protracted and irresolvable with the tools at hand. While the splitters were often wrong, later success in finding genes depended on analyzing families separately. In a way, the splitters were right that there were different forms, although the genetic differences (other than age of onset) did not necessarily refer to the clinical and pathological distinctions. The lesson here is worth keeping in mind: science benefits from a healthy competition between lumpers and splitters.

COMPETITION IN AD GENETICS

AD genetics exhibits some of the pathologies of molecular biological hypercompetition. The molecular biological invasion entailed an expansion of the scope of the science. Small clubs of pioneers — the phage group and the original RNA tie club at the Cavendish Laboratory — gave way to hotly contested international races among gene jockeys, including hunts for Alzheimer genes. Several groups were on the prowl for hundreds of genes. As Pollen (1996) shows, the races became intense, rivalries developed, and rifts appeared. Some of the resulting errant behavior discomfits everyone. The point that is pertinent to the future is that today's research ecosystem is even more heavily populated with competing research groups sustained by larger infusions of public grant moneys and much greater access to private capital. Whereas molecular biology first invaded field after field, now it controls so much territory that competition is mainly between molecular biologists, rather than between them and others. The short distance from genomics to commercial use will likely intensify this competition and make it more complicated.

Observing that a field is bigger, more prestigious, and more potentially lucrative is less a complaint than a caution about the need for continual vigilance. A field like human genetics, including AD genetics, that is now at its apogee faces different challenges than it did earlier in its development. There are at least three areas where trouble could brew: (1) how the science itself is conducted; (2) how genetic discoveries are turned into genetic tests, with the attendant problems of how to use those tests and constrain the flow of private medical information; and (3) how academic science interacts with drug discovery and the quest for commercial applications. As Pollen (1996) raises questions about the first issue, competitive scientific environment, I focus on the second and third issues, genetic testing and the complexities of academic-commercial relations in AD genetics.

THE POWER OF GENETIC MAPS

A decade's investment in genomics has produced amazing results. Instead of the 70 poorly informative chromosomal markers we had two decades ago, we now have almost 18,000 highly informative polymorphisms (GDB 1998). The advent of single nucleotide polymorphisms that are easy to detect will make gene hunting even faster, easier, and more accurate. Technologies are rapidly developing to enable detection of thousands of DNA variations in a single test, either on "DNA chips" or using other physical arrays as will be described later.

Beyond the human genome, we can now draw on other genetic resources to enrich human biology. In the past few years, over a dozen free-living model organisms have been completely sequenced. The search for the Huntington disease gene took a decade from genetic linkage to mutated gene; the lag period between linkage to identifying the chromosome 1 mutation for presenilin 2 was two weeks. The difference in speed came from linkage maps, physical maps, sequencing technology, and availability of genetic resources. Colorado's DOE-funded collection of brain gene-fragment sequences revealed a gene similar to presenilin 1, and sequencing of that gene in affected German Volga families quickly uncovered mutations in those affected with AD. The genome project promised to create tools to make biomedical research move faster, and it has delivered.

Markers, maps, and sequencing techniques are uncovering a flood of new genes both in humans and in other organisms. This will lead to many new ways to improve diagnosis, genetic risk assessment, treatment, and perhaps even prevention or delay of onset. With the transition from discovery to application, we begin to encounter problems of public policy.

Issues in Genetic Testing

Bioethicists and policy analysts have done a good job of anticipating many of the issues that will arise in AD testing within the rare families that have an autosomal dominant gene. Within this framework, which probably accounts for only a few percent of all cases, there is a consensus, although not unanimity, that: (1) testing needs to be linked to counseling; (2) tests need to be proven accurate and reliable before widespread adoption; and (3) most decisions should be left to the individuals affected (or, in the case of reproductive decisions, to prospective parents). There are lingering debates about whether to test children (with most agreeing that the practice is questionable until there is some treatment), about whether it makes any sense to test prenatally (with a somewhat more fragile consensus that late onset makes this hard to justify), and about the need for a firm evidentiary base before use of genetic testing is moved beyond high-risk Mendelian families into other populations. The genetic testing task force has set forth some principles for introducing genetic tests and regulating their use (Task Force on Genetic Testing 1997), and a Stanford project reviews previous statements and makes recommendations about genetic testing for AD (Working Group on Genetic Testing and Alzheimer's Disease 1997). These and other reports and statements go into further detail than is possible here.

Other issues have received less attention, for example, how AD tests will be used outside medical contexts, such as in underwriting for long-term care insurance. Another neglected area concerns the commercial-academic interface.

Social Use of Genetic Information: The Case of Long-term Care Insurance

Genetic testing for AD can be used for more than diagnosis and risk prediction. Most of the debate about ApoE testing has focused on whether it is useful in diagnosis, and when and whether it should ever be used as a diagnostic screen in the absence of symptoms (with consensus that for now it should not be). Those are important questions, but other difficult social policy issues extend beyond medical use.

The problem of private markets for long-term care insurance illustrates the problem. To put it bluntly, genetic risk factor assessments are very likely to stratify private markets for voluntary private long-term care insurance, and could entirely undermine those markets. Dementia accounts for a large fraction of long-term care use of nursing homes, other residential facilities, and adult day care. These are the expensive components of long-term care. AD accounts for most dementia and, consequently, for a high percentage of the need for long-term care. We already have problems of adverse selection and moral hazard in private health insurance markets today, for conditions that account for a smaller fraction of acute care than AD does of long-term care. Now, along come tests that may well detect genetic risk for the most common disorder inducing the need for long-term care.

Insurance actuaries do not need to know that a given individual will or will not develop disease in order to use population risk to set rates or decide eligibility. They are in the business of statistical inference, not diagnosis. If ApoE, chromosome 12 markers, HLA haplotypes, or future genetic factors yet to be discovered correlate with risk for many AD cases, individuals seeking long-term care would be well advised to assess their genetic risk. If individuals can do so, however, then insurers must also have access to the information or face a problem of adverse selection. With so much long-term care attributable to a single disorder, and with genetic susceptibility factors associated with a large fraction of cases, the problem of adverse selection is apt to be severe. It will be too dangerous for private long-term care insurers to create a voluntary market if they do not have the same access to information as individuals have. And because individuals may well wish to assess their risk for reasons other than insurance needs, barring the use of tests entirely may prove unwise.

Insurers can address the problem in several ways. They can offer insurance that is priced to cover high risks (in effect what most first-generation, long-term care policies seem priced to address). In the long run, this should result in a stratified market of those who are quite likely to need insurance seeking it (because they have been tested genetically, know of family risk, have early symptoms, or for some other reason are unusually worried about needing long-term care). They, and the few individuals with resources so ample that price does not much matter, may be the only ones willing to pay the high premiums—in effect, a prepayment scheme with some minimal risk-pooling rather than a true insurance market. Insurers could also offer lower-cost insurance on condition that they have access to the same information as consumers have about risk, which in the future could include information about ApoE and other genetic susceptibility factors. This will again lead to stratification into high-risk-high-premium and low-risk-low-premium market segments.

Market segmentation may offend a moral intuition of fairness, because those at genetic risk have no control over the genetic lottery. Those susceptible to AD did not choose their genes. Given the high risk of need for long-term care attributable to AD and the high risk of AD attributable to genetic risk factors, however, this seems to be where we are headed if long-term care is conceived as a problem to be handled by the market. The other solutions entail direct government intervention into the long-term care market. One obvious solution is universal coverage, perhaps as part of universal access to health care. The United States is further from achieving this goal than any other developed country and actually appears to be retreating from it.

Mandated universal purchase of private insurance is another option. To avoid penalizing those who lose in the genetic lottery, such mandatory insurance would have to offer a single price or allow adjustment only for controllable risk factors. This is how many states have handled automobile insurance. By forcing everyone into the same risk pool, it would, in effect, create a subsidy from those at low genetic risk to those at high risk.

Although universal long-term care programs and mandated insurance may be more just, they both face two serious problems: (1) there is no consensus that long-term care should be an entitlement or part of the social welfare network (if such consensus existed, we would have it); and (2) even if we agreed that universal access to long-term care were desirable, there is no political will to achieve it. If we cannot implement a longstanding broad consensus favoring universal coverage for acute health care, it seems naive to hope we will do so for long-term care. Yet genetic testing could completely undermine or deeply stratify a voluntary insurance market, the most obvious private alternative.

While I cannot speak for other countries, this debate has not even begun in the United States, perhaps because long-term care has drifted to the back burner of national policy. This is ominous because the problem of long-term care is bound to grow enormously throughout the world over the next several decades. In the United States, it is viewed as a "private sector" problem, not because there are promising private sector solutions, but because government programs are off the table and government intrusions inherently suspect.

The future of AD genetics places it at the nexus of a wrenching policy dilemma: unless we find an effective treatment or means of prevention, the prevalence and demand for long-term care will rise steeply for decades to come. Genetic technologies may enable risk prediction that seriously complicates private market solutions at a time when public sector solutions are ideologically out of favor.

COMPLEXITIES IN COMMERCIAL USES OF GENETICS: THE CASE OF MICRO-ARRAYS

A policy storm is brewing on another front. The anticipatory analysis of genetic testing has progressed well over the past several years, in no small part because the Ethical, Legal, and Social Implications programs of the National Institutes of Health and Department of Energy have paid for sound empirical and theoretical analysis. But the technology of genetic analysis is moving very quickly toward micro-array techniques, which will pose ethical and social problems different from the Mendelian framework in which most analysis has proceeded to date. Micro-array techniques may probe hundreds of thousands or millions of alleles in a single experiment. One DNA sample might conceivably be tested for all known disease-associated alleles and genetic risk factor alleles at all known loci. That is, a single micro-array genetic test might (in theory) detect all known mutations for cystic fibrosis; oncogenes and tumor suppressors (breast, colon, prostate, brain tumor, p53, p16, ataxia-telangiectasia, and other cancer-related genes); Huntington disease and myotonic dystrophy; all known Mendelian disease mutations; and all known genetic risk factors for AD, cancer, diabetes, hypertension, atherosclerosis, and other common disorders.

The economics of chip design that characterize microprocessor manufacture are likely to apply to the half-dozen or so micro-array genetic testing technologies. These technologies include "DNA chips" with multiple short-tethered sequences available for hybridization, multiplex hybridization (melding pools systematically), microvolume liquid hybridization borne of ink-jet printer technology, metallic bead-magnetic hybridization schemes, and automated microwell hybridization. The economics dictate high costs of initial setup but low costs of replication. That is, it is hard and costly to develop the process, but if it is used by many, it becomes cheaper and cheaper.

To date, most analyses of genetic testing have used the familiar scenarios from Huntington disease, sickle cell, or cystic fibrosis testing. In these Mendelian scenarios, those at high risk choose whether to seek a genetic test for one disorder. Although prices for testing are generally high, the high risk gives the resulting information high value. Testing for thousands of alleles at once would be entirely different. The incremental cost of testing for a particular disorder would be low, but the likelihood of finding something useful would be quite high because so many alleles would be detected. So the value of the information might still justify the costs.

Such multi-allele, multi-locus testing seems technologically plausible, but it is not getting much policy attention. It should get attention, however, because it matters for at least two reasons. It would dramatically change pretest counseling, which is now directed at those with sufficient risk to justify thinking seriously about a test for a single condition. Its aim is to prepare an individual for the possibility of bad news that might affect one's health, job, self-image, and ability to get insurance. Since it would be impossible to go over all the genetic risks for every condition in micro-array testing, counseling would focus instead on generic risks, with perhaps an explanation of the range of genetic disorders and risk factors being examined. Few individuals today would emerge from a comprehensive gene scan entirely free of genetic risks, and the advance of genetics clearly indicates that in coming years more alleles and more risks will come to light.

The technology would also change post-test counseling, which now concentrates on explaining the result of a single test and putting it into the context of the individual's life and the implications for others in the family. Post-test counseling for a multi-allele genome scan would instead focus on the disorders and risks revealed at the first pass. It might as often feed into subsequent rounds of clinical testing as produce a definitive yes or no answer about inheritance of genetic disease. This shift in framework might limit the prospects for micro-array testing. Yet social norms and new technology have often collided, and sometimes technology wins — particularly if it gets powerful enough or cheap enough.

Multi-allele testing raises another policy conundrum that provides a bridge to some final observations about commercial applications. Suppose inexpensive and widespread micro-array genetic testing proved technically feasible. The identification of each diagnostically useful sequence, however, is based on correlating DNA structure with function or phenotype or both. That knowledge is contributed by thousands of groups, and most of those groups are securing intellectual property rights. For AD alone, for example, one would confront more than a dozen patents on the amyloid precursor protein, presenilin 1 and 2, and ApoE testing for AD risk assessment. More patents will surely follow, because we are only at the beginning of the story. Multiply that by hundreds of patents and trade secrets for breast cancer, colon cancer, diabetes, and other conditions. Will all the relevant intellectual prop-

erty rights be licensed to a single micro-array manufacturer? (This leaves aside for the moment the unpredictable but intense competition among micro-array technologies themselves.) Such a licensing scheme would require reworking the existing licensing arrangements, many of which would be difficult to change.

The cost of a micro-array test might be determined more by the stacked royalties on hundreds of patents than by the cost of the procedure itself. If the information is valuable enough, it might happen anyway, but the cross-licensing task is daunting. Microprocessor chip manufacturers faced a similar problem, as did automobile manufacturers at the turn of the century and aircraft manufacturers during World War I. The differences between these industries and medical diagnostics are substantial, however. Research and development for these manufacturing sectors was far less decentralized at similarly early developmental phases, and they were less dependent on patents. Firms in transportation, aeronautics, communication, microelectronics, and software are more accustomed to cross-licensing and collective action. In biotechnology, pharmaceuticals, and medical diagnostics, patent protection is much stronger; cross-licensing is less pervasive; and collective action, such as industry-wide pooling of intellectual property, has few precedents.

I use the example of micro-array technologies because of parallels with microelectronics, the other transforming technology of our age. It is a cliché that we are progressing into the information age, ushered in by a plethora of telecommunication and computer technologies. We presume that biotechnology will build on this revolution, mainly via its own technologies and the deluge of biological information they are generating. A big part of the story of information technology is commercial development, which is now also becoming a much bigger part of molecular biology. But the industrial development of molecular biology will differ from microelectronics in some important technological and moral respects.

To a growing extent, the future of genetics, including AD genetics, lies in private commerce. No other major industrial sector is as research and development intensive as pharmaceuticals. No other sector is as dependent on strong patent protection. And no other sector is as dependent on academic science. These distinctive features of the pharmaceutical business are corroborated by empirical data: (1) the surveys of economist Edwin Mansfield (1991, 1995) that show four of five pharmaceutical products either depend on academic research or benefit from it (more than twice as high as any other sector); (2) the higher proportion of patents held by academic institutions (Henderson et al. 1994); (3) high citation rates of academic research in pharmaceutical patents and high citation of patents assigned to academic institutions (Narin and Rozek 1988; Narin and Olivastro 1992); (4) the uniquely long time horizon for private pharmaceutical research and development investments (National Academy of Engineering 1992); and (5) the correlation between linkages to academic research, successful innovation, and profitability in pharmaceuticals (Office of Technology Assessment 1993; Gambardella 1995; Cockburn and Henderson 1996). Recent surveys by David Blumenthal and colleagues (1996, 1997a, 1997b) suggest that genetics is even more tightly linked to industry than other fields of biomedical research.

Pharmaceuticals are highly regulated. A drug must prove its safety and efficacy by formal scientific methods before entering the market, a feature not shared by many other sectors except defense contracting. While the rationale for such regulation is public safety, it has the side effect of raising barriers to entry for new firms. The end-market for pharmaceuticals is extraordinarily complex and cannot be characterized as a "free market." Prices across national boundaries vary remarkably, and patent monopolies associated with individual products strongly influence prices. Product monopolies (including those conferred by patents) raise prices, with future vitality at any given firm dependent on using today's cash to search for new agents to open entirely new markets. Markets are influenced by how many other drug or nondrug treatments address the same clinical indication and whether alternatives work as well. Only when there are viable treatment alternatives does price competition become possible. Distribution of pharmaceuticals depends on networks of providers and physicians, elaborate education, and promotional strategies. The costs of constructing such networks are high, and they add to the costs of proving safety and clinical efficacy. The point of this litany is that the drug and diagnostics business is uniquely sensitive to developments in science and that it is very difficult to enter the business anew.

The pharmaceutical sector is sui generis, so the history of technologies in other sectors may be only weakly predictive. Genomics is surely high tech. Its first and most lucrative applications are likely to be in diagnostics and therapeutics, but what that implies about policy is highly uncertain.

Since 1993 private investments in genomics have exceeded federal funding. Private research and development funding is available because investors believe that genomics will lead to products and services. The entry markets are likely to be in diagnostics, which should find faster application but are also less lucrative, and therapeutics, where profitability and revenue potential are both high. Private genomics is now a front end to drug discovery, and we can all benefit from the products and services that result.

But there is a dark side to this academic-industrial synergy. In recent surveys of public opinion about biomedical research, the pharmaceutical industry ranks low in public trust (McInturff 1996). After a decade of enormous and highly conspicuous success in discovering new life-saving drugs, why should the public distrust the industry? The industry does good by producing innovative, life-saving products, and Wall Street corroborates that it has also done well financially. The pharmaceutical business has been one of the most financially rewarding for the past decade (Office of Technology Assessment 1993). I believe the public distrust stems from a prudent skepticism about financial self-interest.

The just distribution of rewards from genetic research could prove a source of policy friction. The interests of family members participating in genetic studies can diverge from those of private firms that extract commercial value from the research. In addition to its unique academic-industrial mutualism and patent dependence, there is a moral difference between biomedical research and work in computers or communication technologies. Biomedical research deals with life and death and depends much more heavily on the voluntary participation of individuals who are not the direct beneficiaries of research. This moral difference should influence biomedical science policy in ways that differ from precedents in physics, chemistry, or industrial sectors. Although developing a new computer or software package obviously entails the contributions of many people, it does not involve intimate clinical information or pieces of the bodies of research volunteers.

In most contexts, biomedical research presumes that research subjects *donate* their information and tissues. Informed consent statements typically state that research participants should not expect benefits for themselves. Investigators mine the donated information and tissues to add value in the form of knowledge and technology. They advance their careers, sometimes become famous, and are well paid. Some of the new knowledge, much of which comes from publicly funded research at academic institutions, can be translated into new products and services. Most of that translation takes place in private firms — either health service providers or drug and device manufacturers. Most of those markets are profit driven. Pharmaceutical research and development is one of the most effective pathways for translating biomedical science into practical applications. Private firms devote extraordinary resources to a few promising leads for new drugs and diagnostic tests. In the end, the people who participated in the biomedical research may benefit by having new products and services — and hence better health — but they pay monopoly rents to obtain those benefits when genes and drugs are patented. Monopolies are conferred to induce investments that keep innovation running forward. That is how we have constructed the system.

The system contains some profound asymmetries, however, in what is assumed to motivate human behavior. Those motivational asymmetries translate to different moral frameworks. Research participants are generally presumed to be altruists who can expect no personal benefit. Academic scientists are generally presumed to be motivated by knowledge, career advancement, and prestige within their fields. As financial rewards from private firms increase, however, the profit motive is now increasingly added to the academic mix. The companies that produce drugs and services are presumed to be crass oligopolists answering to investors. Here we have a system that starts with altruism and ends with private profit. It could be that precedents from electronics, manufacturing, and other high technology sectors will suffice for biomedical research. These nonmedical fields, however, do not include a component of research and development that depends on participation by, and information from, donors. It should thus not surprise us if these wildly different moral frameworks come into conflict. The size of the problem will likely be influenced by how much money is made, how concentrated the wealth becomes, and whether those who profit from innovation, particularly pharmaceutical and biotechnology firms, take steps to promote the interests of research volunteers.

A sense of justice is offended when a relatively short chain of events displays obvious financial asymmetries, especially when health and privacy are risked by those who fail to secure the financial rewards. Some family some day may well complain that a university researcher sold their information to Axys, Myriad, Millennium, Mercator, Human Genome Sciences, Incyte, Genset, DeCope, or some other firm. And they may be right.

Collective action by investigators, pharmaceutical firms, biotechnology firms, and government can address some of the asymmetries by mandating royalty streams to support research to benefit those similar to the donors, contractual sharing of rights to intellectual property with "donors" or surrogates, and licensing arrangements that promote patient interests. The feature shared by these options is a transparent link between those donating information and materials voluntarily, and benefits for people like them. At the least, fairness will entail being at the table when the deal is cut. If this materializes as a policy issue, fairer policies will entail at least minor modifications in the way private pharmaceutical and health-care-service firms operate. Academic institutions are likely to be the focal point if policies do change, because that is where science meets commerce and thus where disparate moral norms collide.

Social norms for universities are not the same as for private pharmaceutical firms. Universities and nonprofit research institutions are expected to be private but dedicated to public good, at least to some extent. Public scrutiny may force universities and nonprofit research centers to manage their intellectual property resources as a public trust as well as a private profit center. In the wake of the 1980 Bayh-Dole statute, which conferred patent rights on inventions arising from federally funded research on universities (Eisenberg 1996), academic patenting has increased dramatically (Henderson et al. 1994). In some fields, this has led to many more academic patents but fewer citations of the average academic patent—a so-called dilution of quality with increased patent numbers. Biotechnology and pharmaceutical patents, however, have increased in number, and citations have not dropped. The trend will likely continue, and virtually every research university and major private nonprofit research institution anticipates more patents and growing patent royalties.

Large and sophisticated technology transfer offices take into account the unique role of universities in advancing knowledge and promoting public good. The mission statement for MIT's Technology Licensing Office, for example, is clear: its mission is "to benefit the public by moving results of MIT research into societal use via technology licensing, through a process which is consistent with academic principles, demonstrates a concern for the welfare of students and faculty, and conforms to the highest ethical standards." Although technology transfer offices want to generate income from patents and industrial sponsorship of research, that interest is constrained by the larger mission of the university. Not all technology transfer offices, however, are so sophisticated. Some lack the capacity to analyze goals beyond income maximization, or they lack the foresight to determine when financial goals conflict with other university roles. Some universities have treated their patents as autonomous profit centers with little regard for broad social impact or fair distribution of benefits. In part because genetics has grown from academic science, and in part because its advance requires direct participation of individuals who donate information and tissues, genetics is likely to shine a light on those institutions that promote their financial self-interest over public good or that unfairly appropriate benefits for themselves and investigators but exclude others who participate in research. If this issue ignites, the sparks will likely come from one of the aggressive universities or nonprofit research centers or from one of the biotechnology firms with which they are linked.

The importance of academic-industrial connections and the dependence of technological advancement on individuals participating in research may make the future of genetics look different from the history of automobiles, oil and mineral extraction, transportation, computers, and software. Even if it is difficult to foresee just how or to what extent it will differ, the future of genetics seems likely to little resemble the past of manufacturing or the present of information technologies. The past decade has taught us at least one important lesson about the future of genetics: Our fate lies not in our genes, but in how we treat them.

References

Blumenthal, D., E. G. Campbell, et al. 1997a. Withholding Research Results in Academic Life Science: Evidence from a National Survey of Faculty. *Journal of the American Medical Association* 277 (April 16): 1224–28.

Blumenthal, D., N. Causino, et al. 1996. Relationships Between Academic Institutions and Industry in the Life Sciences: An Industry Survey. *New England Journal of Medicine* 334 (February 8): 368–73.

———. 1997b. Academic-Industry Research Relationships in Genetics: A Field Apart. *Nature Genetics* 16 (May): 104–8.

Botstein, D., R. L. White, et al. 1980. Construction of a Genetic Linkage Map in Man Using Restriction Fragment Length Polymorphisms. *American Journal of Human Genetics* 32:314–31.

Cockburn, I., and R. Henderson. 1996. Public-Private Interaction in Pharmaceutical Research. *Proceedings of the National Academy of Sciences* 93 (November): 12725–30.

Cook, R. H., S. A. Schneck, et al. 1981. Twins with Alzheimer's Disease. *Archives of Neurology* 38:300–301.

Eisenberg, R. S. 1996. Public Research and Private Development: Patents and

Technology Transfer in Government-Sponsored Research. *Virginia Law Review* 82 (November): 1663–727.

Gambardella, A. 1995. *Science and Innovation: The U.S. Pharmaceutical Industry During the 1980s.* New York: Cambridge University Press.

Genome Database. 1998. On-line database maintained by Johns Hopkins University, Baltimore, Maryland, and currently scheduled for termination and transfer to Oak Ridge National Laboratory, Tennessee. Until then, updated daily and available from http:/www.gdb.org/, Johns Hopkins University.

Henderson, R., A. Jaffe, and Trajtenberg, M. 1994. *Universities as a Source of Commercial Technology: A Detailed Analysis of University Patenting, 1965–1988.* Cambridge, Mass.: National Bureau of Economic Research.

Katzman, Robert. 1976. The Prevalence and Malignancy of Alzheimer's Disease: A Major Killer. *Archives of Neurology* 33:217–18.

Mansfield, E. 1991. Academic Research and Industrial Innovation. *Research Policy* 20 (February): 1–12.

———. 1995. Academic Research Underlying Industrial Innovations: Sources, Characteristics, and Financing. *Review of Economics and Statistics* 77 (February): 55–65.

McInturff, W. D. 1996. What Americans Say about the Nation's Medical Schools and Teaching Hospitals. Report on Focus Groups and Surveys performed by Public Opinion Strategies for the Association of American Medical Colleges. Washington, D.C.

McKusick, V. A. 1966. *Mendelian Inheritance in Man.* Baltimore: Johns Hopkins University Press.

Narin, F., and D. Olivastro. 1992. Status Report: Linkage between Technology and Science. *Research Policy* 21:237–49.

Narin, F., and R. P. Rozek. 1988. Bibliometric Analysis of U.S. Pharmaceutical Industry Research Performance. *Research Policy* 17:139–54.

National Academy of Engineering. 1992. *Time Horizons and Technology Investments.* Washington, D.C.: National Academy Press.

Office of Technology Assessment, U.S. Congress. 1993. *Pharmaceutical R & D: Costs, Risks, and Rewards.* Washington, D.C.: U. S. Government Printing Office.

Pollen, D. 1996. *Hannah's Heirs: The Quest for the Genetic Origins of Alzheimer Disease. New York: Oxford University Press.* Swann, J. P. 1988. *Academic Scientists and the Pharmaceutical Industry: Cooperative Research in Twentieth-Century America.* Baltimore: Johns Hopkins University Press.

Task Force on Genetic Testing. 1997. *Promoting Safe and Effective Genetic Testing in the United States.* Washington, D.C.: U. S. Department of Health and Human Services Task Force on Genetic Testing, created by Ethical Legal, and Social Implications Working Group, jointly sponsored by the National Institutes of Health and the Department of Energy.

Walton, J. N. 1977. *Brain's Diseases of the Nervous System.* New York: Oxford University Press.

Working Group on Genetic Testing and Alzheimer's Disease. 1997. Draft Executive Summary of a Report. Stanford, Calif.: Program on Genomics, Ethics, and Society, Stanford University.

16

History and the Future of Alzheimer Disease

Peter J. Whitehouse

Alzheimer disease (AD) is a malignant threat to the quality of life of affected individuals as well as to the quality of life of the human race in the future. Our ability to recognize the challenges and dangers that lie ahead will be critical in determining whether we can make appropriate personal and social responses to this condition. But just what is the nature of the threat that we perceive to be looming ahead? Surely a clear definition of AD is relevant to both those who search for biological cures and those who seek better ways of delivering care. But the concept of AD has changed in the past, and it is likely to change in the future.

In this chapter I examine the value of studying the history of the concept of AD. I also examine the dominance of the biological sciences in finding better treatments, curatives, and even preventatives. It is the emergence of new biological technologies, I hypothesize, that has been critical in defining the disease and developing solutions to the problems it creates. Trends that may challenge the biological view are examined as well. These trends may, in turn, affect public policy and planning. Finally, I focus on quality of life as an approach for developing new integrated concepts of AD (Whitehouse forthcoming).

THE VALUE OF HISTORICAL STUDY

What is the value of historical study? What is the role of history in helping us to understand or even predict the trends that will determine the future? These questions are relevant for academic historians as well as for those of us who seek guidance in moving forward the boundaries of human knowledge to help solve current and future problems. Should we study history because it does repeat itself and because those who are ignorant of the past will be doomed to repeat those cycles? Or should we study history to attempt to understand the complexities of social forces that may change the very manner in which we perceive reality? It seems reasonable to ask these questions at a time when major forces appear to be at work in reshaping the quest for human wisdom. It also seems reasonable and even intuitive to suggest that reality is an evolving social construction described by limit-setting language and especially metaphor, but also based on the physical world in which we live.

Clearly, few would argue that a knowledge of history has no relevance for the future. What one purchases at the grocery store today contributes to the options for dinner tomorrow. However, as the desire for linking past and future extends further in time in both directions and the complexity of the concepts to be assimilated increases, our confidence in the helpfulness of history may wane. Understanding the desires, concepts, and perceived follies of the people of the past should create both a sense of humility and a list of options for us to consider as elements of our worldview. In this sense, historians are like anthropologists, who can expand our appreciation for the diverse human responses to the need to organize socially and adapt to the environment. More important, historians, like anthropologists, can help us understand that culture is our greatest attribute as an evolved species. We are a part of that culture, and our ability to modify it rationally is limited. However, understanding cultural evolution may help us think critically about our common future.

A view of history that is based on a notion of linear progress (such as, one might argue, science promulgates) would limit our appreciation of history to recording our stages of success and celebrating how much more we know and can do. Molecular biologists recognize the need to respond to the findings of last month or maybe late last year. Lack of interest in distant history (and perhaps also a realistic future) constrains their participation in projects such as those that are represented in this book.

As population and environmental pressures increase, our vision of the future has become a bit less rosy. I believe an understanding of history at least allows us to develop a sense of shared connectivity to the human beings who went before and left us their legacy. With modesty and hope, we will leave ours.

Many future-molding forces are at work in the present computerization, globalization, geriatrization, and certainly molecular genetization of the world. Modern information systems are contributing to dramatic changes in how we learn and share information across national boundaries. The effects of the growth of the world's population, particularly the elderly, on our global ecosystems are frightening. Our understanding of biological sciences, particularly those dealing with genes, offers great potential for controlling nature and our biological selves. It also presents challenges pertaining to the wise use of this power. Making short-term personal or company financial gain from genetic tests too quickly brought to market is not admirable in a time when we really need to think through the cost and effectiveness of new technology.

CHANGE IN HEALTHCARE SYSTEMS

The forces for change are most evident in healthcare systems around the world. The rapid population growth in many parts of the world and changes in age stratification are driving revolutions in these systems. Public attention to the increasing proportion of the elderly is growing in industrialized countries; however, this awareness needs to be global because the rate of aging is actually greater in many developing countries than in the industrial world. China and India will lead this aging tsunami.

This attention to aging creates particular interest in the diseases of elderly people — and one of the most visible is AD. The scientific conception of AD is of a progressive neurological disease in which death of brain cells is associated with senile plaques and neurofibrillary tangles and results in loss of cognitive abilities. The power of biological science has never been greater for understanding the processes that lead to cell death and the resulting clinical dementia (see Braak and Braak, Chapter 3; Altstiel and Paul, Chapter 14).

AD is one of the diseases leading the molecular revolution in medical science. Multiple genetic risk factors have been identified. The consequences of these genetic mutations and susceptibility loci on protein function are being elucidated. Perhaps most exciting is the use of genomic technology and chemistry to create and screen vast numbers of candidate compounds to alter pathogenetic cascades. Combinatorial chemistry and high-throughput screening have dramatically increased our ability to develop candidate molecules (Altstiel and Paul, Chapter 14). Cell cultures and transgenic animal models offer the promise of more rapid preclinical development. Even the costly stage of clinical development is being revolutionized by the use of information systems and new organizational mechanisms for conducting drug trials (Whitehouse forthcoming). Despite these advances, the development of dramatically effective medications to treat chronic diseases such as AD has been slow. Complex issues have been raised about the commercialization of this technology (Cook-Deegan, Chapter 15). The backdrop of aging, with its slow changes in cellular function due to interacting genetic and environmental factors, makes degenerative diseases, especially those of the nervous system, difficult targets for therapeutic advances. In general, we must be careful about being seduced by the power of genes and gene therapy while ignoring the deterioration of the environment and environmental health.

THE CHALLENGES TO SCIENCE

The limitations of technological solutions to complex problems are being recognized in several areas of human problem solving, such as environmental issues. A variety of terms have been applied to the shifts in cultural forces that surround science and society. The term *postmodernism* engenders perhaps the most debate. It is difficult for a single word that crosses so many disciplines to capture the magnitude of changes that are occurring and to create any degree of common understanding about its meaning. By nature, postmodernism is deeply suspicious of "isms," consensus, and all-encompassing metanarratives. Yet the emergence of this word into our lexicon signals important shifts in conceptions of human society, quests for new knowledge, and even the very definition of human personhood.

Science is losing its highly privileged position over the search for knowledge and its application to solving human problems. While science is not being rejected by most and should not be, it is, however, being viewed in a broader context that applies less value to rationality as an approach to human problem solving. The critical modern or postmodern person attempts to look at the interplay between values and facts in different ways and with different methods. Aspects of the AD movement would be an ideal target for deconstruction (i.e., a reexamination of latent values and the distribution of power), a popular method and/or fetish of postmodernism. Elsewhere, we have claimed that AD itself represents a postmodern challenge to modern conceptions of personhood (Whitehouse and Deal 1995). Thus, AD needs to be viewed through conceptual lenses that are more than scientific.

Scientific knowledge may not lead to effective applications; in fact, it may create knowledge that cannot be used wisely or that may even contribute to distress and even more dis-ease. As mentioned earlier, the conception of how scientific knowledge accumulates (e.g., linear progression) can distance and limit the ways in which future problems need to be addressed. Part of the challenge is to recognize that disease entities are as much linguistic labels and social constructions as they are the business of science and medicine. Conceptions of health and disease change with societies themselves. Similarly, the power of different groups (e.g., patients, doctors, or policy makers) to control the discourse surrounding disease shifts through time and culture. By understanding how the conceptions of AD have changed through history and how our beliefs and cognitive schemes of reality can go beyond scientific models, we can help plan for the coming need to care for greater numbers of demented individuals.

THE HISTORY OF THE CONCEPT OF ALZHEIMER DISEASE

This book explores the history of the concept of AD—that is, how we came to develop and use this term. The history of AD itself could easily become a chronology of the scientific and clinical advances that have led to greater knowledge about this condition, beginning with Alois Alzheimer's work. A history of the *concept* of AD requires a broader context in which politics, language, power, and culture all come into play (Dillmann 1990; Fox 1989). A fuller, richer understanding of AD requires a range of disciplines as well as a loosening of discipline—or at least lack of disciplinary structure. A history of concepts should not degenerate into a recounting of the ideas of the scientific greats. It should be a narrative of the shared social concepts and their diversity. Such understanding should lead to better ways of dealing with the current and future problems created by AD. In the following section, I consider nineteenth- and twentieth-century conceptions of AD as well as what we mean by the term "concepts of disease."

Alzheimer and Brain Psychiatry

Older individuals have suffered progressive loss of cognitive abilities throughout human history. Before the late 1800s, dementia was thought to be caused by moral or religious factors. The word *degenerate* referred to a deterioration of character before it meant loss of brain cells. The biological characterization of the disease — namely, senile plaques and neurofibrillary tangles — had to await the development of scientific technology and appropriate imaginative individuals. Alois Alzheimer contributed to many areas of neuropathology besides the disease that bears his name (e.g., descriptions of syphilis, Huntington disease, and vascular conditions) (Hoff and Hippius 1989). Alzheimer was practicing a type of psychiatry that has been referred to as "brain psychiatry" (Ackerknecht 1968).

Pioneers such as Emil Kraepelin and Theodore Meynert proposed that an understanding of mental illness be based on an understanding of brain pathology (Papez 1970). Meynert's classic psychiatry textbook *Psychiatry: A Clinical Treatise on Diseases of the Forebrain* (1885) included mostly neuroanatomy — so much so that Meynert had difficulty being promoted to professor of psychiatry because of his primary focus on neuroscience (as defined then). He eventually succeeded in justifying his anatomical studies as being relevant to the development of psychiatry and received his promotion.

Carl Wernicke trained with Meynert. Together they dissected the arcuate fascicles, a fiber bundle that connects frontal and temporal parts of the brain. Wernicke's ideas became a model for understanding that the brain functions through a series of interconnected centers of activity (Marx 1970). Freud, who also trained with Meynert, made initial attempts to understand agnosia from a biological perspective, but because of his inability to explain complex human behavior in purely anatomical terms, he later abandoned an exclusive focus on brain psychiatry.

Meynert and others pioneered techniques for examining the brain. Microtomes were developed to slice thin sections of tissue that could then be stained with a variety of dyes. Alzheimer's pathological findings were dependent upon the work of Nissl and Bielschowsky, his collaborators and friends, who are remembered principally for the cell stains that they developed. Thus, at the end of the nineteenth century, neuroanatomy and neuropathology became the dominant basic sciences of psychiatry.

Other biological discoveries of ultimate relevance to AD were being made in the late nineteenth and early twentieth centuries. Thudicum pioneered the development of the science of neurochemistry in the late 1800s. The concept of neurotransmitters was developed by Lewii and others; acetylcholine, which later played a much more prominent role in the understanding of AD, was one of the first identified. In the early

1900s, Erlich and others (Tower 1972) developed the concept of neurotransmitter receptor molecules, which has clearly had a tremendous influence on drug discovery in modern times. Finally, the use of arsenic as treatment for syphilis must have caused considerable excitement in psychiatry. It was the first time that this disease, which was a common cause of dementia of the time, could be treated with a so-called magic bullet (although the limitations of the power of the magic is now clear; Brandt 1985). Thus, Alzheimer was practicing in a very rich, biologically flavored environment in which hope for the future was based on an understanding of the pathology of mental illness.

Biological Psychiatry

There are evident parallels between brain psychiatry at the end of the nineteenth century and modern biological psychiatry at the beginning of the twenty-first century. In each case, the biological sciences are viewed as the source of explanatory models and therapeutic interventions. Neurochemical studies of degenerative diseases in the late 1960s and 1970s led to the identification of reductions in specific neurotransmitters in the brains of patients at autopsy. For example, detecting lowered levels of dopamine in Parkinson disease led to effective therapies. Reductions in the concentration of acetylcholine in AD eventually led to treatment with cholinesterase (the enzyme that metabolizes acetylcholine in the brain) inhibitors such as tacrine and donepezil — albeit with less success than that of L-dopa in Parkinson disease.

The dominant and controversial explanatory model for AD centered on the so-called cholinergic hypothesis (Whitehouse 1998a). My colleagues and I characterized the loss of cells in the brain that, in turn, caused the loss of acetylcholine. The cholinergic hypothesis was almost always a political rather than a scientific statement, and it occurred in different variants. The strong hypothesis was that the loss of cholinergic cells explained all of the cognitive dysfunction. The weak hypothesis was that it explained nothing. Clearly, truth lay somewhere in between. One "test" of the hypothesis was that drugs that enhance acetylcholine improved cognition to the extent that many countries have approved them for clinical use (although some will not pay for them). Thus the controversy over the power of acetylcholine in the disease continues.

Throughout this controversy, I clearly experienced the nonrational, nonlinear, social aspects of scientific power relationships. Some understanding of these forces was as helpful to career advancement as any scientific prowess, although luck should certainly be mentioned as well.

I also experienced the waning of interest in neurochemistry as the focus shifted from the brain to the gene. It is also perhaps important to note the fifteen to twenty year gap between identification of the cholinergic deficiency and the approval of cholinergic drugs.

Molecular Biology

To a significant degree, molecular genetics and biology have re-placed neuropathology and even neurochemistry as dominant biolog-ical sciences in the latter part of the twentieth century. The quest for the root biological causes has moved from the study of the human brain to the human (and often animal) gene. Based on these molecular ap-proaches, a dominant and perhaps overly simplistic model of drug de-velopment has emerged. Mapping the human genome (a task that is all but automatic at this point) and identifying the genes associated with specific diseases (also proceeding rapidly) is viewed as foundational to developing new drugs. After the abnormal genes are identified, the re-sultant proteins and the mischief that they cause in the brain need to be characterized. Once an understanding of the critical deficiencies has been achieved, medications can be developed to correct the underlying deficit. Transgenic mice produced at great expense and incorporating new mixed mouse and human genes are seen as key to testing drugs before introduction into humans.

When compared with the power of the gene, the environment in which the disease emerges is not viewed as particularly important. In fact, most epidemiological studies in AD focus on biological factors such as diet and exposure to medications (with notable exceptions such as education) as possible risk or protective factors (Whitehouse 1997). Social factors that might affect the course of AD have been relatively neglected. AD was and is being viewed as a biological condition with clinical manifestations due to brain pathology.

Concepts of Disease

The work of Patrick Fox (1989) and Robert Dillmann (1990) brought explicit focus to an exploration of the concept of AD. Dill-mann's thesis was entitled "Alzheimer's Disease: The Concept of Dis-ease and the Construction of Medical Knowledge" (1990). He begins his philosophical discussion by pointing out the importance of separat-ing object and concept. Dillmann divides the history of AD into three periods in psychiatry and medicine: (1) Kraeplinian psychiatry and neuropathological research; (2) neuropharmacology and attempts to develop drug treatment for AD in the 1970s and 1980s; and (3) molecular genetics and DNA recombinant technology. He gives an extensive discussion of the concept of disease, including its philosophical background. He reviews specific frameworks for understanding disease, including deviation from species design, socially constructed abnormality, and classification based on symbolic logic.

Dillmann's account highlights the biological aspects of the concept of AD. Ballenger, Holstein, Gubrium, and others in this volume have focused on the social construction of AD. Ballenger particularly drew attention to what we might call the middle period of AD (i.e., the period between brain psychiatry and biological psychiatry). In the mid-twentieth century increasing attention was paid to the inadequacies of the biological model as an explanation for all clinical phenomenology. For example, some individuals were found to have dementia without extensive pathology, whereas others have extensive pathology without evidence of significant cognitive impairment. This period of development of the concept of AD focused on psychosocial factors. Interventions focused on environment and included milieu therapy and other nonbiological treatments. Moreover, Ballenger argues that the psychodynamic model of dementia became a way in which psychiatrists and gerontologists in the 1940s and 1950s could explain the entire experience of aging.

Stated simplistically but provocatively, our concepts of AD moved from a social model before the turn of the nineteenth century, to a focus on biology in the early 1900s, to a return to psychosocial aspects in midcentury, and then again to the current biological focus at the end of the twentieth century. It is clear that an important part of the history of AD has been determined by the development of biological technologies. When biologists have a new and creative technique to apply to the disease (e.g., the microscope, microtome, molecular probe), they tend to dominate the discussion and the literature. Perhaps it is not just the scientifically perceived value of the technology but the marketing of it to the rest of society that is at stake. For example, although brain imaging techniques such as positron emission tomography claim great power for understanding dementia, the promises have exceeded the products (at least so far) in this waning decade of the brain.

It will be interesting to see whether the cycle repeats and we move to a stronger psychosocial perspective in the early part of the twenty-first century. My guess is that the balance between biological and nonbiological conceptions will again shift because of the need to consider complex ethical and healthcare delivery issues, as well as to recognize the limitations of molecular concepts and resultant therapies. I am not denying the value of molecular approaches; I am merely suggesting that their power to solve the problems of dementia have been overstated and that biological discoveries sometimes create more ethical and policy questions than they answer. Clearly, finding models of disease and its treatment that integrate biological and social perspectives, and avoiding the polarization that often occurs in scientific and policy debuts, would be ideal.

There are certain historically recurring issues that point out the limitations of the biological disease model. One such issue is the relationship between AD and the cognitive changes of normal aging. A strong view has been promulgated in the United States, particularly by the Reagan Institute of the National Alzheimer's Association, that AD is a curable (or at least preventable) condition (see Fox, Chapter 11). To develop this approach, the proponents attempted to separate AD from normal aging. As originally conceived, AD (i.e., presenile dementia) is easier to differentiate from aging than senile dementia of the Alzheimer type. When a gene is identified in a 45-year-old who becomes progressively demented, it seems reasonable to view the condition as an abnormal disease state. However, when a 95-year-old develops memory difficulties that are slowly progressive, it is more difficult to be convinced that the phenomenon represents a disease. Would we all develop AD if we lived long enough? Age-related cognitive decline is common in individuals in their 80s and 90s, and the biology of this state is perhaps not qualitatively different from presenile dementia in early stages (see Braak and Braak, Chapter 3).

Whether or not AD represents an accelerated form of aging has been both a political debate and a scientific issue — or, perhaps better stated, a political issue that can be informed by scientific data. It has not been considered appropriate by some within the AD community to ask whether AD may be merely "accelerated aging." The proponents of research on AD believe that society will be less likely to support the search for a cure for something that might be viewed as normal. Exaggerated statements about the capacity of biological research to create cures or even significant interventions may preclude serious policy discussions about dealing with AD as a social phenomenon, particularly with respect to current and future needs for community and institutional care. In 1911 Alzheimer himself expressed reservations about whether the disease that now bears his name was in fact a separate entity (Schorer 1985; Maurer, Chapter 1; Förstl, Chapter 4). Even pharmaceutical companies are recognizing that they need to be involved more in so-called disease state management, where the treatment involves more than just a medication. The enhancement of health and quality of life of patient and caregiver requires more than pills. Addressing care as well as cure will require attention to human values and relationships that are not addressed by biological approaches.

PRESENT-DAY TRENDS AFFECTING THE CONCEPT OF ALZHEIMER DISEASE

As mentioned above, the dominant research theme has been that an understanding of the genetic basis of AD will lead to better understanding of pathogenesis and more effective therapies. In complex genetic diseases like AD, dramatically effective therapeutic approaches are perhaps more distant than promised. Gene therapy encompasses a variety of approaches. Most specifically, it means correction or replacement of actual abnormal genetic material. We use it here more generally to mean therapies developed on the basis of genetic information.

Two kinds of genetic risks are associated with AD: autosomal mutations of dominant chromosome 1, 14, and 21; and susceptibility loci on chromosome 19. The autosomal dominant mutations usually result in early-onset disease, with 50 percent of children on average inheriting the disease from an affected parent. Susceptibility loci contribute to increased risk for getting the disease but no known deterministic possibilities. Individuals who carry the apolipoprotein E2 (APOE2) allele are at lower risk than those who are APOE3, who in turn are lower than APOE4, yet the three apolipoproteins differ in only one or two amino acids. A therapeutic hope is the production of a drug that reduces the risk of those who are E4 by understanding the biology of the susceptibility locus. These genetic systems are complicated, however, and the feasibility of such simple approaches is not clear.

The use of genetic testing in AD illustrates an attempt to apply the power of genetic knowledge to the clinic too quickly. In autosomal disease, it is possible to reliably inform an individual at 50 percent chance of inheriting a gene from his or her parent whether or not he or she has the gene. In AD and other related conditions such as Huntington disease, however, the usefulness of this knowledge is not clear. Lower than expected numbers of individuals are availing themselves of presymptomatic testing.

The APOE (chromosome 19) story demonstrates the overselling of the power of genetic-based approaches for diagnostic purposes (see Post and Whitehouse 1998). Commercialized by Athena Neuroscience on the basis of a patent to Duke University, APOE genotyping is available for $195 (presenilin testing involving chromosome 14 costs $895). Dr. Alan Roses, a member of the team that discovered the increased risk for AD associated with the APOE4 type, believes that it is unjust not to provide such testing; his belief is based on the desire of families to have such tests and on the potential for saving money in the diagnostic process. He points to the high frequency of APOE 4 in autopsy-proven cases of AD. While the power of the label "autopsy-confirmed" (hence biologically "proven") is great, those who consider the clinical application of such genetic testing are aware that the average patient does not come from a population of patients that is likely to come to autopsy. Because variations in risk may occur as a function of age, family history, and ethnic background, risk assessment in individual patients is difficult. Moreover, it is not clear from Roses' formulation how it saves money — what "standard" diagnostic tests are omitted. Roses does not recommend the use of APOE for predictive testing. However, he does claim that the identification of additional susceptibility loci (perhaps on chromosome 12) will lead to great ethical problems as predictive power increases with combined loci. Thus, although genetic testing offers promise for improving diagnosis, we need to be more critical in evaluating claims before spending valuable healthcare dollars.

In addition to biological studies, many social factors will affect progress in AD. The creation and manipulation of people's expectations will be key. Overaggressive claims for likely biological solutions may produce a backlash of public opinion. For example, one wonders why there is such great interest in alternative and complementary medicine today. Could it be a sign of dissatisfaction with "Western" (i.e. allopathic) formulations of health and treatment? The increasingly costly demands for more services for current clients with dementia may also compete with the scientific enterprise for attention and resources.

Even the initial genetic and therapeutic discoveries are creating a panoply of ethical challenges. How accurately can we predict AD, and who can use the information wisely? How is it possible to gain informed consent for participation on research from cognitively impaired persons? When might it not be appropriate to use placebos in therapeutic trials? What share of society's resources should be spent on severely demented individuals? Although science can provide data to help us consider these issues, it cannot give us the wisdom to provide the answers in isolation from cultural and spiritual values.

Perhaps the most critical issue is how our concepts of AD can be applied to better understand our therapeutic goals. If AD is a form of aging, albeit often premature, can we try to reverse aging? When is it appropriate to consider AD as a terminal illness and thus palliate symptoms and promote a good death? How can we frame and put into practice attempts to prevent, cure, reverse, or even just slow the progression of disease? How do we balance our goals when we use a medication that might improve behavioral symptoms but make a person's thinking less clear?

Too often those trying to develop more effective healthcare interventions, such as day care programs or special care units, and those attempting to find better drugs do not communicate with each other about therapeutic goals, let alone with patients and caregivers (Whitehouse 1997). A common interest in improving quality of life (QOL) of both client and caregiver seems to be emerging more and more (Whitehouse forthcoming). The assessment of QOL in dementia has been relatively neglected, despite the fact that such studies have become critical in other areas of medicine. However, this situation is changing, and several new approaches are being developed.

QOL is difficult to conceptualize and measure. It is a multidimensional concept that encompasses cognition; behavior; function; and social, economic, and, although not as much considered, spiritual factors. Some believe that QOL is merely the sum of its constituent parts; others believe it has emergent properties. Some view QOL as vague and vacuous; others see it as the key to future improvements in drugs and care. Perhaps exploring the concept of QOL in dementia and focusing on its improvements can serve as goals for bridging the biological/medical and social/welfare worlds that are so often poorly coordinated in the care of patients/clients and their families. My own guess is that attempts to study QOL will lead to a better understanding of the limitations of science and the interface of science and values. Great dangers may arise if the concept of QOL becomes dominated by scientific approaches.

CONCLUSION

The world of scientists and clinicians will be quite different in the future. The breakdown of traditional categories of knowledge will continue to promote interdisciplinary teamwork. Information systems will drive innovation. Better educational approaches, including the use of computers and distance learning, will revolutionize teaching and learning as well as foster flexible adaptation to ongoing changes. For example, intergenerational learning communities may emerge as one innovative approach.

Social resources to deal with the problems of dementia may diminish, thereby increasing demands for improved efficiencies in research and health care. "Consumers" of the products of research and of health systems will gain more power to shape the goals and methods of science and care. These forces for change will drive us to avoid the pursuit of simple answers to complex questions — answers that divorce biological and psychosocial approaches to dementia. Although associated with plaques and tangles, genetic mutations, and loss of cholinergic markers, Alzheimer disease is first and foremost a human concept that shares a name with its discoverer. What defines us as uniquely human can be argued; however, language, good memories of the past, and advanced planning skills for the future are clearly candidates. These are progressively lost in AD.

However the concept of AD changes, the disease will likely play an important role in the future of our world and our conceptions of human personhood. Loss of intellect is perhaps the greatest challenge to the post-Enlightenment person who (over) values cognition (Post, Chapter 13). Neuroscience will play a critical, but not the dominant role in addressing the threat of dementia. As global citizens continue to age and the environment is further threatened by economic progress, we may need to reevaluate the place of the demented in our world. It will take a rich understanding of history, culture, and the human spirit as well as science to meet the challenges of the future.

References

Ackerknecht, E. H. 1968. *A Short History of Psychiatry*, 2d ed. New York and London: Hafner Publishing.

Brandt, A. M. 1985. *No Magic Bullet: A Social History of Venereal Disease in the United States Since 1880*. New York: Oxford University Press.

Dillmann, R. 1990. Medical knowledge and the concept of disease. In *Alzheimer's Disease: The Concept of Disease and the Construction of Medical Knowledge*, 1–32. Amsterdam: Thesis Publishers.

Fox, P. 1989. From senility to Alzheimer's disease: The rise of the Alzheimer's disease movement. *Milbank Quarterly* 67(1): 58–102.

Hoff, P., and H. Hippius. 1989. Alois Alzheimer 1864–1915. *De Nervenarzt* 60:32–37.

Marx, O. M. 1970. Nineteenth-century medical psychology: Theoretical problems in the work of Griesinger, Meynert, and Wernicke. *Isis* 61:355–70.

Meynert, T. 1885. *Psychiatry: A Clinical Treatise on Diseases of the Forebrain Based on Its Structure, Function, and Nutrition.* Trans. Bernard Sachs. New York: Putnam and Sons.

Papez, J. F. 1970. Theodor Meynert. In *The Founders of Neurology*, ed. W. Haymaker and F. Schiller, 57–61. Springfield, Ill.: Charles C. Thomas.

Post, S. G., and P. J. Whitehouse, eds. 1998. *Genetic Testing for Alzheimer's Disease: Ethical and Clinical Issues.* Baltimore: Johns Hopkins University Press.

Schorer, C. E. 1985. Historical essay: Kraepelin's description of Alzheimer's disease. *Intl J Aging and Human Dev* 21(3): 235–38.

Tower, D. B. 1972. Neurochemistry in historical perspective. In *Basic Neurochemistry*, ed. G. J. Siegel, R. W. Albers, B. W. Agranoff, and R. Katzman, 1–16. Boston: Little, Brown and Co.

Whitehouse, P. J. 1985. Theodor Meynert: Foreshadowing modern concepts of neuropsychiatric pathophysiology. *Neurology* 35:389–91.

———. 1997. The genesis of Alzheimer's disease. *Neurology* 48 (Suppl 7): 1–6.

———. 1998a. The cholinergic deficit in Alzheimer's disease. *J Clin Psychiatry* 59:1–20.

———. 1998b. Measurements of quality of life in dementia. In *Health Economics of Dementia*, ed. Wimo, Jonsson, Karlsson, and Windblad, 403–17. Chichester, UK: John Wiley & Sons.

———. 1998. Chapter on Future of Drug Development for Alzheimer Disease. In the *Blue Books of Practical Neurology Series on the Dementias*, ed. Growdon and Rossor. Woburn, Mass.: Butterworth Heinemann.

Whitehouse, P. J., and W. E. Deal. (1995) Situated beyond modernity: Lessons for Alzheimer's disease research. *J Amer Ger Soc* 43:1314–15.

Whitehouse, P. J., and S. G. Post. 1998. Pharmacogenetics. In *Genetic Testing for Alzheimer's Disease: Ethical and Clinical Issues*, ed. S. G. Post and P. J. Whitehouse. Baltimore: Johns Hopkins University Press.

Index

Page numbers in *italics* denote figures; those followed by "t" denote tables.

Library of Congress Cataloging-in-Publication Data

Concepts of Alzheimer disease : biological, clinical, and cultural
  perspectives / edited by Peter J. Whitehouse, Konrad Maurer, and
  Jesse F. Ballenger.
    p. cm.
    Includes bibliographical references and index.
    ISBN 0-8018-6233-7 (alk. paper)
    1. Alzheimer's disease. 2. Alzheimer's disease — Genetic aspects.
  3. Alzheimer's disease — Social aspects. I. Whitehouse, Peter J.
  II. Maurer, Konrad, 1943– . III. Ballenger, Jesse F.
    [DNLM: 1. Alzheimer's Association. 2. Alzheimer Disease —
  genetics. 3. Alzheimer Disease — history. 4. Alzheimer Disease —
  psychology. 5. Neuroscience — history. WT 155 C744 2000]
  RC523.C657 2000
  616.8'31 — dc21
  DNLM/DLC
  for Library of Congress   99-27293
                                                                CIP